Renal Cell Carcinoma: Clinical Management

Renal Cell Carcinoma: Clinical Management

Editor: Tanya Walker

FOSTER ACADEMICS
www.fosteracademics.com

www.fosteracademics.com

FOSTER ACADEMICS

Cataloging-in-Publication Data

Renal cell carcinoma : clinical management / edited by Tanya Walker.
p. cm.
Includes bibliographical references and index.
ISBN 978-1-64646-610-8
1. Renal cell carcinoma. 2. Kidneys--Cancer. 3. Renal cell carcinoma--Diagnosis.
4. Renal cell carcinoma--Treatment. 5. Nephrology. I. Walker, Tanya.
RC280.K5 R46 2023
616.994 61--dc23

Foster Academics,
118-35 Queens Blvd., Suite 400,
Forest Hills, NY 11375, USA

ISBN 978-1-64646-610-8 (Hardback)

Contents

Preface

Every book is a source of knowledge and this one is no exception. The idea that led to the conceptualization of this book was the fact that the world is advancing rapidly; which makes it crucial to document the progress in every field. I am aware that a lot of data is already available, yet, there is a lot more to learn. Hence, I accepted the responsibility of editing this book and contributing my knowledge to the community.

Kidney cancer is a form of cancer that develops when renal cortical tumor is formed in the kidneys due to uncontrollable division of healthy cells. It can be classified into several types including renal cell carcinoma (RCC), urothelial cancer, sarcoma, Wilms tumor and lymphoma. RCC is the most common type of kidney cancer that affects the adults. It develops in the proximal tubules which are a part of the filtration system of kidneys. Haematuria, malaise, tiredness, chronic pain in the back, loss of appetite and fever are some common symptoms of RCC. Factors responsible for escalating the risk of RCC include smoking, old age, hypertension and obesity. Clinical management of RCC includes several tests and procedures. Imaging tests like ultrasound, X-ray, CT and MRI are used to detect any abnormality or tumors in the kidneys. Biopsy is a diagnostic method in which a sample of cells is removed from the suspicious area of kidney to identify the signs of cancer. Treatment of RCC consists of surgical methods like metastasectomy and laparoscopic surgery, and non-surgical methods like cryoablation and radiofrequency ablation. This book contains some path-breaking studies on the clinical management of renal cell carcinoma. It will serve as a reference to a broad spectrum of readers.

While editing this book, I had multiple visions for it. Then I finally narrowed down to make every chapter a sole standing text explaining a particular topic, so that they can be used independently. However, the umbrella subject sinews them into a common theme. This makes the book a unique platform of knowledge.

I would like to give the major credit of this book to the experts from every corner of the world, who took the time to share their expertise with us. Also, I owe the completion of this book to the never-ending support of my family, who supported me throughout the project.

Editor

1

Immunotherapy in Renal Cell Carcinoma: The Future is Now

Antoine Deleuze [1,2], Judikaël Saout [1], Frédéric Dugay [1,3], Benoit Peyronnet [4], Romain Mathieu [1,4], Gregory Verhoest [4], Karim Bensalah [4], Laurence Crouzet [2], Brigitte Laguerre [2], Marc-Antoine Belaud-Rotureau [1,3], Nathalie Rioux-Leclercq [1,5] and Solène-Florence Kammerer-Jacquet [1,5,*]

1 Université Rennes, Inserm, EHESP (Ecole des Hautes Etudes en Santé Publique), IRSET (Institut de recherche en santé, environnement et travail), UMR 1085, 35000 Rennes, France; antoine.deleuze@chu-rennes.fr (A.D.); judikael.saout.1@univ-rennes1.fr (J.S.); frederic.dugay@chu-rennes.fr (F.D.); romain.mathieu@chu-rennes.fr (R.M.); marc-antoine.belaud-rotureau@chu-rennes.fr (M.-A.B.-R.); nathalie.rioux-leclercq@chu-rennes.fr (N.R.-L.)

2 Department of Medical Oncology, Centre Eugene Marquis, 35000 Rennes, France; l.crouzet@rennes.unicancer.fr (L.C.); b.laguerre@rennes.unicancer.fr (B.L.)

3 Department of Cytogenetics, University Hospital, 35000 Rennes, France

4 Department of Urology, University Hospital, 35000 Rennes, France; benoit.peyronnet@chu-rennes.fr (B.P.); gregory.verhoest@chu-rennes.fr (G.V.); karim.bensalah@chu-rennes.fr (K.B.)

5 Department of Pathology, University Hospital, 35000 Rennes, France

* Correspondence: jacquet.sf@gmail.com;

Abstract: Renal cell carcinoma is the third type of urologic cancer and has a poor prognosis with 30% of metastatic patients at diagnosis. The antiangiogenics and targeted immunotherapies led to treatment remodeling emphasizing the role of the tumour microenvironment. However, long-term responses are rare with a high rate of resistance. New strategies are emerging to improve the efficacy and the emerging drugs are under evaluation in ongoing trials. With the different treatment options, there is an urgent need to identify biomarkers in order to predict the efficacy of drugs and to better stratify patients. Owing to the limitations of programmed death-ligand 1 (PD-L1), the most studied immunohistochemistry biomarkers, and of the tumor mutational burden, the identification of more reliable markers is an unmet need. New technologies could help in this purpose.

Keywords: immunotherapy; immune checkpoint inhibitors; renal cell carcinoma; PD-1; PD-L1; ongoing trials; biomarkers; emerging drugs

---

1. Introduction

Renal cell carcinoma is the third urological cancer, representing 3% of all cancers in women and 5% in men with an incidence of around 400,000 cases worldwide [1]. The prognosis is poor: 30% of patients are metastatic at diagnosis and almost 30% of the remaining patients will develop metastases detected during the follow-up [2].

Clear cell renal cell carcinomas (ccRCC) represent the vast majority of RCC (around 75%). The other histologies mainly encompass papillary (20%) and chromophobe RCC (5%). The other entities are very rare including translocation-associated RCC, medullar RCC and collecting duct carcinoma. The histological entities based on distinct pathological features present different molecular alterations. Indeed, ccRCC are hallmarked by a frequent alteration of the *VHL* gene, a tumour suppressor gene, leading to angiogenesis through the transcription of genes regulated by *HIF* such as *VEGF* [3–7].

Non ccRCC (nccRCC) represent a heterogeneous group with papillary, chromophobe RCC and translocation RCC, the most frequent entities. Papillary RCC (pRCC) include tumours with indolent outcome (type 1) and more aggressive tumours (type 2) [8]. Type 1 and type 2 pRCC commonly harbor frequent *MET* alterations. However, alterations of *SETD2, CDKN2A, EGFR, NF2* and *TERT* have been described in type 2 and suggest the activation of MAP kinases pathway, cell cycle and deregulation of chromatin remodeling [9]. Chromophobe RCC (cRCC) are rarely metastatic and characterize mitochondrial alterations, frequently mutated *p53* and activation of mTOR pathway [9]. Translocation RCC (tRCC) harbor gene fusions involve *TFE3* and *TFEB*, members of the MiTF family [10]. These transcription factors have multiple partners, mainly involving messenger RNA splicing [11].

The other entities constitute less than 2% of renal tumours. The collecting duct carcinoma have been described as immunogenic tumours with high lymphocyte infiltration resultingfrom the upregulation of genes involved in T-cell activation and proliferation [12]. Renal medullary carcinoma present a frequent loss *INI1* (*SMARCB1*) implicated in the chromatin remodeling complex [13]. Among familial RCC syndromes, patients with hereditary leiomyomatosis and renal cell carcinoma (HLRCC) syndrome harbor *Fumarate Hydratase* (FH) germline mutation and develop clinical aggressive tumours [14]. The *FH* mutation by inactivating the enzyme alters the function of the Krebs cycle.

The sarcomatoid component can be found in all the histologic subtypes and demonstrates an increased tumour mutation burden (TMB) with high frequency of *p53, CDKN2A* and *NF2* mutations and also genes involved the chromatin remodeling such as *ARID1A* and *BAP1* [15].

The treatment and management of metastatic RCC have radically changed over the past 20 years [16]. Initially, first-generation immunotherapy with cytokines: interleukins or interferon represented standard approaches but with poor results [17,18]. The development of tyrosine kinase inhibitors, mainly vascular endothelial growth factor (VEGF) receptor inhibitors, largely improved the prognosis of both progression free survival (PFS) and overall survival (OS) [19].

The emergence of immune checkpoint inhibitors (ICI) alone or in combination (anti-cytotoxic T-lymphocyte antigen-4 (CTLA4) and anti-programmed death 1 (PD-1)) showed interesting results [20,21]. Targeted immunotherapy is an alternative to antiangiogenics because ccRCC is also considered an immunogenic tumour with high numbers of immune cells such as tumour-infiltrating lymphocytes (TIL) [22–24]. Recent trials proposed antiangiogenics in association with targeted immunotherapy to overcome resistance emphasizing the role of the tumour microenvironment (TME) and this strategy is currently an option in first line treatment [25,26].

Mechanisms of resistance with ICI can be primary or innate and secondary or acquired [27]. They encompass neo-antigen loss, defect of antigen presentation, alternative immune checkpoints and defective interferon signalling. Interferon-γ is a major mechanism of resistance by enhancing programmed death-ligand 1 PD-L1 expression and inducing the expression of immune inhibitory molecules [28]. Other immune checkpoints such as TIM-3, LAG-3 and TIGIT play a role in the resistance by inhibiting antitumour immune response [29]. Novel therapeutic approaches try to overcome these mechanisms of resistance and are under evaluation in ongoing trials.

Identifying biomarkers is the key to better select treatments, reduce costs and improve survival in patients with metastatic kidney cancer. However, the limitations of the most studied biomarkers: PD-L1 immunohistochemistry and TMB make necessary the identification of robust markers. New technologies could help in this purpose.

In this comprehensive review, we will discuss: 1. the specificities of the TME in RCC, 2. the treatment update with the results of recent trials, 3. the emerging drugs used in ongoing trials, 4. the predictive biomarkers and 5. the novel technologies.

2. Specificities of the Tumour Microenvironment in Renal Cell Carcinoma

2.1. Vascular Component

Angiogenesis has been described to play an important role in the progression of RCC and leads to the recruitment of endothelial cells. Recent data suggest that endothelial cells in TME differ from normal endothelial cells [30]. Akino et al. identified aneuploidy in one third of endothelial cells freshly dissociated from RCC [31]. This warrants further investigation as it could impact the response to antiangiogenic drugs. Moreover, Edeline et al. demonstrated two different angiogenic phenotype described as mature and immature. These two patterns could coexist within the same tumour demonstrating the heterogeneity of the vascular component [32]. Dufies et al. demonstrated in experimental tumours that sunitinib stimulated the development of lymphatic vessels. Indeed, these vessels are crucial for the recruitment of immune cells [33].

2.2. Immune Component

The expression of PD-L1 is widely represented in RCC suggesting the important role of PD-1/PD-L1 checkpoint with the aberrant expression of tumour cells. Indeed, PD-L1 expression was reported in 23% of ccRCC, 10% of pRCC, 5.6% of cRCC, 30% of t RCC and 20% in collecting duct carcinoma [34,35]. An amplification of 9p24.1, locus of PD-L1, was recently identify in RCC with sarcomatoid component leading to PD-L1 constitutive expression [36].

The immune compartment mainly include T cells, NK cells, B cells, macrophages and dendritic cells with complex interactions. Recently, Chevrier and colleagues used mass cytometry to compile an atlas of immune cells from 73 RCC identifying 22 T cell and 17 tumour-associated macrophage phenotypes with distinct immune composition between tumours [37]. Some macrophages such as M-11 or M-13 were associated with a worse prognosis and could constitute new targets. The phenotype of T cells (CD8+) regarding the expression of immune checkpoints (PD-1, LAG-3, Tim-3) identified the immune-regulated profile as more aggressive in a cohort of 40 RCC [38]. The role of B cells in the TME is unclear with both anti- and pro-tumoral effects. In ccRCC, the density of B cells identified by immunohistochemistry was associated with poor prognosis [39]. Moreover, the B cell signature was correlated with poor prognosis in The Cancer Genome Atlas (TCGA) ccRCC cohort. B cells could exert pro-tumoral functions through different mechanisms such as secretion of immune-regulatory cytokines that affect T cells and macrophages.

To understand the immunomodulation of nivolumab, Chouieri et al. explored the morphological and molecular changes of mRCC ($n = 91$) at screening and on treatment [40]. Immunohistochemical analysis revealed an increase in CD3+, CD8+ and CD4+ lymphocytes. No consistent change was observe in the expression of PD-L1 in tumour cells. Transcriptional analysis identified the up-regulation of genes stimulated by interferon γ with high levels of related chemokine in peripheral blood. A study case reported a histological complete response after nivolumab in metastatic ccRCC [41]. Only fibrotic changes and CD8+ lymphocytes were detected after treatment.

3. Treatment Update in Renal Cell Carcinoma

3.1. First-Line Treatment

The ICI are the new backbone in the therapeutic landscape of renal cancer alongside tyrosine kinase inhibitors, Figure 1. Innovative combinations of ICI or ICI with TKI are now part of the treatment strategy and based on the results of recently published phase III trials in first line setting, Table 1 [20,25,26,42].

The Checkmate 214 trial confirmed the benefit of the nivolumab and ipilimumab association versus sunitinib in first line metastatic ccRCC among patients with intermediate or poor prognostic risk according to the International Metastatic Database Consortium (IMDC) risk model [20]. The objective response rate (ORR) was 42% versus 27%, and the complete response rate (CRR) was 11% versus 1% ($p < 0.001$). No differences were observed in terms of PFS. A recent update showed an interesting increase in OS after 30 months of follow-up in favor of nivolumab (anti-PD-1) plus ipilimumab (anti-CTLA4) combination (60% vs. 47%; HR: 0.66 ; CI 0.54 to 0.80 ; $p < 0.0001$) [43].

Recent updates also highlighted the benefit of ICI and TKI in combination. In Keynote 426, Pembrolizumab (anti-PD-1) plus axitinib showed a benefit in terms of OS at 12 month follow-up (90% vs. 78% ; HR: 0.53 ; CI: 0.38–0.74 ; $p < 0.0001$) leading to Food and Drug Administration (FDA) approval of the association in first line [26]. The Javelin 101 Renal comparing avelumab (anti-PD-L1) plus axitinib versus sunitinib in the PD-L1 positive population, defined as > 1% of positive immune cells staining within the tumour area, demonstrated a longer PFS, 13.8 months versus 8.4 months (HR = 0.69; 95% CI, 0.56 to 0.84; $p < 0.001$) and an improvement of the ORR (55.2% vs. 25%) [25]. After a 12 month follow-up, OS was not significantly different between the two arms. Similarly, the IMmotion 151 trial explored the atezolizumab (anti-PD-L1) and bevacizumab association regarding PD-L1 expression by immunohistochemistry (IHC) with a 1% cut-off on tumour-infiltrating immune cells [42]. The PFS was 11.2 months versus 8.4 months (HR = 0.74; 98.5% CI, 0.57 to 0.96; $p = 0.02$), but there was no statistical difference in OS at 24 months follow-up.

Among the recent phase III trials released, the distribution of patients in IMDC differed [20,25,26,42]. For instance, Checkmate 214 trial focused on intermediate- and poor-risk populations. The geography of recruitment may have an effect as the Keynote 426 trial had a large proportion of patients from outside the USA and Western Europe. Finally, RR and PFS are not strictly comparable. Moreover, follow-up remains short and it is difficult to formally conclude at this stage.

Considering the differences among trial populations and the lack of mature OS, the choice of first line therapy can be challenging. To date, guidelines for treatment decision rely on the IMDC risk model to stratify patients with untreated mRCC or previously treated with first-line targeted therapies [16,44]. However, the interest of this classification remains unclear with the advent of ICI combination therapies and patient characteristics stay major indicators in the absence of prospectively validated biomarkers. Indeed, a significant number of comorbidities could influence the treatment choice and should be confronted by the safety profile of ICI and TKI.

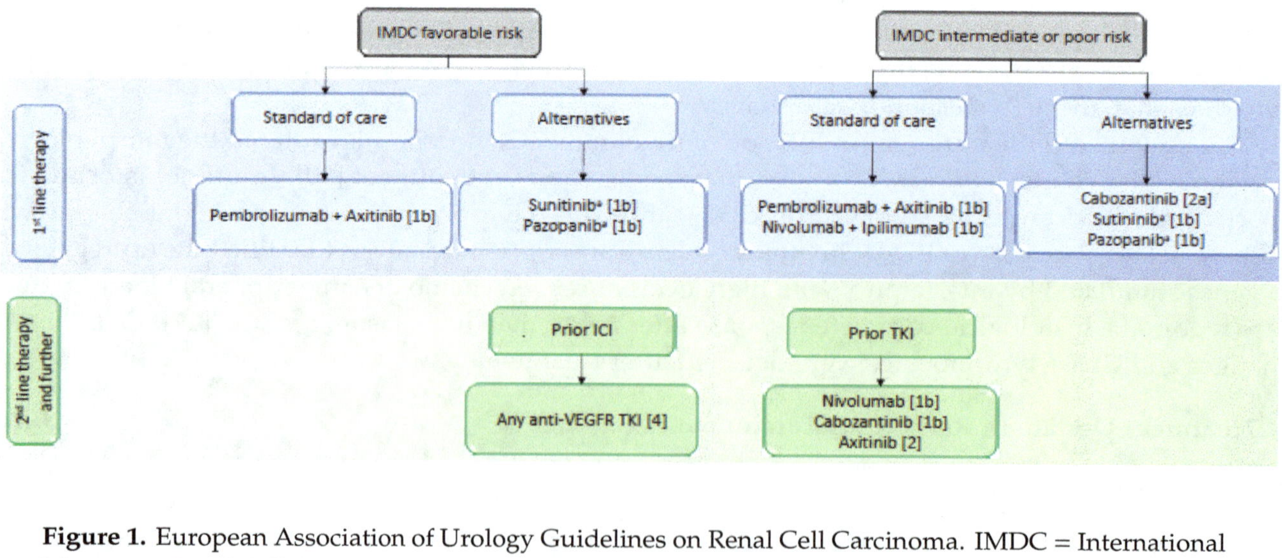

Figure 1. European Association of Urology Guidelines on Renal Cell Carcinoma. IMDC = International Metastatic Renal Cell CarcinomaDatabase Consortium; OS = overall survival; Oxford level of evidence: [1b] = based on one randomised controlled phase 3 trial; [2a] = based on one randomised controlled phase 2 trial; [2b] = subgroup analysis of a randomised controlled phase 3 trial; [4] = expert opinion. a = No OS benefit proven.

Table 1. Comparison of pivotal phase III clinical trials with available results evaluating immune checkpoints inhibitors.

Study Name	Tested Drugs	Comparison	Phase	Histology	Therapy Setting	OS (HR, 95% CI, *p*)	Median PFS (HR, 95% CI)	ORR (%)	CR (%)	Grade 3 (%)
Javelin Renal 101	avelumab + axitinib	sunitinib	III	ccRCC	First line	12-mo: 86% vs. 83% (0.78; 0.55–1.08; $p = 0.14$)	13.8 vs. 7.2 mo (0.61)	55.2 vs. 25,5	3.4 vs. 1.8	71.2 vs. 71.5
Keynote 426	pembrolizumab + axitinib	sunitinib	III	ccRCC	First line	12-mo: 90% vs. 78% (0.53; 0.38–0.74; $p < 0.0001$)	15.1 vs. 11.1 mo (0.69; 0.57–0.84)	59.3 vs. 35.7	5.8 vs. 1.9	75.8 vs. 70.6
CheckMate 214	nivolumab + ipilimumab	sunitinib	III	ccRCC	First line	30-mo : 60% vs, 47% (0.66; 0.54–0.80; $p < 0.0001$)	11.6 vs. 8.4 mo (0.82; 0.64–1,05)	42 vs. 29	9 vs. 1	47 vs. 64
Immotion 151	atezolizumab + bevacizumab	sunitinib	III	ccRCC	First line	24 mo : 63% vs. 60% (0.93; 0.76–1.14; $p = 0·4751$)	11.2 vs. 7.7 mo (0.74; 0.57–0.96)	43 vs. 25	9 vs. 4	40 vs. 54

Abbreviations: OS = overall survival; HR = Hazard Ratio; PFS = progression-free survival; ORR = objective response rate; CR = complete response; ccRCC: clear cell renal cell carcinoma, mo = months.

3.2. *Second-Line Treatment*

The choice of treatment in the second-line setting and beyond depends on the therapy previously received. In case of progression after antiangiogenics, the Checkmate 025 trial comparing nivolumab and everolimus showed an improvement of median OS in the nivolumab arm (25 vs. 19.6 months; HR = 0.73; 98.5% CI, 0.57 to 0.93; $p = 0.0018$) [45]. Notably, PD-L1 expression by IHC was associated with a poorer survival, but was not predictive of nivolumab efficacy. After first line ICI, any anti-angiogenic drug was recommended by the European Association of Urology with a low level of relevance [16]. However, due to the release of recent results, there is no prospectively validated data on the best therapeutic option after ICI and TKI combination in the front-line setting.

3.3. *Adjuvant treatment*

Finally, several ongoing phase III trials are studying the efficacy of ICI alone (atezolizumab, Pembrolizumab, nivolumab and tremelimumab) or in combination (nivolumab + ipilimumab) in the challenging peri-operative and adjuvant settings. Unsurprisingly, there is no combination of ICI plus TKI under evaluation as S-TRAC trial was the only one to show a benefit of adjuvant sunitinib in locally advanced high-risk ccRCC [46].

3.4. *Non-Clear Cell Renal Cell Carcinoma*

Unlike ccRCC, the management of nccRCC remains unclear and clinical trials are preferred [47]. Indeed, few prospective data for nccRCC treatment are available and trials have shown a lower efficacy of anti-angiogenic therapy compared to ccRCC with an impact on the prognosis of both PFS and OS [48]. In a recent retrospective trial including 41 patients, nivolumab seemed to demonstrate its efficacy with a favourable safety profile [49]. Indeed, the ORR was 20% and the median PFS was 3.5 months (95% CI; 1.9–5.0 months). Median OS was not reached, and the overall survival at the 10-month time point from the start of nivolumab treatment was 68%. Behind ccRCC, several trials evaluating ICI targeted drugs alone or in combination with TKI are currently recruiting in nccRCC without distinction of the entities, as shown in Tables 2 and 3. Interestingly, the combination of durvalumab and savolitinib (MET TKI) is specifically evaluated in pRCC. Likewise, nivolumab plus axitinib is studied in tRCC. Of note, ongoing trials using emerging drugs or vaccinal strategies include de facto nccRCC under the non-restrictive RCC inclusion criteria, Table 4.

4. Emerging Drugs in Ongoing Trials Include Renal Cell Carcinoma

4.1. *Inhibitory Immune Checkpoints*

The anergy of T cell is commonly understood as the result of a sequential transduction of signals implicating immune checkpoints in the immune synapse, Figure 2. If CTLA4 and PD-1 are the most common and well-studied, others are emerging and could be implied in resistance to traditional ICI and are evaluated in clinical trials including RCC, as shown in Tables 2 and 3.

Lymphocyte-associated gene 3 (LAG3) is a transmembrane protein mainly expressed in activated T and natural killer (NK) cells, as shown in Figure 2 [29]. LAG3 is located on T cells. It shares a structural homology with CD4 and binds its ligand, the major histocompatibility complex class II (MHCII) with higher affinity. Moreover, the LAG3 blockade leads to an increased production of interferon gamma (INFγ), tumour necrosis factor alpha (TNFα) and pro-inflammatory interleukins [50].

Other ICI are emerging. Among them, T cell immunoglobulin and mucin domain3 (TIM3) expressed on a wide variety of immune cells. TIM3 contributes to immune tolerance by inhibiting T cells activation, mostly by upregulation of apoptosis [51]. Interestingly, there could be a synergistic effect with PD-1-PD-L1 blockade, reversing T cell exhaustion and improving anti-tumoral immune response [52].

T cell immunoglobulin and ITIM domain (TIGIT) is mainly found on TIL and is immunosuppressive through disrupting interleukins production and antigen-presenting cell (APC) maturation [53]. The two ligands Nectin-2 and CD155 are expressed in various cellular types from tumour to immune cells. Similar results in terms of T cells exhaustion were observed in the B7-H3 pathway [54].

The v-domain immunoglobulin suppressor of T cell activation (VISTA) is predominantly expressed on myeloid-derived suppressive cells (MDSC) and APC and down-regulates T cells activation [55]. Remarkably, VISTA blockade seemed to inhibit regulatory T cell immunosuppressive functions [56].

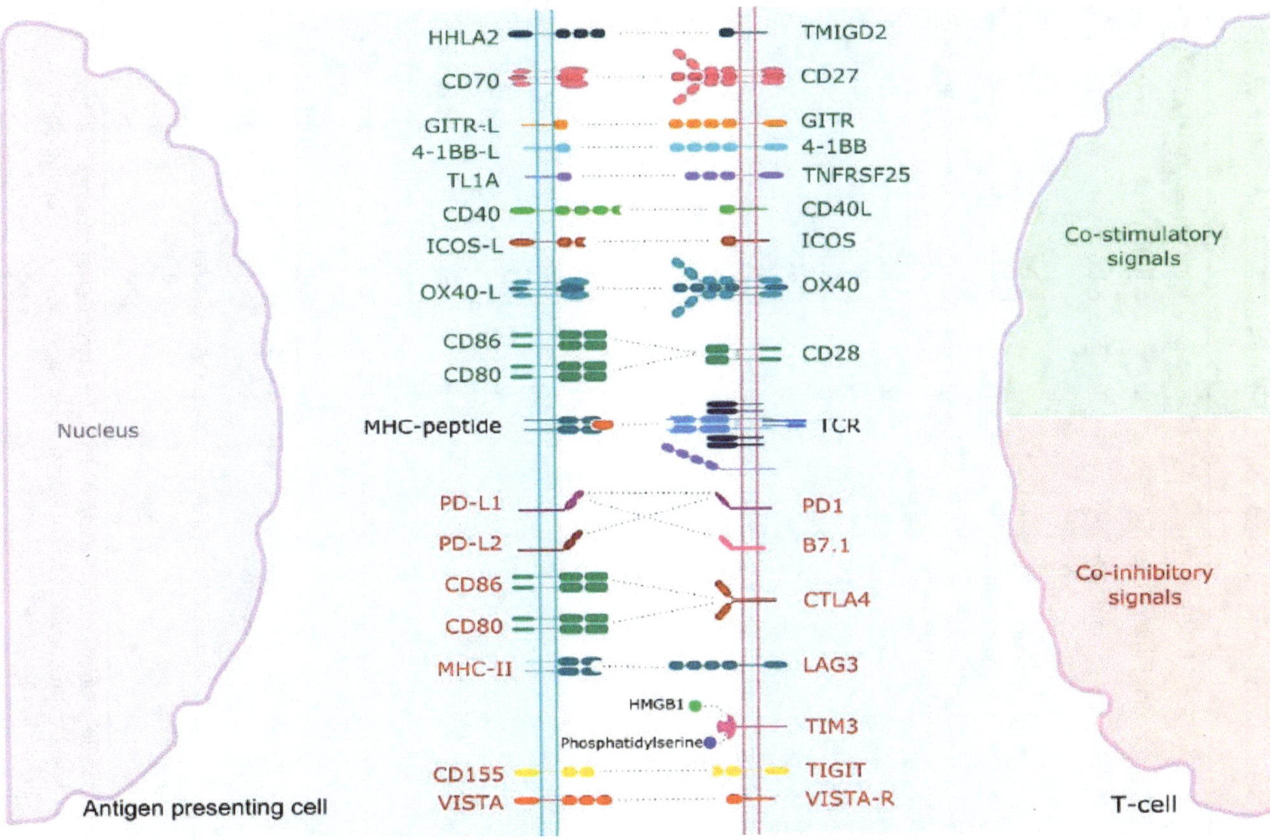

Figure 2. T-cell activation or inhibition is the result of an integrated and sequential intracellular signal cascade after MHC-peptide recognition by TCR. Abbreviations: GITR = Glucocorticoid-Induced TNF Receptor, ICOS = Inducible co-stimulator, OX40 = CD134, TCR = T-Cell Receptor, PD1 = Programmed Death 1, CTLA4 = Cytotoxic T-lymphocyte Antigen-4, LAG3 = Lymphocyte-associated gene 3, TIM3 = Tcell Immunoglobulin and Mucin domain-3, TIGIT = T-cell Immunoglobulin and ITIM domain, VISTA = Vdomain Immunoglobulin Suppressor of T-cell Activation.

Table 2. Clinical trials evaluating immune checkpoint inhibitors in association with tyrosine kinase inhibitors.

NCT Number	Targeting Agents	Comparison	Phase	Histology	Primary Endpoint	Therapy Setting	Status
NCT03260894	pembrolizumab + epacadostat	sunitinib or pazopanib	III	ccRCC	ORR	First line	Active not recruiting
NCT02811861	lenvatinib + everolimus or pembrolizumab	sunitinib	III	ccRCC	PFS	First line	Active not recruiting
NCT03141177	nivolumab + cabozantinib	sunitinib	III	ccRCC	PFS	First line	Active not recruiting
NCT03793166	nivolumab, ipilimumab, cabozantinib	nivolumab or nivolumab + cabozantinib	III	ccRCC	OS	First line	Recruiting
NCT03937219	nivolumab + ipilimumab + cabozantinib	nivolumab + ipilimumab + placebo	III	ccRCC	DFS	First line	Recruiting
NCT03680521	sitravatinib + nivolumab	_	II	ccRCC	ORR	First line	Recruiting
NCT02960906	nivolumab, ipilimumab, VEGFR-TKI	_	II	ccRCC	ORR	First line	Recruiting
NCT03736330	axitinib + pembrolizumab + D-CIK	_	II	ccRCC	ORR	At least second line	Recruiting
NCT02819596	savolitinib, durvalumab, tremelimumab	_	II	ccRCC, pRCC	DLT, ORR	At least second line	Unknown
NCT02964078	pembrolizumab + interleukin-2	_	II	ccRCC	ORR	Any	Active not recruiting
NCT03092856	anti-OX40 agonist antibody + axitinib	_	II	ccRCC	PFS	No standard anymore available	Recruiting
NCT02724878	atezolizumab + bevacizumab	_	II	nccRCC	ORR	Any	Active not recruiting
NCT03635892	nivolumab + cabozantinib	_	II	nccRCC	ORR	Any	Recruiting
NCT03595124	nivolumab + axitinib	_	II	tRCC	PFS	Any	Recruiting
NCT02493751	avelumab + axitinib	_	I/II	ccRCC	DLT	First line	Published
NCT02899078	ibrutinib + nivolumab	_	I/II	ccRCC, nccRCC	PFS	At least second line	Recruiting
NCT02348008	pembrolizumab + bevacizumab	_	I/II	ccRCC	Safety, efficacy	At least second line	Active not recruiting
NCT03172754	nivolumab + axitinib	_	I/II	ccRCC	Safety	At least second line	Recruiting
NCT03024437	atezolizumab + entinostat + bevacizumab	atezolizumab + entinostat	I/II	ccRCC	Safety, ORR	At least second line	Recruiting
NCT02501096	pembrolizumab + lenvatinib	_	I/II	ccRCC	DLT, ORR	No standard anymore available	Active not recruiting
NCT01472081	nivolumab + sunitinib or pazopanib	nivolumab	I	ccRCC	Safety	At least second line	Published
NCT03307785	TSR-022 (anti-TIM3)/niraparib/TSR-042 (anti-PD1)/chemotherapy/bevacizumab	_	I	RCC and others	Safety	At least second line	Active not recruiting
NCT03200587	avelumab + cabozantinib	_	Ib	ccRCC	Safety	Any	Recruiting

Abbreviations: OS = overall survival; HR = Hazard Ratio; PFS = progression-free survival; ORR = objective response rate; CR = complete response; ccRCC = clear cell renal cell carcinoma; nccRCC = non clear cell renal cell carcinoma; DLT = dose-limiting toxicity; DFS = disease-free survival; ICI = immune checkpoint inhibitor; TKI = tyrosine kinase inhibitor; VEGFR: vascular endothelial growth factor receptor; _ = na; SBRT = stereotactic body radiation.

Table 3. Clinical trials evaluating targeted immunotherapies alone or in combination.

NCT Number	Targeting Agents	Comparison	Phase	Histology	Primary Endpoint	Therapy Setting	Status
NCT03729245	NKTR-214 (IL2R agonist) + nivolumab	sunitinib or cabozantinib	III	ccRCC	ORR, OS	First line	Recruiting
NCT03873402	nivolumab + ipilimumab	nivolumab	III	ccRCC	PFS, ORR	First line	Recruiting
NCT01668784	nivolumab	everolimus	III	ccRCC	OS	At least second line	Published
NCT03055013	nivolumab	observation	III	ccRCC	DFS	Peri-operative	Recruiting
NCT03024996	atezolizumab	placebo	III	ccRCC	DFS	Adjuvant	Active not recruiting
NCT03138512	nivolumab + ipilimumab	placebo	III	ccRCC	DFS	Adjuvant	Recruiting
NCT03142334	pembrolizumab	placebo	III	ccRCC	DFS	Adjuvant	Active not recruiting
NCT03288532	nivolumab, tremelimumab	_	III	ccRCC	DFS	Adjuvant	Recruiting
NCT02996110	BMS-986205 (IDO1 oral inhibitor) +/− nivolumab +/− ipilimumab	nivolumab +/− ipilimumab	II	ccRCC, nccRCC	ORR, PFS	First line	Recruiting
NCT03552380	nivolumab + ipilimumab + entinostat	_	II	ccRCC	Safety	At least second line	Recruiting
NCT03501381	entinostat + IL2	IL2	II	ccRCC	PFS	At least second line	Recruiting
NCT03469713	nivolumab + SBRT	_	II	ccRCC	ORR	At least second line	Recruiting
NCT03177239	nivolumab + ipilimumab	_	II	nccRCC	ORR	Any	Active, not recruiting
NCT04262375	oleclumab (anti-CD73 antagonist mAb) + durvalumab	_	II	RCC and others	ORR, PFS	Any	Not yet recruiting
NCT03207867	NIR178 (A2aR antagonist) + spartalizumab (anti-PD1)	_	II	RCC and others	ORR	At least second line	Recruiting
NCT03693612	GSK3359609 (anti-ICOS) + tremelimumab	chemotherapies	II	RCC and others	DLT	No standard anymore available	Recruiting
NCT03693612	anti-ICOS + tremelimumab	_	II	RCC and others	Safety, DLT	No standard anymore available	Recruiting
NCT01038778	entinostat + aldesleukin	_	I/II	ccRCC	Dose, ORR	At least second line	Active, not recruiting
NCT03308396	durvalumab + guadecitabine	_	I/II	ccRCC	Safe dose/ORR	At least second line	Recruiting
NCT02989714	nivolumab + interleukin-2	-	I/II	ccRCC	Safety	Third line	Active not recruiting
NCT02460224	LAG525 (anti-LAG3) + spartalizumab (anti-PD1)	_	I/II	RCC and others	DLT, ORR	At least second line	Active, not recruiting
NCT03652077	anti-TIM3	_	I/II	RCC and others	Safety	No standard anymore available	Recruiting
NCT02608268	MBG453 (anti-TIM3) + spartalizumab (anti-PD1)	spartalizumab anti-PD1	I/II	RCC and others	Safety, ORR, DLT	No standard anymore available	Recruiting
NCT01968109	relatlimab (anti-LAG3) + nivolumab	relatlimab	I/II	RCC and others	Safety, ORR, DLT	No standard anymore available	Recruiting
NCT03126110	INCAGN01876 (anti-GITR) + nivolumab + ipilimumab	_	I/II	RCC and others	Safety, tolerability	No standard anymore available	Recruiting
NCT02335918	varlilumab (anti-CD27) + nivolumab	_	I/II	RCC and others	DLT, ORR	At least second line	Completed

Table 3. *Cont.*

NCT Number	Targeting Agents	Comparison	Phase	Histology	Primary Endpoint	Therapy Setting	Status
NCT02718066	HBI-8000 (HDACi) + nivolumab	–	I/II	RCC and others	RP2D	At least second line	Recruiting
NCT02890069	spartalizumab + LCL16 (IAP inhibitor) + everolimus + panobinostat	–	I/II	RCC and others	DLT	At least second line	Recruiting
NCT02771626	CB-839 (glutaminase inhibitor) + nivolumab	–	I/II	RCC and others	Safety, efficacy	At least second line	Recruiting
NCT02817633	TSR-022 (anti-TIM3)/TSR-042 (anti-PD1)/TSR-033 (anti-LAG3)	–	I	RCC and others	Safety, tolerability	No standard anymore available	Recruiting
NCT03119428	OMP-31M32 (anti-TIGIT) + nivolumab	–	I	RCC and others	DLT	No standard anymore available	Terminated
NCT00351949	IMP321 (anti-LAG3)	–	I	RCC and others	Safety, tolerability	No standard anymore available	Completed
NCT02386111	varlilumab (anti-CD27)	–	I	RCC and others	Safety, tolerability	At least second line	Terminated
NCT03343613	LY3300054 (IDO1 inhibitor) + PD-L1 inhibitor	–	I	RCC and others	DLT	No standard anymore available	Recruiting
NCT02812875	CA-170 (VISTA antagonist)	–	I	RCC and others	DLT	No standard anymore available	Active not recruiting
NCT02655822	ciforadenant (A2aR antagonist) +/- atezolizumab	–	I	RCC and others	DLT	At least second line	Recruiting
NCT04198766	anti-OX40 + pembrolizumab	–	I	RCC and others	Safety	No standard anymore available	Recruiting

Abbreviations: OS = overall survival; HR = Hazard Ratio; PFS = progression-free survival; ORR = objective response rate; CR = complete response; ccRCC = clear cell renal cell carcinoma; nccRCC = non clear cell renal cell carcinoma; DLT = dose-limiting toxicity; DFS = disease-free survival.

Table 4. Vaccinal strategies and CAR T-cells trials.

NCT Number	Targeting Agents	Comparison	Phase	Histology	Primary Endpoint	Therapy Setting	Status
NCT00458536	dendritic cell tumor fusion vaccine + GM-CSF	–	I/II	ccRCC, nccRCC	Safety	Any	Active not recruiting
NCT03633110	GEN-009 Adjuvanted Vaccine + nivolumab + pembrolizumab	–	I/II	RCC and others	Safety	At least second line	Recruiting
NCT00722228	Autologous or Allogeneic tumor cells	–	I/II	RCC and others	Safety, efficacy	At least second line	Recruiting
NCT03393936	anti-ROR2 CAR-T or anti AXL CART-T	–	I/II	ccRCC, nccRCC	Safety	No standard available	Recruiting
NCT02830724	anti-CD70 CAR-T	–	I/II	RCC and others	Safety	At least second line	Recruiting
NCT01218867	anti-VEGFR2 CAR-T	–	I/II	RCC and others	ORR	At least second line	Terminated
NCT03638206	anti-C-MET CAR-T	–	I/II	RCC and others	Safety	At least second line	Recruiting
NCT02950766	neovax vaccine + ipilimumab	–	I	ccRCC	DLT	At least second line	Recruiting
NCT00096629	PSMA DNA vaccine	–	I	ccRCC, nccRCC	Safety	Adjuvant	Completed
NCT03548467	VB10.NEO vaccine +/- bempegaldesleukin (NKTR-214)	–	I	RCC and others	Safety	At least second line	Recruiting
NCT03294083	pexastimogene devacirepvec (Pexa-Vec)	–	I	ccRCC, nccRCC	Safety, efficacy	At least second line	Recruiting
NCT03715985	EVAX-01-CAF09b (peptide-based vaccine) +/- anti-PD1 or anti-PD-L1	–	I	RCC and others	Safety, efficacy	First line	Recruiting

Abbreviations: OS = overall survival; HR = Hazard Ratio; PFS = progression-free survival; ORR = objective response rate; CR = complete response; ccRCC = clear cell renal cell carcinoma; nccRCC = non clear cell renal cell carcinoma; DLT = dose-limiting toxicity; DFS = disease-free survival; ICI = immune checkpoint inhibitor; TKI = tyrosine kinase inhibitor; VEGFR: vascular endothelial growth factor receptor; - = na; SBRT = stereotactic body radiation.

4.2. Co-Activating Immune Checkpoints

Tumour-specific T cell-mediated immune response is balanced by both inhibitory and co-stimulatory signals. If ICI are mainly used to restore immune response, agonist drugs are developed to increase co-stimulatory signals and stimulate immune response, as shown in Figure 2. Like ICI, several co-activating immune checkpoints are used in ongoing trials, Tables 2 and 3.

On T cells, CD28 is known to deliver an activating signal when binding CD80/86 after TCR recognition of major histocompatibility complex (MHC). Inducible co-stimulator (ICOS) mainly located on CD4+ T cells belongs to the immunoglobulin family as well as CD28 and produces inflammatory cytokines. Its intracytoplasmic structure has a strong affinity for phosphoinositide 3-kinase (PI3K) favoring the proliferation signal in lymphocytes [57].

The tumour necrosis factor (TNF) receptor superfamily is represented by a group of both soluble and transmembrane receptors involved in inflammation processes and able to bind a variety of ligands such as TNFα, TNFβ and OX40 ligand [58]. When binding its ligand, OX40 promotes T cells proliferation and survival, particularly CD4+ and CD8+ T cells, by upregulating pro-inflammatory cytokines and anti-apoptotic molecules. Other member TNF receptors such as CD40, CD27 and 4-1BB contribute to increased cytotoxic T cells mediated response through apoptosis or memory-cell differentiation. The glucocorticoid-induced TNF receptor (GITR), located on CD4+ and CD8+ T cells and predominantly on FoxP3+ regulatory T cells, is known to enhance immunity to tumours through the attenuation of the effector activity of immunosuppressive regulatory T cells [59].

4.3. Metabolic Pathways

Metabolic changes influence the TME by providing immunosuppressive metabolites and favoring tumour growth in hypoxic conditions, as shown in Figure 3 [60]. Multiple enzymes have been identified as key regulators of cytotoxic T cells immune response and are under evaluation in clinical trials, as shown in Tables 2 and 3.

Among them, indoleamine 2,3 dioxygenase 1 (IDO1), an intracellular enzyme, catalyses the conversion of tryptophan into kynurenine [61]. Although physiologically expressed in stromal and dendritic cells, it is overexpressed in MDSC and tumour cells. The tryptophan depletion induced by IDO1 expression leads to T cell exhaustion and apoptosis. Moreover, high concentration of kynurenine promotes immune-tolerant dendritic cells and regulatory T cell proliferation [62].

Adenosine is a purine base known to bind G-protein coupled adenosine receptors, upregulated in activated immune cells [63]. Adenosine 2a receptor (A2aR) triggers upregulation of adenylate cyclase activity leading to increased cyclic adenosine monophosphate (cAMP) concentration. It has a profound immunomodulatory effect on immune cells by various mechanisms including ZAP70 inhibition in TCR signalling, IL2 down-regulation, FoxP3 expression enhancement on regulatory T cells and TGFß marked secretion [64].

As previously reported, TME acquires immunosuppressive features by reprogramming metabolic processes. Arginine is an essential amino acid in immune and tumour cells demonstrating a high level of arginase [65]. Arginase inhibitors are currently evaluated in combination with several ICI, Table 3.

4.4. Other Strategies

Various innovative strategies in immunotherapy are applied for RCC. The histone conformation impacts the transcription and is regulated through phosphorylation, sumoylation, ubiquitination, acetylation and deacetylation [66]. Histone deacetylase (HDAC) inhibitors modify the chromatin accessibility and play a crucial role in cycle arrest and apoptosis and could eventually enhance tumour antigens release and indirectly improve antigen presentation by APC and T cells priming [67]. In RCC, entinostat, panobinostat and chidamide are under evaluation in combination with ICI or TKI, as shown in Tables 2 and 3.

Several vaccinal strategies are tested in cancers with the common objective to upregulate tumour neo-antigens exposure to immune system, particularly by T cells priming phase improvement [68]. At this time, three broad vaccine types are under investigation including DNA/RNA-based, peptide-based and cell-based vaccines with encouraging results in RCC. Oncolytic viruses are interesting alternatives, designed to infect tumour cells and hijack cellular machinery to induce transgene expression.

The chimeric Antigen Receptor (CAR) T cells are T cells genetically engineered to produce an artificial T cell receptor that combines both antigen-binding and T cell activating functions. The use of CART cells is hampered in RCC by the tumour heterogeneity. CAR T cells are currently tested in renal cell carcinoma, targeting various antigens such as ROR2, AXL, CD70, VEGFR2, MET or CAIX, as seen in Table 3. Moreover, pre-clinical data suggest the rationale of combining CAR T cells with TKI or radiotherapy [69].

5. Predictive Biomarkers in RCC

5.1. Clinico-Biological Biomarkers

The IMDC risk model includes six clinical and biological variables (poor Karnofsky performance status, less than 1 year between the diagnosis and the treatment, low hemoglobin concentration, high platelet count, high neutrophil count and high serum calcium) and has been validated in ccRCC and nccRCC [70,71]. However, the use of this classification is limited in nccRCC because the group is heterogeneous and samples in each group are small. The guidelines are dichotomized between favorable- and intermediate- or poor-risk disease, as shown in Figure 1 [16]. For instance, the clinical outcome was better in patients with intermediate- or poor-risk disease under nivolumab plus ipilimumab [20]. On the contrary, patients with favorable-risk disease better answered to sunitinib. These results suggest a distinct underlying biology.

5.2. Immunohistochemical Biomarkers

The most studied immunohistochemical biomarker PD-L1 failed to demonstrate a predictive capability in metastatic RCC [20]. If it was demonstrated as a poor prognostic factor in both ccRCC and nccRCC; indeed its ability to discriminate between patients the good responders is questionable [35]. Limitations to the use of PD-L1 have been well described and encompass intra-tumoral heterogeneity, variability of cut-offs and heterogeneous expression between primary and metastatic sites among others [72].

The contradictory and unresolved issue about PD-L1 as a biomarker also reveals the complicated interactions between the tumour and immune response, as shown in Figure 3. A comprehensive immune phenotype including other immunosuppressive factors such as TGFβ or IDO-1 and a better characterization of immune cells could be another step forward in the search of predictive biomarkers. Interestingly, IDO-1 expression was higher in endothelial cells of responders to nivolumab in a cohort of 15 patients with metastatic RCC [73]. This results in a reduced influx of tryptophan in the surrounding tumour tissue leading to a decrease in tumour proliferation.

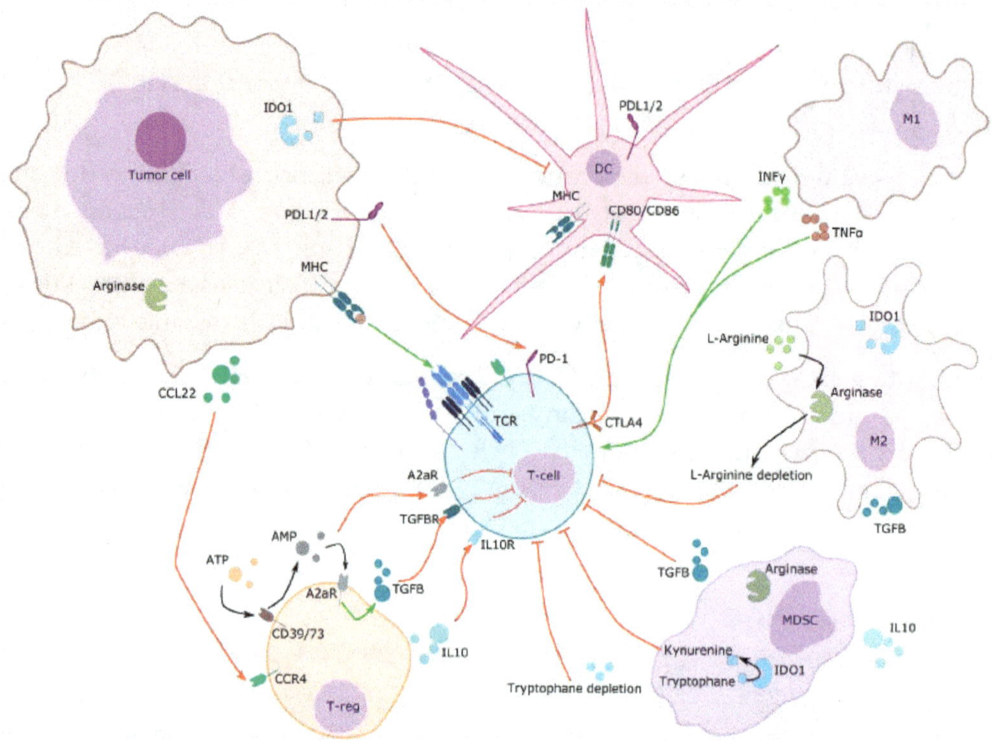

Figure 3. Tumor microenvironment is commonly defined as the co-existence of tumor cells interacting with resident and infiltrating host cells, secreted factors and extracellular matrix proteins. Among them, immunosuppressive cells are recruited in the tumor microenvironment by chemotaxis and are responsible for immunomodulatory cytokines production enhancement and decreased essential amino acids availability, resulting in favorable conditions for tumor growth. MDSC = Myeloïd-derived suppressive cells; T-cell = T lymphocyte; T-reg = Regulator lymphocyte; M2 = Type 2 macrophage; DC = dendritic cell; TGBß = tumor growth factor ß; A2aR = adenosine 2a receptor; ATP = adenosine triphosphate; AMP = adenosine monophosphate; IL10 = interleukin-10; MHC = major histocompatibility complex; PD1 = programmed death protein 1; PDL1 = programmed death ligand 1; IDO1 = indoleamine 2,3 dioxygenase 1; CTLA4 = cytotoxic T-lymphocyte antigen-4; CCL22 = C-C motif chemokine Ligand L22; CCR4 = C-C motif chemokine receptor 4; M1 = type 1 macrophage; INFγ = interferon γ; TNF α = tumor necrosis factor α.

5.3. Transcriptomic Analysis

Beuselink and colleagues first performed clustering transcriptomic analysis in patients with metastatic ccRCC (n = 53) receiving first-line sunitinib [74,75]. Hakimi et al. performed the same analysis in ccRCC of patients included in COMPARZ trial receiving pazopanib or sunitinib (n = 453) and identified four similar clusters [75]. Cluster 3 had the best prognosis with high angiogenic gene expression being associated with a better outcome under antiangiogenic therapy and similar to ccrcc2 cluster reported by Beuselinck et al. [76]. Of note, PBRM1 mutation was frequently associated with angiogenic gene expression. Cluster 4 had a worse prognosis and was similar to ccrcc4 with upregulation of immune pathways. Interestingly, ccrcc4 was enriched in tumours with sarcomatoid differentiation with a frequent expression of PD-L1 [77]. Clusters 1 and 2 were intermediate clusters with a lower expression of angiogenic and immune genes. A consensus classification could emerge from these different studies as proposed in the bladder cancer [78].

McDermott and colleagues explored three gene expression signatures: angiogenesis, T-effector/IFN-γ response, and myeloid inflammatory genes in ccRCC (n = 263) from IMmotion 150 trial: a phase 2 trial before IMmotion 151 of atezolizumab (anti-PD-L1) alone or combined with bevacizumab (anti-VEGF) versus sunitinib [76]. Interestingly, high T effector/IFNγ signature was associated with a better outcome to atezolizumab plus bevacizumab and a high myeloid inflammation signature was associated with reduced survival in the atezolizumab alone arm.

5.4. *Tumour Mutational Burden and Mismatch Repair Deficiency*

The TMB is based on the total number of mutations per coding area of the tumour genome. High mutation burden favors the formation of neo-antigens that enhance the tumour immune response [79]. This biomarker initially failed to identify responders to immunotherapy in ccRCC but is still under evaluation [80,81]. However, Limitations of this marker may be due to technical requirements such as coverage, DNA amount and analysis time and lack of standardization.

Even if RCC are not considered to be in the spectrum of hereditary non-polyposis colon cancer (HNPCC) or Lynch syndrome, loss of mismatch repair (MMR) proteins leading to microsatellite instability is frequently observed [82]. MMR deficient tumours demonstrate a higher rate of mutations but on specific genes. In RCC, data on the response to immunotherapy according to MMR status are also still ongoing.

5.5. *Gut Microbiome*

The gut microbiome, defined by the environmental conditions and the collection of microorganism and host genomes in an ecosystem, seems to influence the response to ICI. Indeed, the use of antibiotics could unfavorably impact the response. Indeed, Derosa et al. demonstrated a shorter survival and higher rates of progressive disease in patients with mRCC who received antibiotics within the month following the beginning of the treatment [83]. Indeed, antibiotics-related dysbiosis impacted the mirobiome and could decrease the activity of ICI. Conversely, they identified that some bacteria such as *B. salyersiae* or *A. muciniphila* could restore the efficacy of ICI.

6. Future Directions

6.1. *Microenvironment Cell Population Counter*

The microenvironment cell population counter (MCP counter) aims to assess the proportion of immune and stromal cells in the TME from transcriptomic data [84]. They classified tumours into four molecular TME subgroups: immune infiltration, T and NK lymphocytes, MCH1 expression and fibroblastic infiltration. This classification could be judiciously applied to previous transcriptomic data.

6.2. *Single-Cell Technologies*

The development and proper use of immunotherapies rely on the detailed understanding of tumour composition. However, this purpose is hampered by intratumour heterogeneity, which was demonstrated to be extensive in ccRCC [85]. With recent developments in single-cell technologies though, we can now circumvent and integrate intratumour heterogeneity into analyses in oncology by characterizing each individual cells within tumours [86]. In RCC, Kim and collaborators performed single-cell RNA sequencing to study the intratumour heterogeneity of paired primary RCC and lung metastasis [87]. A considerable variability between the primary and metastatic sites and among tumour cells was demonstrated by the activation of drug target pathways. This study encourages the use of single-cell RNA sequencing to better characterize cell populations and to favor the discovery of new biomarkers.

6.3. *3D Culture Models*

The 3D culture models of ccRCC could represent good pre-clinical models based on tissue slices preserving the stromal components of the TME [88]. Already used for TKI targeted therapies, these models are increasingly being considered as potential platforms for monitoring immunotherapy responses [89]. Recent studies indeed reported an active immune TME after applying immunomodulatory molecules on tumour slice organotypic cultures, opening the way for their study on 3D ex vivo tumour models [90]. Interestingly, co-cultures of tumour-derived organoids were enriched with lymphocytes, leading Dijkstra and collaborators to recently demonstrate the generation of tumour-reactive T cells by co-culture of peripheral blood lymphocytes and colorectal cancer-derived organoids [91]. These precursor approaches will allow to learn more about immune escape mechanisms and determine associated predictive biomarkers.

6.4. Imaging

Novel methods of imaging are non-invasive and assess RCC at different time points. Bensch et al. demonstrated that positron emission tomography (PET) imaging was able to localize ^{89}Zr-labeled atezolizumab to tumours expressing PD-L1 between primary and metastatic sites [92]. The uptake in tumours was heterogeneous and the clinical response better correlated with the pretreatment PET signal than with PD-L1 immunohistochemistry or T-effector gene expression signature. Moreover, CD8+ T cell infiltration was inferred from computed tomography [93].

6.5. Circulating Tumour Cells

The circulating tumour cells (CTC) is a non-invasive method isolating CTC from blood circulation [94]. The challenge is to detect them because of the rare expression of the usual marker epithelial cell adhesion molecule (EpCAM). This is due to the transdifferentiation of tumour cells through the epithelial mesenchymal transition [95]. The antibodies directed against membrane carbonic anhydrase 9 (CA9) and CD147 largely improved the detection of CTC from 17% with EpcAM to 97% of samples with CA9 and CD147 markers [96]. Other methods are based on RT-PCR targeting VHL gene alteration and size-based blood filtration associated with genetic and morphological analyses [97]. The CTC analyses could be used to select patients for clinical trials guided by biomarkers. The phenotype could evolve under treatment and be timely investigated to adapt the therapeutic strategy.

7. Conclusions

Renal cell carcinoma include distinct entities with specific molecular alterations. Among them, ccRCC, the most frequent, is particularly characterized by its angiogenic and immunogenic TME with complex interactions between stromal and immune cells. Like tumour cells, intratumour heterogeneity is present in the TME with a variable distribution and phenotype and consequently favours resistance to treatment.

Therapeutic options for patients with mRCC have expanded rapidly over the past decade with targeted immunotherapy being the new corner stone. Several emerging drugs are designed to enhance the antitumour immune response and are tested in ongoing trials.

With an increasing number of treatment options available, improved biomarkers are needed to better stratify patients and define the optimal selection of patients and the sequence of treatment to overcome resistance. Promising biomarkers such as gene expression signatures or gut microbiome are under evaluation. It is likely that the future of predictive biomarkers relies on the combination of different approaches reflecting the complexity of the TME.

We hope that, in the future, new technologies such as single-cell technologies contribute to unravel the intratumour heterogeneity, identify predictive biomarkers and discover new treatment targets.

Author Contributions: Conception and design: S.-F.K.-J., N.R.-L.; Collection and assembly of data: S.-F.K.-J., A.D., J.S., L.C., B.L., F.D., M.-A.B.-R., R.M., K.B., G.V.; Manuscript writing: A.D., J.S., S.-F.K.-J.; Final approval of the manuscript: all authors; Accountable for all aspects of the work: all authors. All authors have read and agreed to the published version of the manuscript.

References

1. Siegel, R.L.; Miller, K.D.; Jemal, A. Cancer statistics. *CA Cancer J. Clin.* **2019**, *69*, 7–34. [CrossRef] [PubMed]
2. Ljungberg, B.; Campbell, S.C.; Choi, H.Y.; Jacqmin, D.; Lee, J.E.; Weikert, S.; Kiemeney, L.A. The epidemiology of renal cell carcinoma. *Eur. Urol.* **2011**, *60*, 615–621. [CrossRef] [PubMed]

3. Gossage, L.; Eisen, T.; Maher, E.R. Vhl, the story of a tumour suppressor gene. *Nat. Rev. Cancer* **2015**, *15*, 55–64. [CrossRef] [PubMed]
4. Akaza, H.; Fukuyama, T. Axitinib for the treatment of advanced renal cell carcinoma. *Expert Opin. Pharmacother.* **2014**, *15*, 283–297. [CrossRef]
5. Motzer, R.J.; Hutson, T.E.; Cella, D.; Reeves, J.; Hawkins, R.; Guo, J.; Nathan, P.; Staehler, M.; de Souza, P.; Merchan, J.R.; et al. Pazopanib versus sunitinib in metastatic renal-cell carcinoma. *N. Engl. J. Med.* **2013**, *369*, 722–731. [CrossRef]
6. Choueiri, T.K.; Escudier, B.; Powles, T.; Mainwaring, P.N.; Rini, B.I.; Donskov, F.; Hammers, H.; Hutson, T.E.; Lee, J.L.; Peltola, K.; et al. Cabozantinib versus everolimus in advanced renal-cell carcinoma. *N. Engl. J. Med.* **2015**, *373*, 1814–1823. [CrossRef]
7. Rini, B.I.; Pal, S.K.; Escudier, B.J.; Atkins, M.B.; Hutson, T.E.; Porta, C.; Verzoni, E.; Needle, M.N.; McDermott, D.F. Tivozanib versus sorafenib in patients with advanced renal cell carcinoma (tivo-3): A phase 3, multicentre, randomised, controlled, open-label study. *Lancet Oncol.* **2020**, *21*, 95–104. [CrossRef]
8. Moch, H.; Cubilla, A.L.; Humphrey, P.A.; Reuter, V.E.; Ulbright, T.M. The 2016 who classification of tumours of the urinary system and male genital organs-part a: Renal, penile, and testicular tumours. *Eur. Urol.* **2016**, *70*, 93–105. [CrossRef]
9. Cancer Genome Atlas Research, N.; Linehan, W.M.; Spellman, P.T.; Ricketts, C.J.; Creighton, C.J.; Fei, S.S.; Davis, C.; Wheeler, D.A.; Murray, B.A.; Schmidt, L.; et al. Comprehensive molecular characterization of papillary renal-cell carcinoma. *N. Engl. J. Med.* **2016**, *374*, 135–145. [CrossRef]
10. Argani, P. Mit family translocation renal cell carcinoma. *Semin. Diagn. Pathol.* **2015**, *32*, 103–113. [CrossRef]
11. Malouf, G.G.; Monzon, F.A.; Couturier, J.; Molinie, V.; Escudier, B.; Camparo, P.; Su, X.; Yao, H.; Tamboli, P.; Lopez-Terrada, D.; et al. Genomic heterogeneity of translocation renal cell carcinoma. *Clin. Cancer Res.* **2013**, *19*, 4673–4684. [CrossRef] [PubMed]
12. Malouf, G.G.; Comperat, E.; Yao, H.; Mouawad, R.; Lindner, V.; Rioux-Leclercq, N.; Verkarre, V.; Leroy, X.; Dainese, L.; Classe, M.; et al. Unique transcriptomic profile of collecting duct carcinomas relative to upper tract urothelial carcinomas and other kidney carcinomas. *Sci. Rep.* **2016**, *6*, 30988. [CrossRef] [PubMed]
13. Carlo, M.I.; Chaim, J.; Patil, S.; Kemel, Y.; Schram, A.M.; Woo, K.; Coskey, D.; Nanjangud, G.J.; Voss, M.H.; Feldman, D.R.; et al. Genomic characterization of renal medullary carcinoma and treatment outcomes. *Clin. Genitourin. Cancer* **2017**, *15*, e987–e994. [CrossRef] [PubMed]
14. Chen, Y.B.; Brannon, A.R.; Toubaji, A.; Dudas, M.E.; Won, H.H.; Al-Ahmadie, H.A.; Fine, S.W.; Gopalan, A.; Frizzell, N.; Voss, M.H.; et al. Hereditary leiomyomatosis and renal cell carcinoma syndrome-associated renal cancer: Recognition of the syndrome by pathologic features and the utility of detecting aberrant succination by immunohistochemistry. *Am. J. Surg. Pathol.* **2014**, *38*, 627–637. [CrossRef]
15. Malouf, G.G.; Ali, S.M.; Wang, K.; Balasubramanian, S.; Ross, J.S.; Miller, V.A.; Stephens, P.J.; Khayat, D.; Pal, S.K.; Su, X.; et al. Genomic characterization of renal cell carcinoma with sarcomatoid dedifferentiation pinpoints recurrent genomic alterations. *Eur. Urol.* **2016**, *70*, 348–357. [CrossRef]
16. Albiges, L.; Powles, T.; Staehler, M.; Bensalah, K.; Giles, R.H.; Hora, M.; Kuczyk, M.A.; Lam, T.B.; Ljungberg, B.; Marconi, L.; et al. Updated european association of urology guidelines on renal cell carcinoma: Immune checkpoint inhibition is the new backbone in first-line treatment of metastatic clear-cell renal cell carcinoma. *Eur. Urol.* **2019**, *76*, 151–156. [CrossRef]
17. Motzer, R.J.; Bacik, J.; Murphy, B.A.; Russo, P.; Mazumdar, M. Interferon-alfa as a comparative treatment for clinical trials of new therapies against advanced renal cell carcinoma. *J. Clin. Oncol.* **2002**, *20*, 289–296. [CrossRef]
18. Fyfe, G.; Fisher, R.I.; Rosenberg, S.A.; Sznol, M.; Parkinson, D.R.; Louie, A.C. Results of treatment of 255 patients with metastatic renal cell carcinoma who received high-dose recombinant interleukin-2 therapy. *J. Clin. Oncol.* **1995**, *13*, 688–696. [CrossRef]
19. Motzer, R.J.; Hutson, T.E.; Tomczak, P.; Michaelson, M.D.; Bukowski, R.M.; Rixe, O.; Oudard, S.; Negrier, S.; Szczylik, C.; Kim, S.T.; et al. Sunitinib versus interferon alfa in metastatic renal-cell carcinoma. *N. Engl. J. Med.* **2007**, *356*, 115–124. [CrossRef]
20. Motzer, R.J.; Tannir, N.M.; McDermott, D.F.; Aren Frontera, O.; Melichar, B.; Choueiri, T.K.; Plimack, E.R.; Barthelemy, P.; Porta, C.; George, S.; et al. Nivolumab plus ipilimumab versus sunitinib in advanced renal-cell carcinoma. *N. Engl. J. Med.* **2018**, *378*, 1277–1290. [CrossRef]

21. Motzer, R.J.; Escudier, B.; McDermott, D.F.; George, S.; Hammers, H.J.; Srinivas, S.; Tykodi, S.S.; Sosman, J.A.; Procopio, G.; Plimack, E.R.; et al. Nivolumab versus everolimus in advanced renal-cell carcinoma. *N. Engl. J. Med.* **2015**, *373*, 1803–1813. [CrossRef] [PubMed]
22. Leite, K.R.; Reis, S.T.; Junior, J.P.; Zerati, M.; Gomes Dde, O.; Camara-Lopes, L.H.; Srougi, M. Pd-l1 expression in renal cell carcinoma clear cell type is related to unfavorable prognosis. *Diagn. Pathol.* **2015**, *10*, 189. [CrossRef] [PubMed]
23. Thompson, R.H.; Dong, H.; Kwon, E.D. Implications of b7-h1 expression in clear cell carcinoma of the kidney for prognostication and therapy. *Clin. Cancer Res.* **2007**, *13*, 709s–715s. [CrossRef]
24. Thompson, R.H.; Dong, H.; Lohse, C.M.; Leibovich, B.C.; Blute, M.L.; Cheville, J.C.; Kwon, E.D. Pd-1 is expressed by tumor-infiltrating immune cells and is associated with poor outcome for patients with renal cell carcinoma. *Clin. Cancer Res.* **2007**, *13*, 1757–1761. [CrossRef]
25. Motzer, R.J.; Penkov, K.; Haanen, J.; Rini, B.; Albiges, L.; Campbell, M.T.; Venugopal, B.; Kollmannsberger, C.; Negrier, S.; Uemura, M.; et al. Avelumab plus axitinib versus sunitinib for advanced renal-cell carcinoma. *N. Engl. J. Med.* **2019**, *380*, 1103–1115. [CrossRef]
26. Rini, B.I.; Plimack, E.R.; Stus, V.; Gafanov, R.; Hawkins, R.; Nosov, D.; Pouliot, F.; Alekseev, B.; Soulieres, D.; Melichar, B.; et al. Pembrolizumab plus axitinib versus sunitinib for advanced renal-cell carcinoma. *N. Engl. J. Med.* **2019**, *380*, 1116–1127. [CrossRef]
27. Sharma, P.; Hu-Lieskovan, S.; Wargo, J.A.; Ribas, A. Primary, adaptive, and acquired resistance to cancer immunotherapy. *Cell* **2017**, *168*, 707–723. [CrossRef]
28. Dunn, G.P.; Bruce, A.T.; Ikeda, H.; Old, L.J.; Schreiber, R.D. Cancer immunoediting: From immunosurveillance to tumor escape. *Nat. Immunol.* **2002**, *3*, 991–998. [CrossRef]
29. Anderson, A.C.; Joller, N.; Kuchroo, V.K. Lag-3, tim-3, and tigit: Co-inhibitory receptors with specialized functions in immune regulation. *Immunity* **2016**, *44*, 989–1004. [CrossRef]
30. Lambrechts, D.; Wauters, E.; Boeckx, B.; Aibar, S.; Nittner, D.; Burton, O.; Bassez, A.; Decaluwe, H.; Pircher, A.; Van den Eynde, K.; et al. Phenotype molding of stromal cells in the lung tumor microenvironment. *Nat. Med.* **2018**, *24*, 1277–1289. [CrossRef]
31. Akino, T.; Hida, K.; Hida, Y.; Tsuchiya, K.; Freedman, D.; Muraki, C.; Ohga, N.; Matsuda, K.; Akiyama, K.; Harabayashi, T.; et al. Cytogenetic abnormalities of tumor-associated endothelial cells in human malignant tumors. *Am. J. Pathol.* **2009**, *175*, 2657–2667. [CrossRef] [PubMed]
32. Edeline, J.; Mottier, S.; Vigneau, C.; Jouan, F.; Perrin, C.; Zerrouki, S.; Fergelot, P.; Patard, J.J.; Rioux-Leclercq, N. Description of 2 angiogenic phenotypes in clear cell renal cell carcinoma. *Hum. Pathol.* **2012**, *43*, 1982–1990. [CrossRef] [PubMed]
33. Dufies, M.; Giuliano, S.; Ambrosetti, D.; Claren, A.; Ndiaye, P.D.; Mastri, M.; Moghrabi, W.; Cooley, L.S.; Ettaiche, M.; Chamorey, E.; et al. Sunitinib stimulates expression of vegfc by tumor cells and promotes lymphangiogenesis in clear cell renal cell carcinomas. *Cancer Res.* **2017**, *77*, 1212–1226. [CrossRef] [PubMed]
34. Thompson, R.H.; Kuntz, S.M.; Leibovich, B.C.; Dong, H.; Lohse, C.M.; Webster, W.S.; Sengupta, S.; Frank, I.; Parker, A.S.; Zincke, H.; et al. Tumor b7-h1 is associated with poor prognosis in renal cell carcinoma patients with long-term follow-up. *Cancer Res.* **2006**, *66*, 3381–3385. [CrossRef] [PubMed]
35. Choueiri, T.K.; Fay, A.P.; Gray, K.P.; Callea, M.; Ho, T.H.; Albiges, L.; Bellmunt, J.; Song, J.; Carvo, I.; Lampron, M.; et al. Pd-l1 expression in nonclear-cell renal cell carcinoma. *Ann. Oncol.* **2014**, *25*, 2178–2184. [CrossRef]
36. Gupta, S.; Cheville, J. C.; Jungbluth, A. A.; Zhang, Y.; Zhang, L.; Chen, Y. B.; Tickoo, S. K.; Fine, S. W.; Gopalan, A.; Al-Ahmadie, H. A.; et al. JAK2/PD-L1/PD-L2 (9p24.1) amplifications in renal cell carcinomas with sarcomatoid transformation: Implications for clinical management. *Mod. Pathol.* **2019**, *32*, 1344–1358. [CrossRef] [PubMed]
37. Chevrier, S.; Levine, J.H.; Zanotelli, V.R.T.; Silina, K.; Schulz, D.; Bacac, M.; Ries, C.H.; Ailles, L.; Jewett, M.A.S.; Moch, H.; et al. An immune atlas of clear cell renal cell carcinoma. *Cell* **2017**, *169*, 736–749. [CrossRef]
38. Giraldo, N.A.; Becht, E.; Vano, Y.; Petitprez, F.; Lacroix, L.; Validire, P.; Sanchez-Salas, R.; Ingels, A.; Oudard, S.; Moatti, A.; et al. Tumor-infiltrating and peripheral blood t-cell immunophenotypes predict early relapse in localized clear cell renal cell carcinoma. *Clin. Cancer Res.* **2017**, *23*, 4416–4428. [CrossRef]
39. Sjoberg, E.; Frodin, M.; Lovrot, J.; Mezheyeuski, A.; Johansson, M.; Harmenberg, U.; Egevad, L.; Sandstrom, P.; Ostman, A. A minority-group of renal cell cancer patients with high infiltration of cd20 + b-cells is associated with poor prognosis. *Br. J. Cancer* **2018**, *119*, 840–846. [CrossRef]

40. Choueiri, T.K.; Fishman, M.N.; Escudier, B.; McDermott, D.F.; Drake, C.G.; Kluger, H.; Stadler, W.M.; Perez-Gracia, J.L.; McNeel, D.G.; Curti, B.; et al. Immunomodulatory activity of nivolumab in metastatic renal cell carcinoma. *Clin. Cancer Res.* **2016**, *22*, 5461–5471. [CrossRef]
41. Shirotake, S.; Kaneko, G.; Nagata, K.; Oyama, M.; Nishimoto, K. Histological complete response with nivolumab for renal cell carcinoma with multiple metastases: A case report. *Mol. Clin. Oncol.* **2019**, *10*, 244–248. [CrossRef] [PubMed]
42. Rini, B.I.; Powles, T.; Atkins, M.B.; Escudier, B.; McDermott, D.F.; Suarez, C.; Bracarda, S.; Stadler, W.M.; Donskov, F.; Lee, J.L.; et al. Atezolizumab plus bevacizumab versus sunitinib in patients with previously untreated metastatic renal cell carcinoma (immotion151): A multicentre, open-label, phase 3, randomised controlled trial. *Lancet* **2019**, *393*, 2404–2415. [CrossRef]
43. Motzer, R.J.; Rini, B.I.; McDermott, D.F.; Aren Frontera, O.; Hammers, H.J.; Carducci, M.A.; Salman, P.; Escudier, B.; Beuselinck, B.; Amin, A.; et al. Nivolumab plus ipilimumab versus sunitinib in first-line treatment for advanced renal cell carcinoma: Extended follow-up of efficacy and safety results from a randomised, controlled, phase 3 trial. *Lancet Oncol.* **2019**, *20*, 1370–1385. [CrossRef]
44. Lalani, A.A.; McGregor, B.A.; Albiges, L.; Choueiri, T.K.; Motzer, R.; Powles, T.; Wood, C.; Bex, A. Systemic treatment of metastatic clear cell renal cell carcinoma in 2018: Current paradigms, use of immunotherapy, and future directions. *Eur. Urol.* **2019**, *75*, 100–110. [CrossRef] [PubMed]
45. Tomita, Y.; Fukasawa, S.; Shinohara, N.; Kitamura, H.; Oya, M.; Eto, M.; Tanabe, K.; Kimura, G.; Yonese, J.; Yao, M.; et al. Nivolumab versus everolimus in advanced renal cell carcinoma: Japanese subgroup analysis from the checkmate 025 study. *Jpn. J. Clin. Oncol.* **2017**, *47*, 639–646. [CrossRef]
46. Ravaud, A.; Motzer, R.J.; Pandha, H.S.; George, D.J.; Pantuck, A.J.; Patel, A.; Chang, Y.H.; Escudier, B.; Donskov, F.; Magheli, A.; et al. Adjuvant sunitinib in high-risk renal-cell carcinoma after nephrectomy. *N. Engl. J. Med.* **2016**, *375*, 2246–2254. [CrossRef]
47. Motzer, R.J.; Jonasch, E.; Michaelson, M.D.; Nandagopal, L.; Gore, J.L.; George, S.; Alva, A.; Haas, N.; Harrison, M.R.; Plimack, E.R.; et al. Nccn guidelines insights: Kidney cancer, version 2.2020. *J. Natl. Compr. Cancer Netw.* **2019**, *17*, 1278–1285. [CrossRef]
48. Vera-Badillo, F.E.; Templeton, A.J.; Duran, I.; Ocana, A.; de Gouveia, P.; Aneja, P.; Knox, J.J.; Tannock, I.F.; Escudier, B.; Amir, E. Systemic therapy for non-clear cell renal cell carcinomas: A systematic review and meta-analysis. *Eur. Urol.* **2015**, *67*, 740–749. [CrossRef]
49. Koshkin, V.S.; Barata, P.C.; Zhang, T.; George, D.J.; Atkins, M.B.; Kelly, W.J.; Vogelzang, N.J.; Pal, S.K.; Hsu, J.; Appleman, L.J.; et al. Clinical activity of nivolumab in patients with non-clear cell renal cell carcinoma. *J. Immunother. Cancer* **2018**, *6*, 9. [CrossRef]
50. Benci, J.L.; Xu, B.; Qiu, Y.; Wu, T.J.; Dada, H.; Twyman-Saint Victor, C.; Cucolo, L.; Lee, D.S.M.; Pauken, K.E.; Huang, A.C.; et al. Tumor interferon signaling regulates a multigenic resistance program to immune checkpoint blockade. *Cell* **2016**, *167*, 1540–1554. [CrossRef]
51. Gao, X.; Zhu, Y.; Li, G.; Huang, H.; Zhang, G.; Wang, F.; Sun, J.; Yang, Q.; Zhang, X.; Lu, B. Tim-3 expression characterizes regulatory t cells in tumor tissues and is associated with lung cancer progression. *PLoS ONE* **2012**, *7*, e30676. [CrossRef] [PubMed]
52. Sakuishi, K.; Apetoh, L.; Sullivan, J.M.; Blazar, B.R.; Kuchroo, V.K.; Anderson, A.C. Targeting tim-3 and pd-1 pathways to reverse t cell exhaustion and restore anti-tumor immunity. *J. Exp. Med.* **2010**, *207*, 2187–2194. [CrossRef] [PubMed]
53. Casado, J.G.; Pawelec, G.; Morgado, S.; Sanchez-Correa, B.; Delgado, E.; Gayoso, I.; Duran, E.; Solana, R.; Tarazona, R. Expression of adhesion molecules and ligands for activating and costimulatory receptors involved in cell-mediated cytotoxicity in a large panel of human melanoma cell lines. *Cancer Immunol. Immunother.* **2009**, *58*, 1517–1526. [CrossRef] [PubMed]
54. Inamura, K.; Amori, G.; Yuasa, T.; Yamamoto, S.; Yonese, J.; Ishikawa, Y. Relationship of b7-h3 expression in tumor cells and tumor vasculature with foxp3+ regulatory t cells in renal cell carcinoma. *Cancer Manag. Res.* **2019**, *11*, 7021–7030. [CrossRef] [PubMed]
55. Wang, L.; Rubinstein, R.; Lines, J.L.; Wasiuk, A.; Ahonen, C.; Guo, Y.; Lu, L.F.; Gondek, D.; Wang, Y.; Fava, R.A.; et al. Vista, a novel mouse ig superfamily ligand that negatively regulates t cell responses. *J. Exp. Med.* **2011**, *208*, 577–592. [CrossRef] [PubMed]

56. Le Mercier, I.; Chen, W.; Lines, J.L.; Day, M.; Li, J.; Sergent, P.; Noelle, R.J.; Wang, L. Vista regulates the development of protective antitumor immunity. *Cancer Res.* **2014**, *74*, 1933–1944. [CrossRef]
57. Fos, C.; Salles, A.; Lang, V.; Carrette, F.; Audebert, S.; Pastor, S.; Ghiotto, M.; Olive, D.; Bismuth, G.; Nunes, J.A. Icos ligation recruits the p50alpha pi3k regulatory subunit to the immunological synapse. *J. Immunol.* **2008**, *181*, 1969–1977. [CrossRef]
58. Aspeslagh, S.; Postel-Vinay, S.; Rusakiewicz, S.; Soria, J.C.; Zitvogel, L.; Marabelle, A. Rationale for anti-ox40 cancer immunotherapy. *Eur. J. Cancer* **2016**, *52*, 50–66. [CrossRef]
59. Shevach, E.M.; Stephens, G.L. The gitr-gitrl interaction: Co-stimulation or contrasuppression of regulatory activity? *Nat. Rev. Immunol.* **2006**, *6*, 613–618. [CrossRef]
60. Ramapriyan, R.; Caetano, M.S.; Barsoumian, H.B.; Mafra, A.C.P.; Zambalde, E.P.; Menon, H.; Tsouko, E.; Welsh, J.W.; Cortez, M.A. Altered cancer metabolism in mechanisms of immunotherapy resistance. *Pharmacol. Ther.* **2019**, *195*, 162–171. [CrossRef]
61. Chen, J.Y.; Li, C.F.; Kuo, C.C.; Tsai, K.K.; Hou, M.F.; Hung, W.C. Cancer/stroma interplay via cyclooxygenase-2 and indoleamine 2,3-dioxygenase promotes breast cancer progression. *Breast Cancer Res.* **2014**, *16*, 410. [CrossRef] [PubMed]
62. Cheong, J.E.; Sun, L. Targeting the ido1/tdo2-kyn-ahr pathway for cancer immunotherapy—challenges and opportunities. *Trends Pharmacol. Sci.* **2018**, *39*, 307–325. [CrossRef] [PubMed]
63. Leone, R.D.; Emens, L.A. Targeting adenosine for cancer immunotherapy. *J. Immunother. Cancer* **2018**, *6*, 57. [CrossRef] [PubMed]
64. Linnemann, C.; Schildberg, F.A.; Schurich, A.; Diehl, L.; Hegenbarth, S.I.; Endl, E.; Lacher, S.; Muller, C.E.; Frey, J.; Simeoni, L.; et al. Adenosine regulates cd8 t-cell priming by inhibition of membrane-proximal t-cell receptor signalling. *Immunology* **2009**, *128*, e728–e737. [CrossRef]
65. Ananieva, E. Targeting amino acid metabolism in cancer growth and anti-tumor immune response. *World J. Biol. Chem.* **2015**, *6*, 281–289. [CrossRef]
66. Dawson, M.A.; Kouzarides, T. Cancer epigenetics: From mechanism to therapy. *Cell* **2012**, *150*, 12–27. [CrossRef]
67. Eckschlager, T.; Plch, J.; Stiborova, M.; Hrabeta, J. Histone deacetylase inhibitors as anticancer drugs. *Int. J. Mol. Sci.* **2017**, *18*. [CrossRef]
68. Pan, R.Y.; Chung, W.H.; Chu, M.T.; Chen, S.J.; Chen, H.C.; Zheng, L.; Hung, S.I. Recent development and clinical application of cancer vaccine: Targeting neoantigens. *J. Immunol. Res.* **2018**, *2018*, 4325874. [CrossRef]
69. Li, H.; Ding, J.; Lu, M.; Liu, H.; Miao, Y.; Li, L.; Wang, G.; Zheng, J.; Pei, D.; Zhang, Q. Caix-specific car-t cells and sunitinib show synergistic effects against metastatic renal cancer models. *J. Immunother.* **2020**, *43*, 16–28. [CrossRef]
70. Heng, D.Y.; Xie, W.; Regan, M.M.; Harshman, L.C.; Bjarnason, G.A.; Vaishampayan, U.N.; Mackenzie, M.; Wood, L.; Donskov, F.; Tan, M.H.; et al. External validation and comparison with other models of the international metastatic renal-cell carcinoma database consortium prognostic model: A population-based study. *Lancet Oncol.* **2013**, *14*, 141–148. [CrossRef]
71. Kroeger, N.; Klatte, T.; Chamie, K.; Rao, P.N.; Birkhauser, F.D.; Sonn, G.A.; Riss, J.; Kabbinavar, F.F.; Belldegrun, A.S.; Pantuck, A.J. Deletions of chromosomes 3p and 14q molecularly subclassify clear cell renal cell carcinoma. *Cancer* **2013**, *119*, 1547–1554. [CrossRef] [PubMed]
72. Kammerer-Jacquet, S.F.; Deleuze, A.; Saout, J.; Mathieu, R.; Laguerre, B.; Verhoest, G.; Dugay, F.; Belaud-Rotureau, M.A.; Bensalah, K.; Rioux-Leclercq, N. Targeting the pd-1/pd-l1 pathway in renal cell carcinoma. *Int. J. Mol. Sci.* **2019**, *20*, 1692. [CrossRef] [PubMed]
73. Seeber, A.; Klinglmair, G.; Fritz, J.; Steinkohl, F.; Zimmer, K.C.; Aigner, F.; Horninger, W.; Gastl, G.; Zelger, B.; Brunner, A.; et al. High ido-1 expression in tumor endothelial cells is associated with response to immunotherapy in metastatic renal cell carcinoma. *Cancer Sci.* **2018**, *109*, 1583–1591. [CrossRef] [PubMed]
74. Beuselinck, B.; Job, S.; Becht, E.; Karadimou, A.; Verkarre, V.; Couchy, G.; Giraldo, N.; Rioux-Leclercq, N.; Molinie, V.; Sibony, M.; et al. Molecular subtypes of clear cell renal cell carcinoma are associated with sunitinib response in the metastatic setting. *Clin. Cancer Res.* **2015**, *21*, 1329–1339. [CrossRef] [PubMed]
75. Hakimi, A.A.; Voss, M.H.; Kuo, F.; Sanchez, A.; Liu, M.; Nixon, B.G.; Vuong, L.; Ostrovnaya, I.; Chen, Y.B.; Reuter, V.; et al. Transcriptomic profiling of the tumor microenvironment reveals distinct subgroups of clear cell renal cell cancer—data from a randomized phase iii trial. *Cancer Discov.* **2019**, *9*, 510–525. [CrossRef] [PubMed]

76. McDermott, D.F.; Huseni, M.A.; Atkins, M.B.; Motzer, R.J.; Rini, B.I.; Escudier, B.; Fong, L.; Joseph, R.W.; Pal, S.K.; Reeves, J.A.; et al. Clinical activity and molecular correlates of response to atezolizumab alone or in combination with bevacizumab versus sunitinib in renal cell carcinoma. *Nat. Med.* **2018**, *24*, 749–757. [CrossRef] [PubMed]
77. Joseph, R.W.; Millis, S.Z.; Carballido, E.M.; Bryant, D.; Gatalica, Z.; Reddy, S.; Bryce, A.H.; Vogelzang, N.J.; Stanton, M.L.; Castle, E.P.; et al. Pd-1 and pd-l1 expression in renal cell carcinoma with sarcomatoid differentiation. *Cancer Immunol. Res.* **2015**, *3*, 1303–1307. [CrossRef]
78. Kamoun, A.; de Reynies, A.; Allory, Y.; Sjodahl, G.; Robertson, A.G.; Seiler, R.; Hoadley, K.A.; Groeneveld, C.S.; Al-Ahmadie, H.; Choi, W.; et al. A consensus molecular classification of muscle-invasive bladder cancer. *Eur. Urol.* **2019**, *77*, 420–433. [CrossRef]
79. Chalmers, Z.R.; Connelly, C.F.; Fabrizio, D.; Gay, L.; Ali, S.M.; Ennis, R.; Schrock, A.; Campbell, B.; Shlien, A.; Chmielecki, J.; et al. Analysis of 100,000 human cancer genomes reveals the landscape of tumor mutational burden. *Genome Med.* **2017**, *9*, 34. [CrossRef]
80. de Velasco, G.; Miao, D.; Voss, M.H.; Hakimi, A.A.; Hsieh, J.J.; Tannir, N.M.; Tamboli, P.; Appleman, L.J.; Rathmell, W.K.; Van Allen, E.M.; et al. Tumor mutational load and immune parameters across metastatic renal cell carcinoma risk groups. *Cancer Immunol. Res.* **2016**, *4*, 820–822. [CrossRef]
81. Miao, D.; Margolis, C.A.; Gao, W.; Voss, M.H.; Li, W.; Martini, D.J.; Norton, C.; Bosse, D.; Wankowicz, S.M.; Cullen, D.; et al. Genomic correlates of response to immune checkpoint therapies in clear cell renal cell carcinoma. *Science* **2018**, *359*, 801–806. [CrossRef] [PubMed]
82. Dudley, J.C.; Lin, M.T.; Le, D.T.; Eshleman, J.R. Microsatellite instability as a biomarker for pd-1 blockade. *Clin. Cancer Res.* **2016**, *22*, 813–820. [CrossRef] [PubMed]
83. Derosa, L.; Hellmann, M.D.; Spaziano, M.; Halpenny, D.; Fidelle, M.; Rizvi, H.; Long, N.; Plodkowski, A.J.; Arbour, K.C.; Chaft, J.E.; et al. Negative association of antibiotics on clinical activity of immune checkpoint inhibitors in patients with advanced renal cell and non-small-cell lung cancer. *Ann. Oncol.* **2018**, *29*, 1437–1444. [CrossRef] [PubMed]
84. Becht, E.; Giraldo, N.A.; Lacroix, L.; Buttard, B.; Elarouci, N.; Petitprez, F.; Selves, J.; Laurent-Puig, P.; Sautes-Fridman, C.; Fridman, W.H.; et al. Estimating the population abundance of tissue-infiltrating immune and stromal cell populations using gene expression. *Genome Biol.* **2016**, *17*, 218. [CrossRef]
85. Gerlinger, M.; Catto, J.W.; Orntoft, T.F.; Real, F.X.; Zwarthoff, E.C.; Swanton, C. Intratumour heterogeneity in urologic cancers: From molecular evidence to clinical implications. *Eur. Urol.* **2015**, *67*, 729–737. [CrossRef]
86. Suva, M.L.; Tirosh, I. Single-cell rna sequencing in cancer: Lessons learned and emerging challenges. *Mol. Cell* **2019**, *75*, 7–12. [CrossRef]
87. Kim, K.T.; Lee, H.W.; Lee, H.O.; Song, H.J.; Jeong da, E.; Shin, S.; Kim, H.; Shin, Y.; Nam, D.H.; Jeong, B.C.; et al. Application of single-cell rna sequencing in optimizing a combinatorial therapeutic strategy in metastatic renal cell carcinoma. *Genome Biol.* **2016**, *17*, 80. [CrossRef]
88. Roelants, C.; Pillet, C.; Franquet, Q.; Sarrazin, C.; Peilleron, N.; Giacosa, S.; Guyon, L.; Fontanell, A.; Fiard, G.; Long, J.A.; et al. Ex-vivo treatment of tumor tissue slices as a predictive preclinical method to evaluate targeted therapies for patients with renal carcinoma. *Cancers (Basel)* **2020**, *12*, 232. [CrossRef]
89. Meijer, T.G.; Naipal, K.A.; Jager, A.; van Gent, D.C. Ex vivo tumor culture systems for functional drug testing and therapy response prediction. *Future Sci. OA* **2017**, *3*, FSO190. [CrossRef]
90. Seo, Y.D.; Jiang, X.; Sullivan, K.M.; Jalikis, F.G.; Smythe, K.S.; Abbasi, A.; Vignali, M.; Park, J.O.; Daniel, S.K.; Pollack, S.M.; et al. Mobilization of cd8(+) t cells via cxcr4 blockade facilitates pd-1 checkpoint therapy in human pancreatic cancer. *Clin. Cancer Res.* **2019**, *25*, 3934–3945. [CrossRef]
91. Dijkstra, K.K.; Cattaneo, C.M.; Weeber, F.; Chalabi, M.; van de Haar, J.; Fanchi, L.F.; Slagter, M.; van der Velden, D.L.; Kaing, S.; Kelderman, S.; et al. Generation of tumor-reactive t cells by co-culture of peripheral blood lymphocytes and tumor organoids. *Cell* **2018**, *174*, 1586–1598. [CrossRef] [PubMed]
92. Bensch, F.; van der Veen, E.L.; Lub-de Hooge, M.N.; Jorritsma-Smit, A.; Boellaard, R.; Kok, I.C.; Oosting, S.F.; Schroder, C.P.; Hiltermann, T.J.N.; van der Wekken, A.J.; et al. (89)zr-atezolizumab imaging as a non-invasive approach to assess clinical response to pd-l1 blockade in cancer. *Nat. Med.* **2018**, *24*, 1852–1858. [CrossRef] [PubMed]

93. Sun, R.; Limkin, E.J.; Vakalopoulou, M.; Dercle, L.; Champiat, S.; Han, S.R.; Verlingue, L.; Brandao, D.; Lancia, A.; Ammari, S.; et al. A radiomics approach to assess tumour-infiltrating cd8 cells and response to anti-pd-1 or anti-pd-l1 immunotherapy: An imaging biomarker, retrospective multicohort study. *Lancet Oncol.* **2018**, *19*, 1180–1191. [CrossRef]
94. Gradilone, A.; Iacovelli, R.; Cortesi, E.; Raimondi, C.; Gianni, W.; Nicolazzo, C.; Petracca, A.; Palazzo, A.; Longo, F.; Frati, L.; et al. Circulating tumor cells and "suspicious objects" evaluated through cellsearch(r) in metastatic renal cell carcinoma. *Anticancer. Res.* **2011**, *31*, 4219–4221. [PubMed]
95. He, H.; Magi-Galluzzi, C. Epithelial-to-mesenchymal transition in renal neoplasms. *Adv. Anat. Pathol.* **2014**, *21*, 174–180. [CrossRef] [PubMed]
96. Liu, S.; Tian, Z.; Zhang, L.; Hou, S.; Hu, S.; Wu, J.; Jing, Y.; Sun, H.; Yu, F.; Zhao, L.; et al. Combined cell surface carbonic anhydrase 9 and cd147 antigens enable high-efficiency capture of circulating tumor cells in clear cell renal cell carcinoma patients. *Oncotarget* **2016**, *7*, 59877–59891. [CrossRef] [PubMed]
97. Santoni, M.; Cimadamore, A.; Cheng, L.; Lopez-Beltran, A.; Battelli, N.; Massari, F.; Scarpelli, M.; Galosi, A.B.; Bracarda, S.; Montironi, R. Circulating tumor cells in renal cell carcinoma: Recent findings and future challenges. *Front. Oncol.* **2019**, *9*, 228. [CrossRef]

2

A Precision Strategy to Cure Renal Cell Carcinoma by Targeting Transglutaminase 2

Soo-Youl Kim [1,*] and Jeffrey W. Keillor [2]

1 Division of Cancer Biology, National Cancer Center, Goyang 10408, Korea
2 Department of Chemistry and Biomolecular Sciences, University of Ottawa, Ottawa, ON K1N 6N5, Canada; jkeillor@uottawa.ca
* Correspondence: kimsooyoul@gmail.com;

Abstract: In a recent report, no significance of transglutaminase 2 (TGase 2) was noted in the analyses of expression differences between normal and clear cell renal cell carcinoma (ccRCC), although we found that knock down of TGase 2 induced significant p53-mediated cell death in ccRCC. Generally, to find effective therapeutic targets, we need to identify targets that belong specifically to a cancer phenotype that can be differentiated from a normal phenotype. Here, we offer precise reasons why TGase 2 may be the first therapeutic target for ccRCC, according to several lines of evidence. TGase 2 is negatively regulated by von Hippel-Lindau tumor suppressor protein (pVHL) and positively regulated by hypoxia-inducible factor 1-α (HIF-1α) in renal cell carcinoma (RCC). Therefore, most of ccRCC presents high level expression of TGase 2 because over 90% of ccRCC showed *VHL* inactivity through mutation and methylation. Cell death, angiogenesis and drug resistance were specifically regulated by TGase 2 through p53 depletion in ccRCC because over 90% of ccRCC express wild type p53, which is a cell death inducer as well as a HIF-1α suppressor. Although there have been no detailed studies of the physiological role of TGase 2 in multi-omics analyses of ccRCC, a life-long study of the physiological roles of TGase 2 led to the discovery of the first target as well as the first therapeutic treatment for ccRCC in the clinical field.

Keywords: clear cell renal cell carcinoma (ccRCC); transglutaminase 2 (TGase 2); p53; therapeutic target

---

1. Introduction

Renal cell carcinoma (RCC) is known to comprise a number of different types of cancers in the kidney, including clear cell renal cell carcinoma (ccRCC), papillary RCC, and chromophobe RCC. Among them, ccRCC represents 75% of all RCC cases [1]. Much of what is known about the genetic basis of this disease was learned from the study of inherited forms of RCC [1]. To date, germline mutations of genes have been associated with an increased risk of kidney cancer and have provided the foundation for mapping the genetic pathways altered in RCC [2]. Mutation of these genes such as von Hippel-Lindau (*VHL*) tumor suppressor gene can activate the hypoxia-inducible factor (HIF) pathway [3] and upregulate the phosphoinositide 3-kinase (PI3K)/ mammalian target of rapamycin (mTOR) pathway [4]. Inactivation of pVHL through protein modification also induces signaling of HIF-1α [5] and NF-κB [6]. Those activated pathways have been targeted for treatment, although there are no RCC-specific drugs with a specific therapeutic target. The first line of RCC treatment was selected by targeting universal cancer characteristics, such as the fast growth of cancer, based on growth signaling including mTOR, vascular endothelial growth factor (VEGF), and platelet-derived growth factor (PDGF) pathways. Temsirolimus [7] and everolimus [8] were selected for mammalian target of rapamycin complex 1 (mTORC1) inhibition. Cabozantinib [9], pazopanib [10], and axitinib [11] were selected for VEGFR inhibition by targeting HIF signaling. Sorafenib [12] and sunitinib were selected for PDGFR inhibition [13]. However, the most important limit for therapeutic outcome in ccRCC is recurrent phenotypes with drug resistance [1]. Due to drug resistance, it is difficult to achieve complete tumor remission [14]. There are two major categories of drug resistance, involving mTORC1 inhibition and receptor tyrosine kinase (RTK) (VEGFRs, PDGF-R) inhibition-induced drug resistance. Rapamycin targeting mTORC1 induces mTORC2, which promotes cancer cell survival through Akt activation [15]. Sunitinib targeting RTK induces autophagy through mTORC1 inhibition, which promotes biosynthetic intermediates for cancer survival [16]. Recently it has been shown that a combination treatment of immune-oncologic drugs, such as nivolumab targeting programmed death receptor-1 and ipilimumab targeting cytotoxic T lymphocytes antigen-4 inhibitors, led to a three-month increase of median progression-free survival compared to sunitinib [17]. Although a combination treatment of immune-oncologic drugs improved survival rate, it did not achieve complete tumor remission.

Recently, the clinical proteomic tumor analysis consortium (CPTAC) study on ccRCC was published, including molecular profiling data on 103 ccRCC tumor cases, as well as 83 samples of normal adjacent tissue [18]. The ccRCC proteomics data set included over 11,000 total proteins and over 40,000 phosphopeptides [18]. In addition to that, other analyses applied to these samples included whole exome and genome sequencings, as well as RNA sequencing [18]. Although this ensemble of data regarding ccRCC may explain why ccRCC shows resistance to therapeutics, it did not identify any specific therapeutic target for ccRCC. Although transglutaminase 2 (TGase 2) expression is reported to be high in ccRCC, and TGase 2 inhibition showed significant potential for a therapeutic approach for ccRCC in a series of past studies [19–23], the CPTAC study did not reveal any significance of TGase 2 in ccRCC [18]. These analytical results did not seem to fit, in the overall effort to find a cure for ccRCC. On the contrary, the discovery of TGase 2 as a therapeutic target for ccRCC may indeed be a breakthrough in the search for a cure of this disease. Analysis of ccRCC mutation from the COSMIC database revealed that less than 4% of total ccRCC patients have a p53 mutation [21]. This suggests that p53 is suppressed, even though 96% of ccRCC patients present wild type functional p53. In this review, TGase 2 is analyzed as a precise therapeutic target for ccRCC, considering how TGase 2 expression is increased, why the increase of TGase 2 is specifically related to ccRCC, and what the role of TGase 2 is that makes it critical to ccRCC survival. A key conclusion of this review article is that TGase 2 is a valid target for ccRCC because TGase 2 is the major regulator of functional p53 in ccRCC, and inhibitors that interfere with binding between TGase 2 and p53 show therapeutic potential.

2. Currently Suggested Role of TGase 2 in ccRCC—An Overview

2.1. TGase 2 in Normal Tissue

TGase 2 has been known as a cross-linking enzyme for about 50 years. Dr. Folk discovered transglutaminase C (TGase C, later *TGM2* gene renamed to TGase 2) from liver cytosol, at a time when Factor XIII was the only known cross-linking enzyme [24]. Cross-linking activity by TGase 2 was considered as a form of inactivation of substrate proteins [25]. Therefore, an increase of TGase 2 activity in tissues was thought to be responsible for an increase of apoptosis for decades [26] until a TGase 2 knock out mouse was shown to also be able to induce apoptosis [27,28]. In fact, the TGase 2 knock out mouse showed normal phenotype unless it was challenged with allergens. The TGase 2 knock out mouse showed significantly reduced inflammation in a unilateral ureteral obstruction model [29]. It also showed a reversal of allergic asthma induced by ovalbumin [30], pulmonary inflammation induced by bleomycin [31], and nephropathy induced by IgA1 [32]. These phenotypic responses suggested that an increase of TGase 2 expression was responsible for defensive mechanisms against foreign material infiltration [33,34]. Drosophila larvae with TGase knock out showed increased mortality after septic injury [35]. TGase 2 is an important effector of early innate immunity, which helps to promote survival against infection. Under this concept, cancer cells may promote survival during anticancer treatment by adopting an advantage from the defensive mechanism role of TGase 2.

2.2. TGase 2 in Cancer Tissue

The general role of TGase 2 in cancer may be difficult to clarify because various roles of increased TGase 2 expression have been reported in various cancers, including pancreatic cancer [36], breast cancer [37,38], ovarian cancer [38], and colon cancers [39]. Although the roles of TGase 2 may be diverse in different contexts of cancers, the role of TGase 2 is commonly related to cancer promotion in growth and migration. TGase 2 is induced in cancer cells, which may promote cancer progression by increases of cell growth [6], epithelial–mesenchymal transition (EMT) [40], drug resistance [41–43], and cell signaling (reviewed in [44]). There are a numbers of reports that TGase 2 is involved in cancer progression through activity on the cell surface and in the extracellular matrix (ECM), including its role in the regulation of cell-extracellular matrix (ECM) interactions by complex formation with several types of transmembrane receptors such as integrins β1, β3, and fibronectin (reviewed in [45]). TGase 2 plays the role of a co-receptor for integrin-mediated cell binding to fibronectin in cancer cells. Therefore, TGase 2 knock down reduced the cell attachment, migration and invasion in cancer, showing the same effect produced by knock down of fibronectin [46].

TGase 2 regulates cell signaling directly in the signaling by NF-κB [47], HIF-1α [6], and VEGF [48] by regulation of I-κBα, pVHL, and VEGF, respectively. NF-κB activation is commonly observed in cancer cells, where it promotes drug resistance and cell survival [49] and also recruits tumor associated cells by producing inflammatory molecules [50]. In liver cancer cells, TGase 2 induction was observed by TNF-α treatment, which was induced through NF-κB activation [51]. Indeed, the TGase 2 promoter contains binding sites for the NF-κB response element [52]. Later, we were surprised by the opposite regulation, in that TGase 2 was also able to activate NF-κB through I-κBα depletion via polymerization in immortalized glial cells [47] and breast cancer cells [42].

pVHL is a well-known tumor suppressor. *VHL* mutation is often observed in cancer, which results in an increase of the HIF-1α protein level [53] and IGF-1R transcription level [54]. It has been reported that TGase 2 was induced by hypoxia through HIF heterodimer (HIF-1α and HIF-1β) binding at promoter regions of HIF-1α response molecule [55]. However, an increase of TGase 2 expression was also able to induce HIF-1α through pVHL depletion by direct polymerization activity in ovarian cancer and breast cancer cells [6]. As we know that HIF-1α is the master controller of angiogenesis, it follows that TGase 2 mediated HIF-1α stabilization may contribute to angiogenesis promotion.

TGase 2 has also been reported to be involved in EMT in cancer cells through β-catenin activation by c-Src activation through complex formation with fibronectin, TGase 2, and c-Src [56]. This implies that different roles of TGase 2 may arise from differential effects in a context-dependent manner because TGase 2 is expressed in all type of tissues, including cancer, as well as immune cells, extra matrix cells, and endothelial cells. TGase 2 has a specific role in each context (reviewed in [57]). At a biochemical level, the differentiated roles of TGase 2 in a context-dependent manner can be explained by the relative affinity and reactivity of alternative physiological substrates (reviewed in [58]). TGase 2 can recognize a wide variety of substrates having different K_M values. When two glutamine donor substrates are present, having low and high K_M values, TGase 2 preferentially reacts with the substrate having the lower K_M value. For example, in the presence of many proteins in the extracellular matrix, TGase 2 readily reacts with fibronectin, which is bound with high affinity [59]. Once TGase 2 reacts with the glutamine donor substrate protein, the resulting acyl-enzyme intermediate binds an acyl-acceptor substrate, depending on the relative affinity of available amines [60]. For example, when two TGase 2 substrates such as histamine (K_M: 0.38 mM) [61] and ornithine (K_M: 1.35 mM) [62] are present in the same concentration, TGase 2 will bind and react preferentially with histamine. In addition to this general control at the molecular kinetic level, TGase 2 reactivity is regulated by many activity effectors, including GTP, ATP, calcium, and conditions including pH and temperature, all of which may affect substrate preference in different cancer types. Taking all these factors into account, it can be seen that TGase 2 may promote different cancers by reaction with different biological targets that are dictated by a precisely designated environment. In ccRCC, TGase 2 specifically interacts with p53 to promote oncogenesis. Although the roles of TGase 2 in cancer are well studied, the subgroup of TGase 2-positive patients in specific cancer types is small [63]. Therefore, from a therapeutic point of view, TGase 2 is commonly considered a chemo-sensitizing target instead of an anti-cancer therapeutic target [42]. However, in ccRCC, TGase 2 is over 90% positive and plays a major role in suppressing wild type p53 [21]. The impact of this correlation is significant, as it indicates that TGase 2 can be a specific target for ccRCC therapy and that inhibitors such as GK921 and streptonigrin, which inhibit binding between TGase 2 and p53, can be an anti-cancer therapeutics [23,64].

2.3. TGase 2 in ccRCC

Recently the role of TGase 2 in ccRCC was reviewed, revealing the importance of its role (reviewed in [44]). Clinical data analysis regarding TGase 2 expression in ccRCC patients from The Cancer Genome Atlas showed increased expression of TGase 2 in RNA and protein levels in ccRCC [23,65]. Meta-analysis of ccRCC patients showed that an increased level of TGase 2 was inversely correlated with five-year disease free survival [66]. Furthermore, this study showed that an increase of TGase 2 expression was correlated with an increase of metastatic potential, as well as worse prognosis [65].

It has been shown that TGase 2 knock down induced p53-mediated cell death [19] and that inhibition of TGase 2 by a single treatment of 0.2 mg/kg of streptonigrin showed almost a complete response of therapeutic effect [23] in ccRCC xenograft models. A series of reports showed that in ccRCC cell lines, cell death was induced by TGase 2 knock down using siRNA of TGase 2, while TGase 2 knock down did not lead to any cell death effect in the normal immortalized cell HEK293 [19–21,23,67]. This implies that ccRCC specifically employs TGase 2 for survival. TGase 2 acts as a chaperone protein in addition to a cross-linking enzyme [22]. TGase 2 forms a ternary complex wherein the N-terminus of p53 binds to the N-terminus of TGase 2 while the C-terminus of TGase 2 binds the N-terminus of p62 [21].

Additionally, p53 inactivation in cancer is associated with aggressive growth and poor prognosis. Many cancer types have a high level of p53 mutation that abrogates p53's tumor suppressive role. However, less than 5% of ccRCCs show p53 mutations [21], even though p53 levels are down-regulated [1]. TGase 2 expression depletes p53 by direct binding and transferring to the autophagosome, which results in increased tumor cell survival [19]. TGase 2 targets the DNA-binding domain (residue 102–292 of p53) [21]. Upon deletion of this region, p53 completely loses its capacity to bind to TGase 2 [19]. p53-TGase 2-p62 complexes are specifically transported to the autophagosome and are degraded by the autophagic process [19]. TGase 2-mediated autophagic degradation of p53 is a novel mechanism that does not require TGase 2 catalytic activity, as demonstrated in Figure 1.

TGase 2 inhibitors targeting its catalytic activity did not induce p53 mediated apoptosis in ccRCC. This result concurs with the mechanism of action of streptonigrin, which is bound at the N-terminus of TGase 2, resulting in prevention of p53 binding by competition in the same site and induction of p53-mediated apoptosis by the released p53.

It is known that over 90% of ccRCC shows pVHL inactivation, which leads to an increase of HIF-1α activity [3]. TGase 2 is also induced under hypoxic stress in cancer cells by HIF-1α activation [55]. The TGase 2 promoter region contains a HIF binding region and an NF-κB binding region [52]. It is clear that hypoxia and/or pVHL inactivity are major contributors to TGase 2 induction in ccRCC through HIF-1α activity [55]. Interestingly, pVHL was found to be a target of TGase 2, which can be depleted by cross-linking [6]. This suggests an amplified cycle of HIF-1α signaling, because induced TGase 2 suppresses the pVHL feedback mechanism.

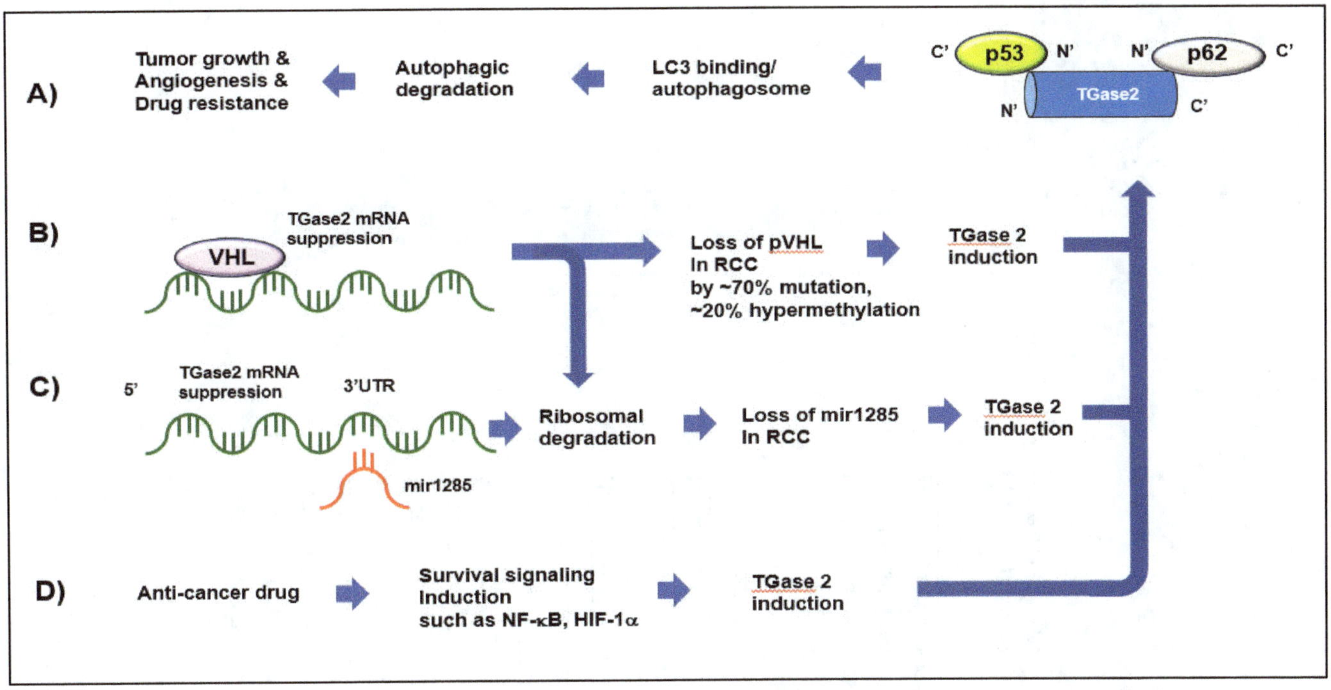

Figure 1. Various pathways inducing TGase 2 expression, as well as the major role of TGase 2 in ccRCC. (**A**) TGase 2 can form a complex by binding p53 and p62 simultaneously, which is then transferred to the autophagosome [21,22]. (**B**) *VHL* inactivation in about 90% of ccRCC induces TGase 2 expression, which can potentiate suppressing p53 signaling [68]. (**C**) Universal decrease of mir1285 level in RCC induces TGase 2 expression, which correlates with RCC proliferation [69]. TGase 2 mRNA expression is suppressed by mir1285 binding at 3′UTR of TGase 2. (**D**) TGase 2 expression is also induced by anti-cancer drug treatment along with drug resistance through NF-κB activation [42,70]. All of these pathways can be reversed by a single treatment of GK921 [71] or streptonigrin [23], which binds to the N-terminus of TGase 2 where p53 would bind, prior to transfer to the autophagosome in ccRCC [64].

2.4. *Anti-Cancer Effect of TGase 2 Inhibition in ccRCC*

The Keillor group recently reported the TGase 2 inhibitor VA4, optimized from hit compound NC9. This inhibitor blocks the transamidation activity of TGase 2, as well as its GTP binding ability, through an allosteric mechanism [72]. VA4 was reported to be the best lead compound among the sulfonamide and piperazinyl amide derivatives designed to interact with the active site of TGase 2 [72]. We investigated whether these specific irreversible inhibitors for TGase 2 might also block TGase 2—p53 binding and p53 depletion in RCC cells. Our results showed that these inhibitors have no effect on RCC survival (Figure 2). Although these inhibitors were reported to induce a conformational change of TGase 2 that affects GTP binding to TGase 2, the binding of these inhibitors to TGase 2 did not apparently block p53 binding to TGase 2. This result corroborates previous reports regarding p53 binding to TGase 2, in that it is specifically the N-terminus of p53 that interacted with the N-terminus of TGase 2 [21–23,64]. This suggests indirectly that streptonigrin induced p53 activation by competing with p53 for binding to TGase 2 [23].

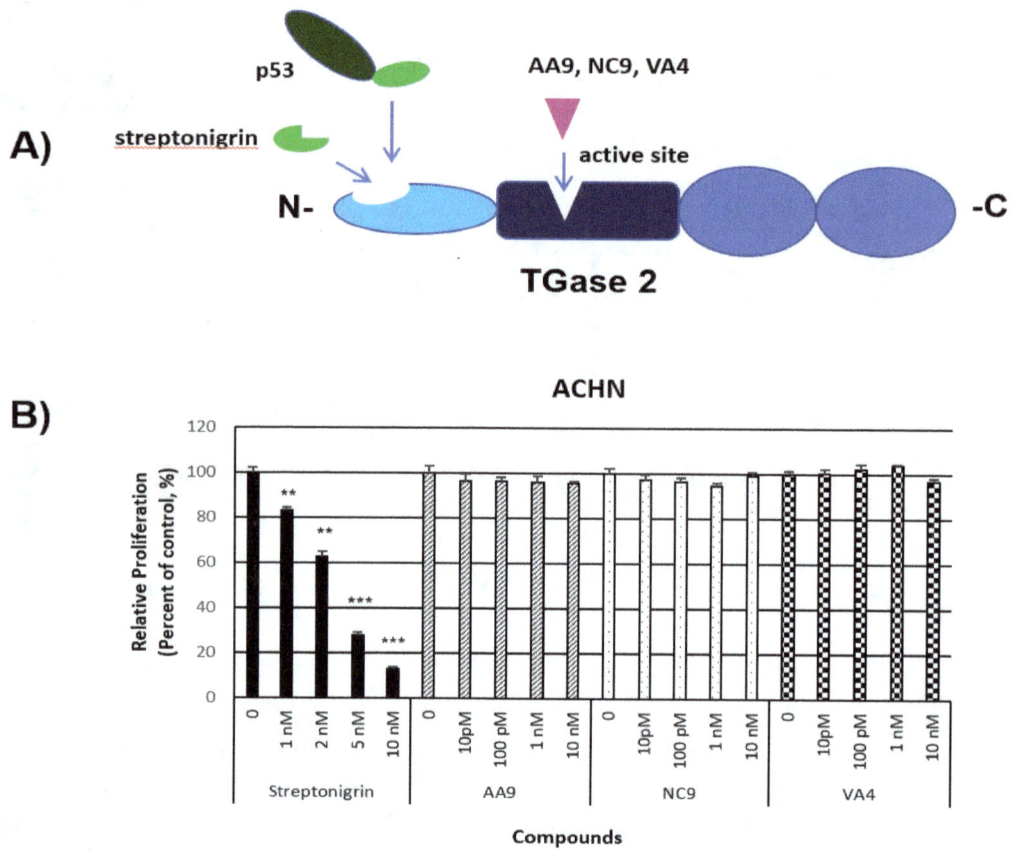

Figure 2. Inhibitor targeting the N-terminus p53 binding region of transglutaminase 2 (TGase 2) shows an anti-cancer effect in clear cell renal cell carcinoma (ccRCC), cell line ACHN. (**A**) Streptonigrin binding to N-terminus of TGase 2 stabilized p53, which induced apoptosis in ccRCC. AA9, NC9, and VA4 binding to active site of TGase 2 caused inactivation of TGase 2. (**B**) Cells were tested for proliferation assay using sulforhodamine B assay as reported [23] for 48 h with the indicated concentrations of streptonigrin, AA9, NC9 and VA4 compounds. Streptonigrin showed an anti-cancer effect in a dose-dependent manner, while TGase 2 active site inhibitors such as AA9, NC9, and VA4 [72] did not show an anti-cancer effect in ccRCC. This suggests that TGase 2 mediated p53 depletion is not dependent on enzyme activity but related to an N-terminal binding chaperone effect to the autophagosome. (mean ± SD, n = 3) ** $p < 0.01$, and *** $p < 0.001$.

3. Precision Strategy for Targeting TGase 2 in RCC

3.1. TGase 2 Is a Major VHL-Repressible Gene

Somatic mutation or inactivation via gene modification of both *VHL* tumor suppressor alleles is commonly observed in ccRCC [73]. The gene product pVHL has a ubiquitin ligase activity that targets the HIF-1α subunit by oxygen dependent proteolysis [74]. Therefore, pVHL inactive cells induce HIF-1α stabilization leading to the activation of specific target genes, such as pyruvate kinase or VEGF, involved in the increase of glycolysis or angiogenesis, respectively [75,76]. More than 60 putative direct HIF-1 target genes have been identified. Among them, TGase 2 was observed in the category of amino-acid metabolism [77]. It was also observed in cancer cells that TGase 2 was induced by HIF-1α under hypoxia [55].

There is an interesting report about analysis of *VHL* target genes suppressed by oxygen regulation in ccRCC. In the report, TGase 2 was shown to be induced over 5-fold by hypoxia in ccRCC cells with pVHL expression [68]. This suggests that TGase 2 is one of the top targets of *VHL*. Therefore, the high level of *VHL* inactivation in ccRCC was primarily responsible for the induction of TGase 2 expression (Figure 1).

3.2. *mir1285 Directly Regulating TGase 2 Suppresses RCC*

A group investigating non-coding RNA in cancer investigated microRNA (miRNA) expression signatures and searched for tumor suppressive miRNAs in RCC [69]. They found that the level of *miR-1285* was extensively decreased in RCC. Transfection of *miR-1285* showed a strong inhibitory effect on RCC proliferation [69]. The report showed that 11 genes had target sites for *miR-1285* in their 3′-untranslated regions. Among them, TGase 2 was a target of *miR-1285*. TGase 2 expression was down regulated 4–8 fold by *miR-1285* transfection in RCC (Figure 1) [69]. Furthermore, this report showed that TGase 2 knock down significantly reduced cell proliferation and invasion in RCC cells [69], which corroborates other reports that TGase 2 knock down induced cell death [19,21,23].

3.3. *TGase 2 Is Induced by mTOR Inhibition*

Targeting the mechanistic target of rapamycin complex 1 (mTORC1) raises great concern of drug resistance after treatment, although this treatment may have an anti-proliferative effect on cancer cells. mTORC1 is almost the last signaling kinase in the process of biosynthesis (anabolism), which is absolutely required for cell proliferation [78]. FDA-approved mTORC1 inhibitors, such as Temsirolimus and Everolimus, showed only limited anti-cancer effects and recurrence after treatment because rapamycin and rapalogs are generally cytostatic instead of cytotoxic [78]. There was a report about identification of rapamycin-enhanced transcription changes using a public GEO dataset focusing on rapamycin-treated tuberous sclerosis complex (TSC)-deficient cells. One of the markedly increased transcripts was the *TGM2* gene (TGase 2 protein), which occurred five times in the top 20 probes among 39,000 probed genes [70]. TGase 2 was induced by rapamycin treatment in a time dependent manner (Figure 1) [70]. Although this report did not show the mechanism by which TGase 2 was induced by mTOR inhibition, it showed that combined inhibition of TGase 2 and mTOR reversed mTOR resistance in cancer cell. Autophagy induction by mTOR inhibition or AMPK activation has been reported to have a therapeutic effect in cancer [79]. However, it is also known that mTOR inhibition induces drug resistance through autophagy induction in cancer cells [80]. Interestingly, an increase of TGase 2 is correlated with an increase of autophagy by increase of LC3 levels in various cancer cells [81]. This report suggests that TGase 2 induces drug resistance by potentiating autophagy through LC3 induction via p53 depletion in cancer [81].

4. Conclusions

TGase 2 is not critical for normal life because the TGase 2 knock out mouse showed a normal phenotype under normal conditions [28,29,82]. However, the TGase 2 knock out mouse behaved differently from a wild type mouse under stress—including allergic reaction, septic shock, and cancer growth [33]. Loss of TGase 2 expression causes great damage in sepsis but conversely, it helps with evading inflammation in an allergic reaction [29]. In cancer, TGase 2 knock down causes down regulation of cancer progression because the roles of TGase 2 in cancer converge, promoting cancer progression by way of adhesion, proliferation, and EMT (reviewed in [44,83]). TGase 2 knock down or inhibition by single targeting specifically induces an anti-cancer effect in ccRCC through stabilization of p53, because p53 binds directly to TGase 2 and is thus chaperoned to the autophagosome for degradation [19–21,23,67,71]. This is only possible in ccRCC because over 90% of p53 in ccRCC is wild type. Thus, collectively these observations represent a breakthrough for the clinical field because they identify TGase 2 as a specific therapeutic target for ccRCC, and the marked potential for binding inhibitors between TGase 2 and p53 such as GK921 [71] and streptonigrin [23] to become the first therapeutics for ccRCC (reviewed in [64]).

Author Contributions: Conceptualization and major writing, S.-Y.K.; experimental advice, discussion of conceptualization, and proof-reading, J.W.K. All authors have read and agreed to the published version of the manuscript.

Abbreviations

ccRCC	clear cell renal cell carcinoma
ECM	extracellular matrix
EMT	epithelial–mesenchymal transition
mTOR	mammalian target of rapamycin
TGase 2	Transglutaminase 2
VEGF	vascular endothelial growth factor
PDGF	platelet-derived growth factor

References

1. Cancer Genome Atlas Research Network. Comprehensive molecular characterization of clear cell renal cell carcinoma. *Nature* **2013**, *499*, 43–49. [CrossRef] [PubMed]
2. Linehan, W.M. Genetic basis of kidney cancer: Role of genomics for the development of disease-based therapeutics. *Genome Res.* **2012**, *22*, 2089–2100. [CrossRef] [PubMed]
3. Kaelin, W.G., Jr. The von Hippel-Lindau tumour suppressor protein: O_2 sensing and cancer. *Nat. Rev. Cancer* **2008**, *8*, 865–873. [CrossRef] [PubMed]
4. Pantuck, A.J.; An, J.; Liu, H.; Rettig, M.B. NF-kappaB-dependent plasticity of the epithelial to mesenchymal transition induced by Von Hippel-Lindau inactivation in renal cell carcinomas. *Cancer Res.* **2010**, *70*, 752–761. [CrossRef]
5. Tedesco, L.; Elguero, B.; Pacin, D.G.; Senin, S.; Pollak, C.; Garcia Marchinena, P.A.; Jurado, A.M.; Isola, M.; Labanca, M.J.; Palazzo, M.; et al. von Hippel-Lindau mutants in renal cell carcinoma are regulated by increased expression of RSUME. *Cell Death Dis.* **2019**, *10*, 266. [CrossRef]
6. Kim, D.S.; Choi, Y.B.; Han, B.G.; Park, S.Y.; Jeon, Y.; Kim, D.H.; Ahn, E.R.; Shin, J.E.; Lee, B.I.; Lee, H.; et al. Cancer cells promote survival through depletion of the von Hippel-Lindau tumor suppressor by protein crosslinking. *Oncogene* **2011**, *30*, 4780–4790. [CrossRef]
7. Rini, B.I. Temsirolimus, an inhibitor of mammalian target of rapamycin. *Clin. Cancer Res.* **2008**, *14*, 1286–1290. [CrossRef]
8. Atkins, M.B.; Yasothan, U.; Kirkpatrick, P. Everolimus. *Nat. Rev. Drug Discov.* **2009**, *8*, 535–536. [CrossRef]
9. Al-Salama, Z.T.; Keating, G.M. Cabozantinib: A Review in Advanced Renal Cell Carcinoma. *Drugs* **2016**, *76*, 1771–1778. [CrossRef]
10. Frampton, J.E. Pazopanib: A Review in Advanced Renal Cell Carcinoma. *Target Oncol.* **2017**, *12*, 543–554. [CrossRef]
11. Keating, G.M. Axitinib: A review in advanced renal cell carcinoma. *Drugs* **2015**, *75*, 1903–1913. [CrossRef] [PubMed]
12. Harrison, C. Angiogenesis: A deeper understanding of VEGFR inhibitors. *Nat. Rev. Cancer* **2012**, *12*, 735. [CrossRef] [PubMed]
13. Papaetis, G.S.; Syrigos, K.N. Sunitinib: A multitargeted receptor tyrosine kinase inhibitor in the era of molecular cancer therapies. *BioDrugs* **2009**, *23*, 377–389. [CrossRef] [PubMed]
14. Rini, B.I.; Campbell, S.C.; Escudier, B. Renal cell carcinoma. *Lancet* **2009**, *373*, 1119–1132. [CrossRef]
15. Sparks, C.A.; Guertin, D.A. Targeting mTOR: Prospects for mTOR complex 2 inhibitors in cancer therapy. *Oncogene* **2010**, *29*, 3733–3744. [CrossRef]
16. White, E. Deconvoluting the context-dependent role for autophagy in cancer. *Nat. Rev. Cancer* **2012**, *12*, 401–410. [CrossRef]
17. Motzer, R.J.; Tannir, N.M.; McDermott, D.F.; Aren Frontera, O.; Melichar, B.; Choueiri, T.K.; Plimack, E.R.; Barthelemy, P.; Porta, C.; George, S.; et al. Nivolumab plus Ipilimumab versus Sunitinib in Advanced Renal-Cell Carcinoma. *N. Engl. J. Med.* **2018**, *378*, 1277–1290. [CrossRef]
18. Clark, D.J.; Dhanasekaran, S.M.; Petralia, F.; Pan, J.; Song, X.; Hu, Y.; da Veiga Leprevost, F.; Reva, B.; Lih, T.M.; Chang, H.Y.; et al. Integrated Proteogenomic Characterization of Clear Cell Renal Cell Carcinoma. *Cell* **2019**, *179*, 964–983 e31. [CrossRef]
19. Ku, B.M.; Kim, D.S.; Kim, K.H.; Yoo, B.C.; Kim, S.H.; Gong, Y.D.; Kim, S.Y. Transglutaminase 2 inhibition found to induce p53 mediated apoptosis in renal cell carcinoma. *FASEB J.* **2013**, *27*, 3487–3495. [CrossRef]

20. Ku, B.M.; Kim, S.J.; Kim, N.; Hong, D.; Choi, Y.B.; Lee, S.H.; Gong, Y.D.; Kim, S.Y. Transglutaminase 2 inhibitor abrogates renal cell carcinoma in xenograft models. *J. Cancer Res. Clin. Oncol.* **2014**, *140*, 757–767. [CrossRef]
21. Kang, J.H.; Lee, J.S.; Hong, D.; Lee, S.H.; Kim, N.; Lee, W.K.; Sung, T.W.; Gong, Y.D.; Kim, S.Y. Renal cell carcinoma escapes death by p53 depletion through transglutaminase 2-chaperoned autophagy. *Cell Death Dis.* **2016**, *7*, e2163. [CrossRef]
22. Kang, J.H.; Lee, S.H.; Kim, S.Y. Discovery of a novel target for renal cell carcinoma: Transglutaminase 2. *Cell Death Dis.* **2016**, *7*, e2200. [CrossRef] [PubMed]
23. Lee, S.H.; Lee, W.K.; Kim, N.; Kang, J.H.; Kim, K.H.; Kim, S.G.; Lee, J.S.; Lee, S.; Lee, J.; Joo, J.; et al. Renal Cell Carcinoma Is Abrogated by p53 Stabilization through Transglutaminase 2 Inhibition. *Cancers (Basel)* **2018**, *10*, 455. [CrossRef] [PubMed]
24. Folk, J.E. Mechanism of action of guinea pig liver transglutaminase. VI. Order of substrate addition. *J. Biol. Chem.* **1969**, *244*, 3707–3713. [PubMed]
25. Fesus, L.; Tarcsa, E.; Kedei, N.; Autuori, F.; Piacentini, M. Degradation of cells dying by apoptosis leads to accumulation of epsilon(gamma-glutamyl)lysine isodipeptide in culture fluid and blood. *FEBS Lett.* **1991**, *284*, 109–112. [CrossRef]
26. Fesus, L.; Madi, A.; Balajthy, Z.; Nemes, Z.; Szondy, Z. Transglutaminase induction by various cell death and apoptosis pathways. *Experientia* **1996**, *52*, 942–949. [CrossRef]
27. Szondy, Z.; Sarang, Z.; Molnar, P.; Nemeth, T.; Piacentini, M.; Mastroberardino, P.G.; Falasca, L.; Aeschlimann, D.; Kovacs, J.; Kiss, I.; et al. Transglutaminase 2-/- mice reveal a phagocytosis-associated crosstalk between macrophages and apoptotic cells. *Proc. Natl. Acad. Sci. USA* **2003**, *100*, 7812–7817. [CrossRef]
28. De Laurenzi, V.; Melino, G. Gene disruption of tissue transglutaminase. *Mol. Cell Biol.* **2001**, *21*, 148–155. [CrossRef]
29. Kim, D.S.; Kim, B.; Tahk, H.; Kim, D.H.; Ahn, E.R.; Choi, C.; Jeon, Y.; Park, S.Y.; Lee, H.; Oh, S.H.; et al. Transglutaminase 2 gene ablation protects against renal ischemic injury by blocking constant NF-kappaB activation. *Biochem. Biophys. Res. Commun.* **2010**, *403*, 479–484. [CrossRef]
30. Hong, G.U.; Park, B.S.; Park, J.W.; Kim, S.Y.; Ro, J.Y. IgE production in CD40/CD40L cross-talk of B and mast cells and mediator release via TGase 2 in mouse allergic asthma. *Cell. Signal.* **2013**, *25*, 1514–1525. [CrossRef]
31. Oh, K.; Park, H.B.; Byoun, O.J.; Shin, D.M.; Jeong, E.M.; Kim, Y.W.; Kim, Y.S.; Melino, G.; Kim, I.G.; Lee, D.S. Epithelial transglutaminase 2 is needed for T cell interleukin-17 production and subsequent pulmonary inflammation and fibrosis in bleomycin-treated mice. *J. Exp. Med.* **2011**, *208*, 1707–1719. [CrossRef] [PubMed]
32. Berthelot, L.; Papista, C.; Maciel, T.T.; Biarnes-Pelicot, M.; Tissandie, E.; Wang, P.H.; Tamouza, H.; Jamin, A.; Bex-Coudrat, J.; Gestin, A.; et al. Transglutaminase is essential for IgA nephropathy development acting through IgA receptors. *J. Exp. Med.* **2012**, *209*, 793–806. [CrossRef] [PubMed]
33. Yoo, H.; Ahn, E.R.; Kim, S.J.; Lee, S.H.; Oh, S.H.; Kim, S.Y. Divergent results induced by different types of septic shock in transglutaminase 2 knockout mice. *Amino Acids* **2013**, *44*, 189–197. [CrossRef] [PubMed]
34. Kim, S.Y. Transglutaminase 2 in inflammation. *Front. Biosci.* **2006**, *11*, 3026–3035. [CrossRef]
35. Wang, Z.; Wilhelmsson, C.; Hyrsl, P.; Loof, T.G.; Dobes, P.; Klupp, M.; Loseva, O.; Morgelin, M.; Ikle, J.; Cripps, R.M.; et al. Pathogen entrapment by transglutaminase–a conserved early innate immune mechanism. *PLoS Pathog.* **2010**, *6*, e1000763. [CrossRef]
36. Iacobuzio-Donahue, C.A.; Ashfaq, R.; Maitra, A.; Adsay, N.V.; Shen-Ong, G.L.; Berg, K.; Hollingsworth, M.A.; Cameron, J.L.; Yeo, C.J.; Kern, S.E.; et al. Highly expressed genes in pancreatic ductal adenocarcinomas: A comprehensive characterization and comparison of the transcription profiles obtained from three major technologies. *Cancer Res.* **2003**, *63*, 8614–8622.
37. Hettasch, J.M.; Bandarenko, N.; Burchette, J.L.; Lai, T.S.; Marks, J.R.; Haroon, Z.A.; Peters, K.; Dewhirst, M.W.; Iglehart, J.D.; Greenberg, C.S. Tissue transglutaminase expression in human breast cancer. *Lab. Investig.* **1996**, *75*, 637–645.
38. Singer, C.F.; Hudelist, G.; Walter, I.; Rueckliniger, E.; Czerwenka, K.; Kubista, E.; Huber, A.V. Tissue array-based expression of transglutaminase-2 in human breast and ovarian cancer. *Clin. Exp. Metastasis* **2006**, *23*, 33–39. [CrossRef]

39. Miyoshi, N.; Ishii, H.; Mimori, K.; Tanaka, F.; Hitora, T.; Tei, M.; Sekimoto, M.; Doki, Y.; Mori, M. TGM2 is a novel marker for prognosis and therapeutic target in colorectal cancer. *Ann. Surg. Oncol.* **2010**, *17*, 967–972. [CrossRef]
40. Shao, M.; Cao, L.; Shen, C.; Satpathy, M.; Chelladurai, B.; Bigsby, R.M.; Nakshatri, H.; Matei, D. Epithelial-to-mesenchymal transition and ovarian tumor progression induced by tissue transglutaminase. *Cancer Res.* **2009**, *69*, 9192–9201. [CrossRef]
41. Park, K.S.; Kim, H.K.; Lee, J.H.; Choi, Y.B.; Park, S.Y.; Yang, S.H.; Kim, S.Y.; Hong, K.M. Transglutaminase 2 as a cisplatin resistance marker in non-small cell lung cancer. *J. Cancer Res. Clin. Oncol.* **2010**, *136*, 493–502. [CrossRef] [PubMed]
42. Kim, D.S.; Park, S.S.; Nam, B.H.; Kim, I.H.; Kim, S.Y. Reversal of drug resistance in breast cancer cells by transglutaminase 2 inhibition and nuclear factor-kappaB inactivation. *Cancer Res.* **2006**, *66*, 10936–10943. [CrossRef] [PubMed]
43. Herman, J.F.; Mangala, L.S.; Mehta, K. Implications of increased tissue transglutaminase (TG2) expression in drug-resistant breast cancer (MCF-7) cells. *Oncogene* **2006**, *25*, 3049–3058. [CrossRef] [PubMed]
44. Nezir, A.E.; Ulukan, B.; Telci, D. Transglutaminase 2: The Maestro of the Oncogenic Mediators in Renal Cell Carcinoma. *Med. Sci. (Basel)* **2019**, *7*, 24. [CrossRef]
45. Belkin, A.M. Extracellular TG2: Emerging functions and regulation. *FEBS J.* **2011**, *278*, 4704–4716. [CrossRef]
46. Chen, S.H.; Lin, C.Y.; Lee, L.T.; Chang, G.D.; Lee, P.P.; Hung, C.C.; Kao, W.T.; Tsai, P.H.; Schally, A.V.; Hwang, J.J.; et al. Up-regulation of fibronectin and tissue transglutaminase promotes cell invasion involving increased association with integrin and MMP expression in A431 cells. *Anticancer Res.* **2010**, *30*, 4177–4186.
47. Lee, J.; Kim, Y.S.; Choi, D.H.; Bang, M.S.; Han, T.R.; Joh, T.H.; Kim, S.Y. Transglutaminase 2 induces nuclear factor-kappaB activation via a novel pathway in BV-2 microglia. *J. Biol. Chem.* **2004**, *279*, 53725–53735. [CrossRef]
48. Feng, Q.; Zhang, C.; Lum, D.; Druso, J.E.; Blank, B.; Wilson, K.F.; Welm, A.; Antonyak, M.A.; Cerione, R.A. A class of extracellular vesicles from breast cancer cells activates VEGF receptors and tumour angiogenesis. *Nat. Commun.* **2017**, *8*, 14450. [CrossRef]
49. Karin, M.; Greten, F.R. NF-kappaB: Linking inflammation and immunity to cancer development and progression. *Nat. Rev. Immunol.* **2005**, *5*, 749–759. [CrossRef]
50. Ji, Z.; He, L.; Regev, A.; Struhl, K. Inflammatory regulatory network mediated by the joint action of NF-kB, STAT3, and AP-1 factors is involved in many human cancers. *Proc. Natl. Acad. Sci. USA* **2019**, *116*, 9453–9462. [CrossRef]
51. Kuncio, G.S.; Tsyganskaya, M.; Zhu, J.; Liu, S.L.; Nagy, L.; Thomazy, V.; Davies, P.J.; Zern, M.A. TNF-alpha modulates expression of the tissue transglutaminase gene in liver cells. *Am. J. Physiol.* **1998**, *274*, G240–G245. [PubMed]
52. Gundemir, S.; Colak, G.; Tucholski, J.; Johnson, G.V. Transglutaminase 2: A molecular Swiss army knife. *Biochim. Biophys. Acta* **2012**, *1823*, 406–419. [CrossRef] [PubMed]
53. Kapitsinou, P.P.; Haase, V.H. The VHL tumor suppressor and HIF: Insights from genetic studies in mice. *Cell Death Differ.* **2008**, *15*, 650–659. [CrossRef] [PubMed]
54. Yuen, J.S.; Cockman, M.E.; Sullivan, M.; Protheroe, A.; Turner, G.D.; Roberts, I.S.; Pugh, C.W.; Werner, H.; Macaulay, V.M. The VHL tumor suppressor inhibits expression of the IGF1R and its loss induces IGF1R upregulation in human clear cell renal carcinoma. *Oncogene* **2007**, *26*, 6499–6508. [CrossRef]
55. Jang, G.Y.; Jeon, J.H.; Cho, S.Y.; Shin, D.M.; Kim, C.W.; Jeong, E.M.; Bae, H.C.; Kim, T.W.; Lee, S.H.; Choi, Y.; et al. Transglutaminase 2 suppresses apoptosis by modulating caspase 3 and NF-kappaB activity in hypoxic tumor cells. *Oncogene* **2010**, *29*, 356–367. [CrossRef]
56. Condello, S.; Cao, L.; Matei, D. Tissue transglutaminase regulates beta-catenin signaling through a c-Src-dependent mechanism. *FASEB J.* **2013**, *27*, 3100–3112. [CrossRef]
57. Tabolacci, C.; De Martino, A.; Mischiati, C.; Feriotto, G.; Beninati, S. The Role of Tissue Transglutaminase in Cancer Cell Initiation, Survival and Progression. *Med. Sci. (Basel)* **2019**, *7*, 19. [CrossRef]
58. Facchiano, F.; Facchiano, A.; Facchiano, A.M. The role of transglutaminase-2 and its substrates in human diseases. *Front. Biosci.* **2006**, *11*, 1758–1773. [CrossRef]
59. Akimov, S.S.; Belkin, A.M. Cell-surface transglutaminase promotes fibronectin assembly via interaction with the gelatin-binding domain of fibronectin: A role in TGFbeta-dependent matrix deposition. *J. Cell. Sci.* **2001**, *114 Pt 16*, 2989–3000.

60. Keillor, J.W.; Clouthier, C.M.; Apperley, K.Y.P.; Akbar, A.; Mulani, A. Acyl transfer mechanisms of tissue transglutaminase. *Bioorg. Chem.* **2014**, *57*, 186–197. [CrossRef]

61. Ikura, K.; Tsuchiya, Y.; Sasaki, R.; Chiba, H. Expression of guinea-pig liver transglutaminase cDNA in Escherichia coli. Amino-terminal N alpha-acetyl group is not essential for catalytic function of transglutaminase. *Eur. J. Biochem.* **1990**, *187*, 705–711. [CrossRef] [PubMed]

62. Delcros, J.G.; Roch, A.M.; Quash, G. The competitive inhibition of tissue transglutaminase by alpha-difluoromethylornithine. *FEBS Lett.* **1984**, *171*, 221–226. [CrossRef]

63. Choi, C.M.; Jang, S.J.; Park, S.Y.; Choi, Y.B.; Jeong, J.H.; Kim, D.S.; Kim, H.K.; Park, K.S.; Nam, B.H.; Kim, H.R.; et al. Transglutaminase 2 as an independent prognostic marker for survival of patients with non-adenocarcinoma subtype of non-small cell lung cancer. *Mol. Cancer* **2011**, *10*, 119. [CrossRef] [PubMed]

64. Kim, S.Y. New Insights into Development of Transglutaminase 2 Inhibitors as Pharmaceutical Lead Compounds. *Med. Sci. (Basel)* **2018**, *6*, 87. [CrossRef] [PubMed]

65. Park, M.J.; Baek, H.W.; Rhee, Y.Y.; Lee, C.; Park, J.W.; Kim, H.W.; Moon, K.C. Transglutaminase 2 expression and its prognostic significance in clear cell renal cell carcinoma. *J. Pathol. Transl. Med.* **2015**, *49*, 37–43. [CrossRef] [PubMed]

66. Erdem, S.; Yegen, G.; Telci, D.; Yildiz, I.; Tefik, T.; Issever, H.; Kilicaslan, I.; Sanli, O. The increased transglutaminase 2 expression levels during initial tumorigenesis predict increased risk of metastasis and decreased disease-free and cancer-specific survivals in renal cell carcinoma. *World J. Urol.* **2015**, *33*, 1553–1560. [CrossRef]

67. Kang, J.H.; Lee, S.H.; Cheong, H.; Lee, C.H.; Kim, S.Y. Transglutaminase 2 Promotes Autophagy by LC3 Induction Through p53 Depletion in Cancer Cell. *Biomol. Ther. (Seoul)* **2018**, *1*, 3. [CrossRef]

68. Wykoff, C.C.; Pugh, C.W.; Maxwell, P.H.; Harris, A.L.; Ratcliffe, P.J. Identification of novel hypoxia dependent and independent target genes of the von Hippel-Lindau (VHL) tumour suppressor by mRNA differential expression profiling. *Oncogene* **2000**, *19*, 6297–6305. [CrossRef]

69. Hidaka, H.; Seki, N.; Yoshino, H.; Yamasaki, T.; Yamada, Y.; Nohata, N.; Fuse, M.; Nakagawa, M.; Enokida, H. Tumor suppressive microRNA-1285 regulates novel molecular targets: Aberrant expression and functional significance in renal cell carcinoma. *Oncotarget* **2012**, *3*, 44–57. [CrossRef]

70. Cao, J.; Huang, W. Compensatory Increase of Transglutaminase 2 is Responsible for Resistance to mTOR Inhibitor Treatment. *PLoS ONE* **2016**, *11*, e0149388. [CrossRef]

71. Kim, N.; Kang, J.H.; Lee, W.K.; Kim, S.G.; Lee, J.S.; Lee, S.H.; Park, J.B.; Kim, K.H.; Gong, Y.D.; Hwang, K.Y.; et al. Allosteric inhibition site of transglutaminase 2 is unveiled in the N terminus. *Amino Acids* **2018**, *50*, 1583–1594. [CrossRef] [PubMed]

72. Akbar, A.; McNeil, N.M.R.; Albert, M.R.; Ta, V.; Adhikary, G.; Bourgeois, K.; Eckert, R.L.; Keillor, J.W. Structure-Activity Relationships of Potent, Targeted Covalent Inhibitors That Abolish Both the Transamidation and GTP Binding Activities of Human Tissue Transglutaminase. *J. Med. Chem.* **2017**, *60*, 7910–7927. [CrossRef] [PubMed]

73. Gnarra, J.R.; Tory, K.; Weng, Y.; Schmidt, L.; Wei, M.H.; Li, H.; Latif, F.; Liu, S.; Chen, F.; Duh, F.M.; et al. Mutations of the VHL tumour suppressor gene in renal carcinoma. *Nat. Genet.* **1994**, *7*, 85–90. [CrossRef] [PubMed]

74. Maxwell, P.H.; Wiesener, M.S.; Chang, G.W.; Clifford, S.C.; Vaux, E.C.; Cockman, M.E.; Wykoff, C.C.; Pugh, C.W.; Maher, E.R.; Ratcliffe, P.J. The tumour suppressor protein VHL targets hypoxia-inducible factors for oxygen-dependent proteolysis. *Nature* **1999**, *399*, 271–275. [CrossRef]

75. Shweiki, D.; Itin, A.; Soffer, D.; Keshet, E. Vascular endothelial growth factor induced by hypoxia may mediate hypoxia-initiated angiogenesis. *Nature* **1992**, *359*, 843–845. [CrossRef]

76. Semenza, G.L.; Roth, P.H.; Fang, H.M.; Wang, G.L. Transcriptional regulation of genes encoding glycolytic enzymes by hypoxia-inducible factor 1. *J. Biol. Chem.* **1994**, *269*, 23757–23763.

77. Semenza, G.L. Targeting HIF-1 for cancer therapy. *Nat. Rev. Cancer* **2003**, *3*, 721–732. [CrossRef]

78. Li, J.; Kim, S.G.; Blenis, J. Rapamycin: One drug, many effects. *Cell Metab.* **2014**, *19*, 373–379. [CrossRef]

79. Harrison, D.E.; Strong, R.; Sharp, Z.D.; Nelson, J.F.; Astle, C.M.; Flurkey, K.; Nadon, N.L.; Wilkinson, J.E.; Frenkel, K.; Carter, C.S.; et al. Rapamycin fed late in life extends lifespan in genetically heterogeneous mice. *Nature* **2009**, *460*, 392–395. [CrossRef]

80. Jung, C.H.; Ro, S.H.; Cao, J.; Otto, N.M.; Kim, D.H. mTOR regulation of autophagy. *FEBS Lett.* **2010**, *584*, 1287–1295. [CrossRef]

81. Kang, J.H.; Lee, S.H.; Cheong, H.; Lee, C.H.; Kim, S.Y. Transglutaminase 2 Promotes Autophagy by LC3 Induction through p53 Depletion in Cancer Cell. *Biomol. Ther. (Seoul)* **2019**, *27*, 34–40. [CrossRef]
82. Nanda, N.; Iismaa, S.E.; Owens, W.A.; Husain, A.; Mackay, F.; Graham, R.M. Targeted inactivation of Gh/tissue transglutaminase II. *J. Biol. Chem.* **2001**, *276*, 20673–20678. [CrossRef]
83. Zemskov, E.A.; Janiak, A.; Hang, J.; Waghray, A.; Belkin, A.M. The role of tissue transglutaminase in cell-matrix interactions. *Front. Biosci.* **2006**, *11*, 1057–1076. [CrossRef]

3

Cytoreductive Nephrectomy and Overall Survival of Patients with Metastatic Renal Cell Carcinoma Treated with Targeted Therapy—Data from the National Renis Registry

Alexandr Poprach [1,2,*], Milos Holanek [1,2], Renata Chloupkova [3], Radek Lakomy [1,2], Michal Stanik [4], Ondrej Fiala [5], Bohuslav Melichar [6,7], Katerina Kopeckova [8], Milada Zemanova [9], Igor Kiss [1,2], Igor Penka [10], Julia Bohosova [11] and Tomas Buchler [12]

1 Department of Comprehensive Cancer Care, Masaryk Memorial Cancer Institute, 656 53 Brno, Czech Republic; holanek@mou.cz (M.H.); lakomy@mou.cz (R.L.); kiss@mou.cz (I.K.)
2 Department of Comprehensive Cancer Care, Faculty of Medicine, Masaryk University, 625 00 Brno, Czech Republic
3 Institute of Biostatistics and Analyses, Faculty of Medicine, Masaryk University, 625 00 Brno, Czech Republic; chloupkova@iba.muni.cz
4 Department of Urologic Oncology, Masaryk Memorial Cancer Institute and Masaryk University, 656 53 Brno, Czech Republic; stanik@mou.cz
5 Department of Oncology, University Hospital, 323 00 Pilsen, Czech Republic; ondrej.fiala@fnplzen.cz
6 Department of Oncology, Palacky University Medical School and Teaching Hospital, 779 00 Olomouc, Czech Republic; Bohuslav.melichar@upol.cz
7 University Hospital in Hradec Kralove, 500 05 Hradec Kralove, Czech Republic
8 Department of Oncology, Motol University Hospital and 2nd Faculty of Medicine Charles University, 150 06 Prague, Czech Republic; katerina.kopeckova@fnmotol.cz
9 Department of Oncology, First Faculty of Medicine Charles University and General University Hospital, 120 00 Prague, Czech Republic; milada.zemanova@vfn.cz
10 Department of Surgery, University Hospital Bohunice, Faculty of Medicine, Masaryk University, 625 00 Brno, Czech Republic; penka.igor@fnbrno.cz
11 Central European Institute of Technology (CEITEC), University Campus Bohunice, Masaryk University, 625 00 Brno, Czech Republic; julia.bohosova@ceitec.muni.cz
12 Department of Oncology, First Faculty of Medicine, Thomayer Hospital and Charles University, 140 59 Prague, Czech Republic; tomas.buchler@ftn.cz
* Correspondence: poprach@mou.cz;

Simple Summary: The treatment of metastatic renal cell carcinoma is traditionally initiated with the removal of the diseased kidney with the tumor in many patients. However, there is ongoing controversy about the benefit of kidney removal if targeted therapy is used. The present paper analyses a large cohort of patients, and the results indicate that primary tumor removal should still be strongly considered in patients who are treated with targeted therapies.

Abstract: The role of cytoreductive nephrectomy (CN) in treatment of locally advanced or metastatic renal cell carcinoma (mRCC) in the era of targeted therapies (TT) is still not clearly defined. The study population consisted of 730 patients with synchronous mRCC. The RenIS (Renal carcinoma Information System) registry was used as the data source. The CN/TT cohort included patients having CN within 3 months from the mRCC diagnosis and subsequently being treated with TT, while the TT cohort included patients receiving TT upfront. Median progression-free survival from the first intervention was 6.7 months in the TT arm and 9.3 months in the CN/TT patients ($p < 0.001$). Median overall survival was 14.2 and 27.2 months, respectively ($p < 0.001$). Liver metastasis, high-grade tumor, absence of CN, non-clear cell histology, and MSKCC (Memorial Sloan-Kettering Cancer Center) poor prognosis status were associated with adverse treatment outcomes. According to the results of this retrospective study, patients who underwent CN and subsequently were treated with TT had better outcomes compared to patients treated with upfront TT. The results of the study support the use of CN in the treatment algorithm for mRCC.

Keywords: metastatic renal cell carcinoma; targeted therapy; cytoreductive nephrectomy; overall survival

1. Introduction

Cytoreductive nephrectomy (CN) is one of the most controversial interventions in the treatment of metastatic renal cell carcinoma (mRCC). In the cytokine therapy era, CN was considered a mainstay of treatment for fit patients in cases where it led to substantial reduction of total tumor mass [1–3]. CN was even reported to result in spontaneous regression of metastases in rare cases [4,5].

The role of CN is less clear if targeted therapies (TT) are used as systemic agents for mRCC. CARMENA, the only prospective phase III trial studying CN in the context of TT, showed that the omission of CN and upfront initiation of sunitinib therapy in patients with synchronous mRCC is non-inferior compared to CN followed by sunitinib [6]. However, the CARMENA trial has been criticized and the conclusions have not been universally accepted [7], partly because of the contradiction with large retrospective studies [8–11] and meta-analyses [12–14]. The CARMENA study suffered from slow accrual that led to premature closure after the second interim analysis. Subsequently, the Steering Committee approved the results of the first interim analysis to be used as the overall trial results. In addition, as many as 44% of patients in the CN-sunitinib arm and 41.5% of patients in the sunitinib-only arm had poor risk features as defined by the Memorial Sloan Kettering Cancer Center (MSKCC) prognostic criteria [15], whereas the benefit of CN had only been postulated for intermediate-prognosis patients in previous reports [9,16,17]. Importantly, the majority of patients enrolled in CARMENA had a relatively high metastatic burden with the median of two metastatic sites. Furthermore, 17% of patients randomized to the sunitinib-only arm eventually underwent CN and, in the other study arm, in 7% of patients, CN was planned but not carried out. All these patients were included in the published analysis [6].

In the present retrospective study using data from the RenIS registry, we analyzed data of patients with de-novo mRCC treated with TT who underwent CN within three months of diagnosis and compared their progression-free survival (PFS) and OS (overall survival) with patients who did not have CN and were treated with TT only. In addition, intermediate-risk patients were analyzed per number of MSKCC risk factors.

2. Results

2.1. Patient Population and Baseline Characteristics

There were 458 patients with synchronous metastatic disease and CN ≤ 3 months post-mRCC diagnosis followed by TT (CN/TT arm) and 272 patients without CN (TT arm). Median age at diagnosis was 64 and 62 years in the CN/TT and TT cohorts, respectively, and 95% of patients had clear cell renal cell carcinoma histology. Table 1 shows patient baseline characteristics. The site of metastasis is shown in Table S1.

Table 1. Baseline patient's characteristics.

Characteristic	Cohort		*p*-Value [(1)]
	CN/TT (*n* = 458)	TT (*n* = 272)	
Sex, *n* (%)			
Male	338 (73.8)	200 (73.5)	0.931
Female	120 (26.2)	72 (26.5)	
Age at diagnosis (years)			
median (range)	62 (25–83)	64 (35–85)	**0.006**
Histology, *n* (%)			
Clear cell carcinoma	431 (94.1)	261 (96.0)	
Papillary cell carcinoma	22 (4.8)	8 (2.9)	
Chromophobe cell carcinoma	2 (0.4)	2 (0.7)	0.581
Bellini duct carcinoma	2 (0.4)	0 (0.0)	
Unknown	1 (0.2)	1 (0.4)	
Primary tumor grade, *n* (%)			
G1–2 well/moderately differentiated	160 (34.9)	161 (59.2)	**<0.001**
G3–4 poorly/non differentiated	298 (65.1)	111 (40.8)	
MSKCC score			
good prognosis	3 (0.7)	7 (2.6)	
intermediate prognosis	417 (91.0)	215 (79.0)	**<0.001**
poor prognosis	38 (8.3)	50 (18.4)	
MSKCC score—2 categories			
good or intermediate prognosis	420 (91.7)	222 (81.6)	**<0.001**
poor prognosis	38 (8.3)	50 (18.4)	
ECOG PS			
PS < 2	433 (94.5)	258 (94.9)	0.999
PS ≥ 2	25 (5.5)	14 (5.1)	
Calcium			
≤2.5 mmol/L	422 (92.1)	231 (84.9)	**0.003**
>2.5 mmol/L	36 (7.9)	41 (15.1)	
Hemoglobin			
normal	273 (59.6)	147 (54.0)	0.163
<lower limit of normal	185 (40.4)	125 (46.0)	
Time from diagnosis to target treatment			
≥1 year	3 (0.7)	10 (3.7)	**0.006**
<1 year	455 (99.3)	262 (96.3)	
LDH			
≤1.5× upper limit of norm	428 (93.4)	229 (84.2)	**<0.001**
>1.5× upper limit of norm	30 (6.6)	43 (15.8)	
Type of first target treatment, *n* (%)			
sunitinib	361 (78.8)	210 (77.2)	0.643
pazopanib	97 (21.2)	62 (22.8)	
Age at first target treatment initiation (years)			
median (range)	63 (25–83)	64 (36–85)	**0.006**
ECOG PS at first target treatment initiation, *n* (%)			
PS 0	174 (38.0)	49 (18.0)	**<0.001**
PS 1	259 (56.6)	209 (76.8)	
PS 2	23 (5.0)	14 (5.1)	
PS 3	2 (0.4)	0 (0.0)	

CN/TT, cytoreductive nephrectomy followed by targeted therapy. TT, targeted therapy only; MSKCC, Memorial Sloan Kettering Cancer Center; ECOG, Eastern Cooperative Oncology Group; PS, performance status; LDH, Lactate dehydrogenase. [(1)] Fisher exact test or Mann–Whitney test. Bold: statistically significant.

2.2. *Treatment Outcomes*

While the overall response rate (ORR) was similar for the two analyzed cohorts, the disease control rate (DCR) favored the CN/TT patients. In the TT arm, overall response rate (ORR) was 19%, with complete response (CR) and partial response (PR) observed in 0.4% and 18.5% of patients, respectively. In the CN/TT, ORR was 24.4% CR (CR 2.9%, PR 21.4%). However, the difference in ORR was not statistically significant ($p = 0.116$). Stable disease was observed in 30.2% and 35.4% of patients in the TT and CN/TT arms, respectively. The disease control rate (DCR) was significantly higher in CN patients, reaching 49.2% and 59.8% for the TT and CN/TT arm, respectively ($p = 0.011$).

Median PFS was 6.7 months (95% CI: 5.5–7.8) in the TT arm and 9.3 months (95%: CI 8.3–10.4) in the CN/TT patients ($p < 0.001$). The median OS was 14.2 months (95% CI: 12.1–16.2) and 27.2 months (95% CI: 22.3–32.1), respectively ($p < 0.001$) (Figure 1).

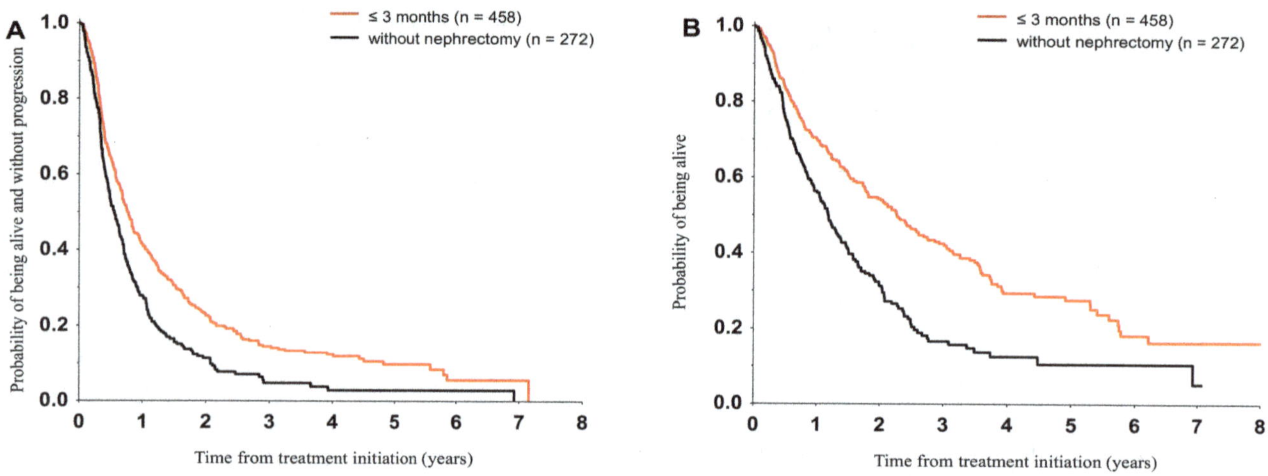

Figure 1. Progression-free (**A**) and overall survival (**B**) from first treatment strategy. All the differences were statistically significant at $p < 0.001$.

2.3. Subgroup Analysis

The benefit of CN on PFS and OS was evident irrespective of age. Patients ≤65 years had a median PFS of 7.6 months (95% CI: 5.9–7.3) in the TT arm and 8.8 months (95% CI: 7.3–9.3) in the CN/TT arm. Median OS was 15 months (95% CI: 12.7–17.2) and 28.7 months (95% CI: 19.4–38.0) for the TT and CN/TT, respectively. In patients >65 years of age, median PFS was 5.8 months (95% CI: 4.3–7.3) and 10.1 months (95% CI: 8.0–12.2) and median OS was 12.5 months (8.3–16.6) and 26.3 months (95% CI: 20.0–32.5) for the TT and CN/TT cohorts, respectively. All the above differences were statistically significant at $p < 0.001$. Age at TT initiation had no statistically significant impact on PFS or OS in the multivariate analysis (Table 2).

Table 2. Progression-free and overall survival results: multivariable Cox-proportional hazards model.

Variable	Category	*n*	Progression-Free Survival		Overall Survival	
			HR (95% CI)	Wald Test *p*-Value	HR (95% CI)	Wald Test *p*-Value
Nephrectomy	TT	271	1.000	-	1.000	-
	CN/TT	457	0.629 (0.525–0.755)	**<0.001**	0.553 (0.449–0.681)	**<0.001**
Sex	female	191	1.000	-	1.000	-
	male	537	0.881 (0.730–1.063)	0.185	0.892 (0.717–1.109)	0.305
Histology	clear cell	692	1.000	-	1.000	-
	other histology types	36	1.961 (1.335–2.879)	**0.001**	1.810 (1.170–2.801)	**0.008**
Primary tumor grade	G1–2	319	1.000	-	1.000	-
	G3–4	409	1.300 (1.093–1.545)	**0.003**	1.453 (1.184–1.783)	**<0.001**
MSKCC	good or intermediate	640	1.000	-	1.000	-
	poor	88	1.359 (1.049–1.761)	**0.020**	1.931 (1.455–2.563)	**<0.001**
Age at first target treatment initiation	≤65 years	425	1.000	-	1.000	-
	>65 years	303	0.956 (0.806–1.135)	0.609	1.101 (0.903–1.344)	0.341
First targeted treatment	sunitinib	570	1.000	-	1.000	-
	pazopanib	158	0.788 (0.640–0.970)	**0.024**	0.825 (0.645–1.054)	0.123

CN/TT, cytoreductive nephrectomy followed by targeted therapy. TT, targeted therapy only; MSKCC, Memorial Sloan Kettering Cancer Center; HR, hazard ratio; CI, confidence interval. Bold: statistically significant.

Similarly, tumor grade was not a factor that significantly altered the benefit of nephrectomy. Patients with low-grade tumors had PFS of 8.1 months (95% CI: 6.7–9.5) versus 12 months (95% CI: 9.0–15.0) and an OS of 19.0 months (95% CI: 13.2–24.8) versus 31.0 months (95% CI: 22.1–39.9), while patients with high-grade tumors had PFS of 4.4 months (95% CI: 3.3–5.6) and 8.3 months (95% CI: 6.9–9.7), and an OS of 10.1 (95% CI: 7.6–12.7) and 23.6 months (95% CI: 17.8–29.4), for the TT and CN/TT cohorts, respectively. All the differences were statistically significant at $p < 0.001$).

There was a major difference in outcomes between intermediate-risk patients with one versus two risk factors, but both subgroups derived benefit from CN (Table 3).

Table 3. Progression-free survival and overall survival from first treatment strategy.

Number of Risk Factors (MSKCC)	Median PFS and OS	Cohort		Log-Rank Test p-Value
		CN/TT	TT	
MSKCC 1 risk factor patients, $n = 328$		$n = 222$	$n = 106$	
	Median PFS (95% CI)	10.2 months (7.8–12.5)	7.7 months (6.2–9.2)	**0.002**
	Median OS (95% CI)	37.9 months (28.1–47.7)	17.5 months (11.2–23.8)	**<0.001**
MSKCC 2 risk factors patients, $n = 304$		$n = 195$	$n = 109$	
	Median PFS (95% CI)	8.5 months (6.7–10.4)	5.8 months (4.7–6.8)	**<0.001**
	Median OS (95% CI)	21.9 months (16.2–27.5)	10.3 months (7.8–12.8)	**<0.001**

CN/TT, cytoreductive nephrectomy followed by targeted therapy. TT, targeted therapy only; MSKCC, Memorial Sloan Kettering Cancer Center; OS, overall survival; PFS, progression-free survival. The factors associated with adverse outcome in a multivariate analysis included the presence of liver metastases, grade 3 or 4 tumor, absence of CN, non-clear cell histology, and MSKCC poor prognosis (Table 2). Bold: statistically significant.

3. Discussion

The present analysis strongly suggests that CN is an independent, favorable predictive factor for treatment outcomes in patients with synchronous mRCC treated with TT. We conducted a subanalysis of the effect of CN on survival in the MSKCC intermediate-risk patients with one or two risk factors. The findings indicate that the benefit of CN is maintained in patients with adverse risk factors, regardless of age.

The present data are in accordance with other retrospective studies. Heng et al. analyzed 1658 patients with synchronous mRCC treated with TT. Median OS was 9.5 months and 20.6 months in the TT-only and TT/CN patients, respectively. However, the results might have been affected by a more favorable prognostic profile in the CN/TT patients. The study also showed that patients with four or more International Metastatic Renal Cell Carcinoma Database Consortium (IMDC) prognostic factors did not benefit from CN [9]. Choueiri et al. showed in a similar retrospective study of 314 patients that CN patients had better OS than non-CN patients (19.8 vs. 9.4 months, respectively). However, again there were imbalances in patient characteristics: CN patients were younger and had better performance status, lower levels of corrected calcium, and a lower number of metastatic sites. Patients ≥75 years did not benefit from CN, in contrast with present findings suggesting similar benefits from CN in younger and older patients. Choueiri et al. also confirmed that poor-risk patients as defined by the MSKCC or the IMDC criteria did not benefit from CN [18]. The results of our study further support findings published by Zhao et al. that patients with both high- and low-grade tumors benefit from CN [19].

Important updates to the CARMENA study after a median follow-up of 61.5 months were presented at the American Society of Clinical Oncology 2019 Annual Meeting. The authors conducted a sub-analysis of IMDC intermediate prognosis patients, focusing on the difference in OS between patients with one versus two prognostic factors, and they explored whether the number of metastatic sites affected patient survival. In an update analysis of the CARMENA trial, patients with one prognostic factor benefited from CN, with the median OS of 31.4 months versus 25.2 months without

CN [20], but patients with two IMDC risk factors did not, with median OS of 16.6 months and 31.2 months for patients with versus without CN, respectively. As the interval from RCC diagnosis to the initiation of treatment of less than year is a risk factor in both MSKCC and IMDC models, this is necessarily the single risk factor present in intermediate-risk patients and one risk factor. The first version of MSKCC criteria included previous nephrectomy instead of the treatment-free interval [21]. Thus, nephrectomy "converts" these patients into favorable-risk patients according the original MSKCC model. Patients with two risk factors remain intermediate-risk even after CN according to the older version of MSKCC classification. Therefore, this result from a prospective study seems to validate the older version of MSKCC if CN is considered.

SURTIME was another prospective trial, a phase II study aiming to determine whether a period of sunitinib therapy before CN improves the outcome compared with immediate CN followed by the same agent. Although the study was underpowered and eventually closed due to poor accrual, the results indicated that deferred CN may be superior to early CN followed by sunitinib, with median OS of 32.4 months versus 15.1 months, respectively. In addition, a recent pooled analysis suggested that in intermediate-risk patients, deferred CN in patients not progressing on first-line vascular endothelial growth factor (VEGF)-directed therapy is superior to immediate CN followed by systemic treatment [22].

These results are in accordance with a post-hoc analysis of 40 patients in the sunitinib only arm of CARMENA, who, for different reasons, underwent nephrectomy. The OS of the CN patients was 48.5 months, while it reached 15.7 months in non-CN patients [20].

To summarize, the results of prospective studies suggest that CN still plays a role in patients with one IMDC risk factor and that patients not progressing on anti-VEGF therapy may benefit from later CN, although the question of upfront versus deferred CN remains unresolved and deserves a prospective trial.

Several biological hypotheses have been put forward to explain the apparent benefit of cytoreductive nephrectomy in patients with metastatic disease. RCC is the prime model for spatial tumor heterogeneity. Gerlinger et al. clearly showed that most genetic driver mutations in RCC are subclonal, and only approximately one-third are present in all regions of the primary tumor and metastases [23,24]. Therefore, volume reduction may result in removal or limitation of tumor clones that may be resistant to the therapy and represent foci of future progressive disease. Immunological mechanisms may play a role in superior survival of patients with mRCC after CN, which is associated with decreased systemic inflammation and reversal of cellular immunity abnormalities [25,26]. These improvements may be especially advantageous in patients receiving immunotherapies but also play a role with VEGF-targeted therapies [27].

Finally, despite adjustments for established risk factors and the prognostic score, some unmeasurable variables may result in selection bias. These include the physician's subjective view of the patient's general condition and comorbidities, as well as primary tumor properties, the extent and volume of metastatic disease, and surgical variables which are imperfectly represented by the prognostic models [28].

In our opinion supported by the results of the present analysis, patients with good performance status and one to two risk factors should be considered for CN. The case for CN is further strengthened after the inclusion of novel immunotherapies in mRCC treatment algorithms. In a phase II study analyzing survival and response rates in patients with mRCC treated with checkpoint inhibitors with/without CN, the treatment response rate and survival were clearly superior in patients after CN [29]. Few patients in the present cohort were defined as good prognosis, i.e., the interval from the diagnosis to the initiation of therapy was more than one year. These patients obviously had a more indolent disease that might have allowed for waiting on the decision to initiate therapy. However, a slight imbalance in the number of these patients in both cohorts probably had limited impact on the results that actually indicated a better outcome in the CN cohort that had only three of such patients.

Single-agent VEGF inhibitors are no longer the first-line treatment of choice for most patients with mRCC. Nevertheless, many issues identified in these studies, including delayed initiation of systemic therapy in exchange for tumor volume reduction, and delaying the emergence of treatment resistance by reducing tumor heterogeneity using CN, remain relevant in the immunotherapy era.

The limitations of our study include the retrospective nature and associated potential bias. The population was not balanced according to the prognostic factors, similar to other retrospective studies, as demonstrated by Bex et al. [17]. Furthermore, inclusion of patients treated in higher lines with checkpoint inhibitors might have affected the survival results. Complete IMDC scoring could be calculated only in about 50% of patients. Therefore, full analysis of data based on IMDC was not possible. In addition, as pazopanib and sunitinib were not reimbursed by the public health insurance in the Czech Republic for the treatment of poor risk patients, few were included in the present analysis.

4. Materials and Methods

4.1. Study Design and Data Source

The data were obtained from the RenIS Registry that represents a database of about 95% of all patients with mRCC treated with TT in the Czech Republic from 2007 to 2018 [30,31]. The database included a total of 4034 patients treated with targeted therapy for mRCC between 2006 and the end of January 2018. Patients with synchronous metastatic disease subsequently treated with first-line TT with pazopanib or sunitinib were included in the analysis. The CN/TT cohort included patients having CN within 3 months from the mRCC diagnosis and subsequently treated with TT, while the TT cohort included patients receiving TT upfront.

The RenIS registry contains information on the baseline patient characteristics, diagnosis, extent of the disease, baseline laboratory parameters, and type, outcome, and toxicity of treatments. The data were updated twice a year. Further details on the RenIS Registry were published elsewhere [20]. The project has been approved by the Multicenter Ethics Committee of the University Hospital and the Masaryk Memorial Cancer Institute in Brno, Czech Republic.

4.2. Statistical Analysis

Descriptive statistics and frequency tables were used to characterize the sample data set. The statistical significance of differences between subgroups was assessed using the Fisher exact test or the Mann–Whitney test.

Overall survival (OS) is defined as the time from the date of first treatment intervention to death due to any cause (i.e., for patients without nephrectomy, OS is computed from the date of the first line target therapy initiation, and for patients with nephrectomy OS is computed from the date of nephrectomy).

Progression-free survival (PFS) is defined as the time from the date of first treatment strategy (analogously to OS) to the date of the first documented progression or death due to any cause.

PFS and OS were estimated using the Kaplan–Meier method, and all point estimates include 95% confidence intervals (95% CI). Statistical significance of differences in survival among subgroups was assessed using the log-rank test.

Multivariable Cox proportional hazards models were used to evaluate the effect of all potential prognostic factors on the survival measures. Statistical significance of hazard ratios was assessed by mean of the Wald test. All statistical tests were performed at a significance level of $\alpha = 0.05$.

5. Conclusions

According to the results of this retrospective study, good and intermediate prognosis mRCC patients clearly benefited from CN. The benefit was particularly pronounced in patients with a single risk factor. CN was beneficial irrespective of tumor grade and age.

Author Contributions: Conceptualization: A.P., T.B., R.L.; Methodology: A.P., T.B.; Formal Analysis: R.C.; Investigation A.P., M.H., R.C., R.L., M.S., O.F., B.M., K.K., M.Z., I.K., I.P., J.B., T.B.; Resources: A.P., M.H., R.C., R.L., M.S., O.F., B.M., K.K., M.Z., I.K., I.P., J.B., T.B.; Data Curation, A.P., T.B.; Writing—Original Draft Preparation, A.P.; Writing—Review and Editing: all authors; Supervision: A.P., T.B.; Funding Acquisition: A.P., M.H., I.K. All authors have read and agreed to the published version of the manuscript.

Acknowledgments: We would like to thank the following heads of the comprehensive cancer centers for the permission to use data of patients from their respective regional networks: Martina Chodacka, Chomutov Hospital and Masaryk Hospital in Usti nad Labem; Vaclav Janovsky, Ceske Budejovice Hospital; Otakar Bednarik, University Hospital, Brno; Jana Prausova, Motol University Hospital, Prague; David Feltl, University Hospital, Ostrava; Jindrich Finek, University Hospital, Pilsen; Jiri Petera, University Hospital, Hradec Kralove; Lubomir Slavicek, Jihlava Hospital; Jana Katolicka, St Anna University Hospital, Brno; Rostislav Vyzula, Masaryk Memorial Institute of Oncology, Brno; Jiri Bartos, County Hospital, Liberec; Martin Safanda, Na Homolce Hospital, Prague; Renata Soumarova, Novy Jicin Hospital; Jitka Abrahamova, Thomayer Hospital, Prague; Lubos Petruzelka, General University Hospital, Prague; Milan Kohoutek, T Bata Memorial Hospital, Zlin. We are also indebted to all physicians who provided data for the RenIS registry.

References

1. Flanigan, R.C.; Salmon, S.E.; Blumenstein, B.A.; Bearman, S.I.; Roy, V.; McGrath, P.C.; Caton, J.R.J.; Munshi, N.; Crawford, E.D. Nephrectomy followed by interferon alfa-2b compared with interferon alfa-2b alone for metastatic renal-cell cancer. *N. Engl. J. Med.* **2001**, *345*, 1655–1659. [CrossRef] [PubMed]
2. Mickisch, G.H.; Garin, A.; van Poppel, H.; de Prijck, L.; Sylvester, R. Radical nephrectomy plus interferon-alfa-based immunotherapy compared with interferon alfa alone in metastatic renal-cell carcinoma: A randomised trial. *Lancet (Lond. Engl.)* **2001**, *358*, 966–970. [CrossRef]
3. Flanigan, R.C.; Mickisch, G.; Sylvester, R.; Tangen, C.; Van Poppel, H.; Crawford, E.D. Cytoreductive nephrectomy in patients with metastatic renal cancer: A combined analysis. *J. Urol.* **2004**, *171*, 1071–1076. [CrossRef] [PubMed]
4. Marcus, S.G.; Choyke, P.L.; Reiter, R.; Jaffe, G.S.; Alexander, R.B.; Linehan, W.M.; Rosenberg, S.A.; Walther, M.M. Regression of metastatic renal cell carcinoma after cytoreductive nephrectomy. *J. Urol.* **1993**, *150*, 463–466. [CrossRef]
5. Melichar, B.; Vanecková, J.; Morávek, P.; Urminská, H.; Podhola, M. Spontaneous regression of renal cell carcinoma lung metastases in a patient with psoriasis. *Acta Oncol.* **2009**, *48*, 925–927. [CrossRef]
6. Mejean, A.; Ravaud, A.; Thezenas, S.; Colas, S.; Beauval, J.-B.; Bensalah, K.; Geoffrois, L.; Thiery-Vuillemin, A.; Cormier, L.; Lang, H.; et al. Sunitinib Alone or after Nephrectomy in Metastatic Renal-Cell Carcinoma. *N. Engl. J. Med.* **2018**. [CrossRef]
7. Massari, F.; Di Nunno, V.; Gatto, L.; Santoni, M.; Schiavina, R.; Cosmai, L.; Brunocilla, E.; Ardizzoni, A.; Porta, C. Should CARMENA Really Change our Attitude Towards Cytoreductive Nephrectomy in Metastatic Renal Cell Carcinoma? A Systematic Review and Meta-Analysis Evaluating Cytoreductive Nephrectomy in the Era of Targeted Therapy. *Target. Oncol.* **2018**, *13*, 705–714. [CrossRef]
8. Hanna, N.; Sun, M.; Meyer, C.P.; Nguyen, P.L.; Pal, S.K.; Chang, S.L.; de Velasco, G.; Trinh, Q.-D.; Choueiri, T.K. Survival Analyses of Patients with Metastatic Renal Cancer Treated with Targeted Therapy with or without Cytoreductive Nephrectomy: A National Cancer Data Base Study. *J. Clin. Oncol. Off. J. Am. Soc. Clin. Oncol.* **2016**, *34*, 3267–3275. [CrossRef]
9. Heng, D.Y.C.; Wells, J.C.; Rini, B.I.; Beuselinck, B.; Lee, J.-L.; Knox, J.J.; Bjarnason, G.A.; Pal, S.K.; Kollmannsberger, C.K.; Yuasa, T.; et al. Cytoreductive nephrectomy in patients with synchronous metastases from renal cell carcinoma: Results from the International Metastatic Renal Cell Carcinoma Database Consortium. *Eur. Urol.* **2014**, *66*, 704–710. [CrossRef]
10. Conti, S.L.; Thomas, I.-C.; Hagedorn, J.C.; Chung, B.I.; Chertow, G.M.; Wagner, T.H.; Brooks, J.D.; Srinivas, S.; Leppert, J.T. Utilization of cytoreductive nephrectomy and patient survival in the targeted therapy era. *Int. J. Cancer* **2014**, *134*, 2245–2252. [CrossRef]
11. Abern, M.R.; Scosyrev, E.; Tsivian, M.; Messing, E.M.; Polascik, T.J.; Dudek, A.Z. Survival of patients undergoing cytoreductive surgery for metastatic renal cell carcinoma in the targeted-therapy era. *Anticancer Res.* **2014**' *34*, 2405–2411.

12. García-Perdomo, H.A.; Zapata-Copete, J.A.; Castillo-Cobaleda, D.F. Role of cytoreductive nephrectomy in the targeted therapy era: A systematic review and meta-analysis. *Investig. Clin. Urol.* **2018**, *59*, 2–9. [CrossRef] [PubMed]
13. Klatte, T.; Fife, K.; Welsh, S.J.; Sachdeva, M.; Armitage, J.N.; 'Aho, T.; Riddick, A.C.; Matakidou, A.; Eisen, T.; Stewart, G.D. Prognostic effect of cytoreductive nephrectomy in synchronous metastatic renal cell carcinoma: A comparative study using inverse probability of treatment weighting. *World J. Urol.* **2018**, *36*, 417–425. [CrossRef]
14. Petrelli, F.; Tomasello, G.; Borgonovo, K.; Ghidini, M.; Turati, L.; Dallera, P.; Passalacqua, R.; Sgroi, G.; Barni, S. Prognostic Survival Associated With Left-Sided vs Right-Sided Colon Cancer. *JAMA Oncol.* **2017**, *3*. [CrossRef] [PubMed]
15. Motzer, R.J.; Bacik, J.; Murphy, B.A.; Russo, P.; Mazumdar, M. Interferon-alfa as a comparative treatment for clinical trials of new therapies against advanced renal cell carcinoma. *J. Clin. Oncol.* **2002**, *20*, 289–296. [CrossRef]
16. Mathieu, R.; Pignot, G.; Ingles, A.; Crepel, M.; Bigot, P.; Bernhard, J.C.; Joly, F.; Guy, L.; Ravaud, A.; Azzouzi, A.R.; et al. Nephrectomy improves overall survival in patients with metastatic renal cell carcinoma in cases of favorable MSKCC or ECOG prognostic features. *Urol. Oncol.* **2015**, *33*, 339.e9–339.e15. [CrossRef] [PubMed]
17. Bex, A.; Ljungberg, B.; van Poppel, H.; Powles, T. The Role of Cytoreductive Nephrectomy: European Association of Urology Recommendations in 2016. *Eur. Urol.* **2016**, *70*, 901–905. [CrossRef] [PubMed]
18. Choueiri, T.K.; Xie, W.; Kollmannsberger, C.; North, S.; Knox, J.J.; Lampard, J.G.; McDermott, D.F.; Rini, B.I.; Heng, D.Y.C. The impact of cytoreductive nephrectomy on survival of patients with metastatic renal cell carcinoma receiving vascular endothelial growth factor targeted therapy. *J. Urol.* **2011**, *185*, 60–66. [CrossRef]
19. Zhao, Z.; Wu, W.; Duan, X.; Zeng, G.; Liu, Y. The value of cytoreductive nephrectomy on the survival of metastatic renal carcinoma patients based on the number of site-specific metastases. *PLoS ONE* **2019**, *14*, e0215861. [CrossRef]
20. Mejean, A.; Thezenas, S.; Chevreau, C.; Bensalah, K.; Geoffrois, L.; Thiery-Vuillemin, A.; Cormier, L.; Lang, H.; Guy, L.; Gravis, G.; et al. Cytoreductive nephrectomy (CN) in metastatic renal cancer (mRCC): Update on Carmena trial with focus on intermediate IMDC-risk population. *J. Clin. Oncol.* **2019**, *37*, 4508. [CrossRef]
21. Motzer, R.J.; Mazumdar, M.; Bacik, J.; Berg, W.; Amsterdam, A.; Ferrara, J. Survival and prognostic stratification of 670 patients with advanced renal cell carcinoma. *J. Clin. Oncol. Off. J. Am. Soc. Clin. Oncol.* **1999**, *17*, 2530–2540. [CrossRef] [PubMed]
22. Bex, A.; Mulders, P.; Jewett, M.; Wagstaff, J.; van Thienen, J.V.; Blank, C.U.; van Velthoven, R.; Del Pilar Laguna, M.; Wood, L.; van Melick, H.H.E.; et al. Comparison of Immediate vs Deferred Cytoreductive Nephrectomy in Patients With Synchronous Metastatic Renal Cell Carcinoma Receiving Sunitinib: The SURTIME Randomized Clinical Trial. *JAMA Oncol.* **2019**, *5*, 164–170. [CrossRef] [PubMed]
23. Gerlinger, M.; Rowan, A.J.; Horswell, S.; Math, M.; Larkin, J.; Endesfelder, D.; Gronroos, E.; Martinez, P.; Matthews, N.; Stewart, A.; et al. Intratumor heterogeneity and branched evolution revealed by multiregion sequencing. *N. Engl. J. Med.* **2012**, *366*, 883–892. [CrossRef] [PubMed]
24. Gerlinger, M.; Horswell, S.; Larkin, J.; Rowan, A.J.; Salm, M.P.; Varela, I.; Fisher, R.; McGranahan, N.; Matthews, N.; Santos, C.R.; et al. Genomic architecture and evolution of clear cell renal cell carcinomas defined by multiregion sequencing. *Nat. Genet.* **2014**, *46*, 225–233. [CrossRef] [PubMed]
25. Dadian, G.; Riches, P.G.; Henderson, D.C.; Taylor, A.; Moore, J.; Atkinson, H.; Gore, M.E. Immunological parameters in peripheral blood of patients with renal cell carcinoma before and after nephrectomy. *Br. J. Urol.* **1994**, *74*, 15–22. [CrossRef]
26. Renner, A.; Samtani, S.; Marín, A.; Burotto, M. Is Cytoreductive Nephrectomy Still a Standard of Care in Metastatic Renal Cell Carcinoma? *J. Kidney Cancer VHL* **2019**, *6*, 1–7. [CrossRef]
27. Shrimali, R.K.; Yu, Z.; Theoret, M.R.; Chinnasamy, D.; Restifo, N.P.; Rosenberg, S.A. Antiangiogenic agents can increase lymphocyte infiltration into tumor and enhance the effectiveness of adoptive immunotherapy of cancer. *Cancer Res.* **2010**, *70*, 6171–6180. [CrossRef]
28. Bex, A.; Haanen, J. Do targeted agents offer clinical benefit as presurgical therapy? *World J. Urol.* **2014**, *32*, 3–8. [CrossRef]

29. Gao, J.; Karam, J.A.; Tannir, N.M.; Campbell, M.T.; Slack Tidwell, R.; Ahrar, K.; Rao, P.; Ng, C.S.; Jonasch, E.; Matin, S.F.; et al. A pilot randomized study evaluating nivolumab (nivo) or nivo + bevacizumab (bev) or nivo + ipilimumab (ipi) in patients with metastatic renal cell carcinoma (MRCC) eligible for cytoreductive nephrectomy, metastasectomy or post-treatment biopsy (Bx). *J. Clin. Oncol.* **2019**, *37*, 4501. [CrossRef]
30. Buchler, T.; Klapka, R.; Melichar, B.; Brabec, P.; Dušek, L.; Vyzula, R.; Abrahamova, J. Sunitinib followed by sorafenib or vice versa for metastatic renal cell carcinoma-data from the Czech registry. *Ann. Oncol.* **2012**, *23*, 395–401. [CrossRef]
31. Poprach, A.; Bortlíček, Z.; Büchler, T.; Melichar, B.; Lakomý, R.; Vyzula, R.; Brabec, P.; Svoboda, M.; Dušek, L.; Gregor, J. Patients with advanced and metastatic renal cell carcinoma treated with targeted therapy in the Czech Republic: Twenty cancer centres, six agents, one database. *Med. Oncol.* **2012**, *29*, 3314–3320. [CrossRef] [PubMed]

4

Clinical Studies Applying Cytokine-Induced Killer Cells for the Treatment of Renal Cell Carcinoma

Ying Zhang [1], Jörg Ellinger [2], Manuel Ritter [2] and Ingo G. H. Schmidt-Wolf [1,*]

1 Department of Integrated Oncology, CIO Bonn, University Hospital Bonn, Venusberg-Campus 1, D 53127 Bonn, Germany; Ying.Zhang@ukbonn.de

2 Department of Urology, University Hospital Bonn, Venusberg-Campus 1, D 53127 Bonn, Germany; joerg.ellinger@ukbonn.de (J.E.); mritter@ukbonn.de (M.R.)

* Correspondence: Ingo.Schmidt-Wolf@ukbonn.de;

Simple Summary: Cytokine-induced killer (CIK) cells are a heterogeneous population of polyclonal T effector cells expanded ex vivo. Here, we updated our last review published in 2012 and provided a synopsis of current 15 clinical studies, including 382 patients with renal cell carcinoma (RCC) enrolled in CIK cell immunotherapy. CIK cells exhibited promising synergistic anti-tumor effects when combined with conventional therapies and showed mild adverse effects in patients with RCC. Preclinical researches also identified potential molecular targets that augmented CIK cell cytotoxicity against renal carcinoma cells. In future, large randomized clinical trials should be organized to further evaluate the clinical efficacy and optimize the treatment modality of CIK cells in RCC.

Abstract: There is growing interest in cytokine-induced killer (CIK) cells on the integrated therapy of patients with RCC, especially those in the late stage or refractory to conventional chemotherapy and radiotherapy. In this review, a total of 15 clinical studies including 681 patients enrolled in CIK cell immunotherapy were outlined. Three-hundred-and-eighty-two patients with RCC were treated with CIK cells alone or in combination with DC vaccination, targeted agents sunitinib or sorafenib, and the PD-1 inhibitor pembrolizumab. Significantly improved 3-year overall survival rate was reported in four trials, whereas remarkably longer median progression-free survival was observed in three studies. Adverse reactions were mild and usually controllable fever and fatigue. Besides, preclinical research progresses were reviewed to increase our understanding about the underlying mechanisms of CIK cell cytotoxicity and identify potential targets to enhance their anti-tumor activity. These studies suggest that CIK cell-based immunotherapy has potential clinical benefits with a good safety profile and could become a promising approach in the combined therapies of RCC patients. However, further large-scale studies are required to evaluate the clinical efficacy of CIK cells and more efforts should be performed to identify the optimal CIK cell-based therapeutic regimen for RCC patients.

Keywords: cytokine-induced killer cells; clinical study; renal cell carcinoma; immunotherapy; preclinical research

1. Introduction

Renal cell carcinoma (RCC), among the 10 most frequently diagnosed cancers, acts as one of the most lethal urological malignancies worldwide [1]. The highest age-standardized incidence rate is in North America (11.7 per 100,000), with Western Europe ranking the second (9.8 per 100,000) [1].

Lots of patients with renal masses remain asymptomatic until the late stages and over 60% of RCCs are detected incidentally with abdominal imaging performed for other reasons [2]. Although most detected lesions are small tumors at the time of diagnosis, locally advanced disease continues to be diagnosed in a notable proportion of patients, with distant metastases present in up to 17% of patients [3].

Surgery is the only curative treatment for localized RCC, but metastatic RCC (mRCC) is usually refractory to conventional therapies [4]. For most patients with mRCC, systemic therapy, including targeted therapy and immunotherapy, is necessarily required [2]. There are several targeted drugs that have been approved for the treatment of mRCC. They mainly consist of inhibitors targeting vascular endothelial growth factor (VEGF) and its receptors (bevacizumab, sunitinib, sorafenib, pazopanib, axitinib, tivozanib and cabozantinib) and mammalian target of rapamycin (mTOR) (everolimus and temsirolimus) [5,6]. Until targeted therapies were introduced in 2006, the first-line treatment strategy for mRCC was immunotherapies based on interleukin-2 (IL-2) combined with interferon-α (IFN-α) [7]. In 2018, the CheckMate 214 study reported superiority of the programmed cell death-1(PD-1) inhibitor nivolumab and cytotoxic T-lymphocyte-associated antigen 4 (CTLA-4) inhibitor ipilimumab over sunitinib in intermediate- and poor-risk patients. A significantly higher overall survival (OS) and objective response rates were achieved with nivolumab plus ipilimumab than with sunitinib [8]. These findings resulted in an updated recommendation of the first-line management for mRCC patients.

In the past decades, there has been growing interest in adoptive cell-based immunotherapy as a therapeutic option in patients with RCC [9–11]. Cytokine-induced killer (CIK) cells, one of the main adoptive cell-based strategies, are a heterogeneous cell population comprising the main effector subset of double positive CD3 and CD56 cells. Schmidt-Wolf et al. first reported the generation of CIK cells ex vivo from peripheral blood mononuclear cells (PBMCs) in 1991, by adding IFN-γ on day 0 and monoclonal antibody against CD3 (anti-CD3 mAb), human recombinant IL-2 and IL-1 on the next day. An increased cytotoxicity of CIK cells against lymphoma was observed in a SCID mouse/human lymphoma model [12]. CIK cells exert a potent major histocompatibility complex (MHC)-unrestricted cytotoxicity against both hematological and solid malignancies with CD3+CD56+ cells as the main effectors. The natural killer group 2 member D (NKG2D) receptor appears to play the most important role in tumor recognition by CIK cells (Figure 1) [13]. NKG2D, a member of the c-type lectin-activating receptor family, recognizes the MHC-class I-like molecules, MICA and MICB and members of the ULBP family (ULPB1-4) that are restrictedly expressed on malignant tissues and mediates subsequently granzyme release [14]. It is also indicated that NK-like structures, including DNAX accessory molecule-1 (DNAM-1) and NKp30 are expressed on CIK cells and involved in the recognition and killing of tumor targets [15]. Furthermore, CIK cells showed reduced allo-reactive potential and minimal graft-versus-host disease (GVHD) activity in several in vitro and in vivo models, compared with conventional T cells [16,17]. This advantage makes CIK cells an appealing and promising alternative to classic donor lymphocyte infusion (DLI) after hematopoietic stem cell trans-plantation (HSCT).

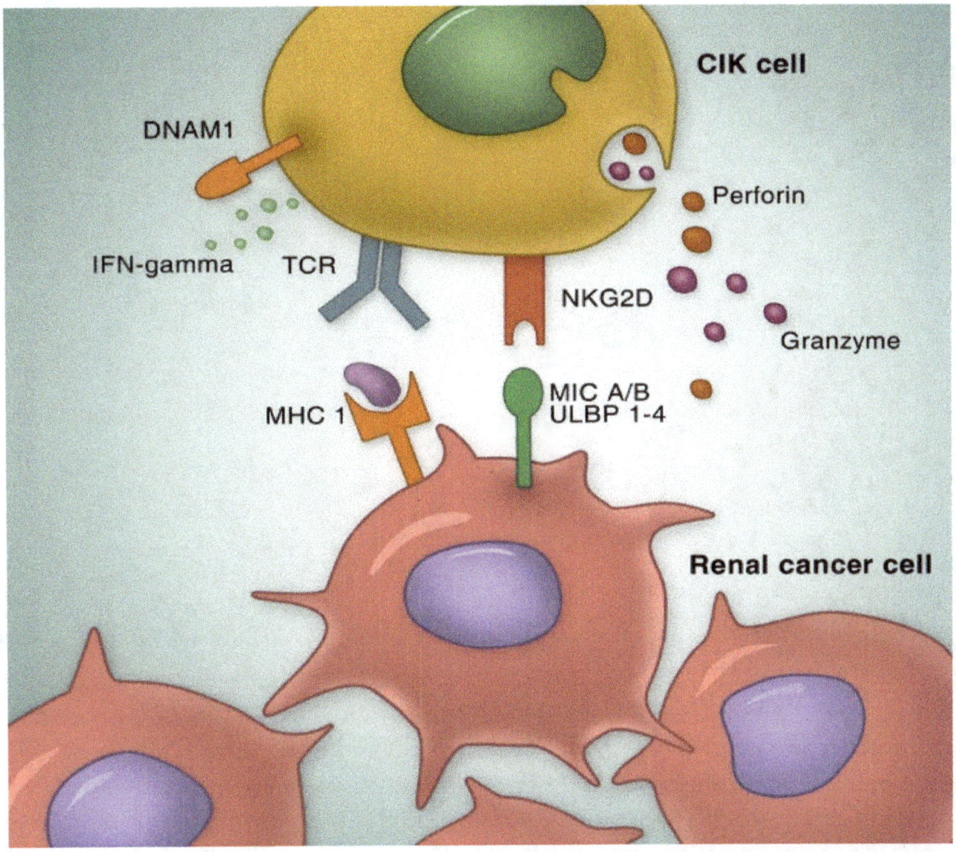

Figure 1. Mechanisms of CIK cell anti-tumor activity. The majority of CIK cell cytotoxicity is exerted through the interaction between NKG2D and its ligand MIC A/B and ULPB 1–4, resulting in granule exocytosis and secretion of cytokines like IFN-γ. NK-like structures, such as DNAM-1, is also involved in the recognition and killing of tumor targets. Besides, CIK cells can eradicate tumors in an MHC-restricted manner by TCR engagement, which is the so-called "dual-functional capability". CIK cell, cytokine induced killer cells; NKG2D, natural killer group 2 member D; MIC A/B, MHC class I polypeptide-related sequence A/B; ULPB 1–4, UL16 binding protein 1–4. DNAM-1, DNAX accessory molecule-1; TCR, T-cell receptor; MHC 1, major histocompatibility complex 1; IFN-γ, interferon-γ.

In our last review published in 2012, we summarized eight clinical studies utilizing CIK cells for the treatment of RCC [18]. These studies showed that the combination of CIK cell therapy and standard therapy was superior to standard therapy alone. Since 2012, more efforts have been put to optimize the anti-tumor potency and treatment regimen of CIK cell-based therapies. In the following sections, we will provide an update on our former review by outlining new clinical results of RCC (Figure 2) and presenting progress of adoptive immunotherapy strategies based on CIK cells.

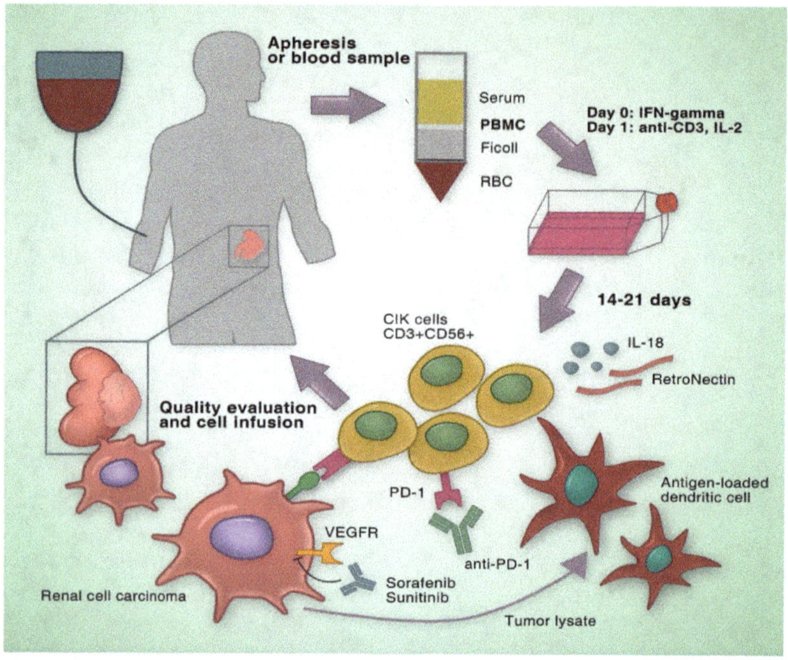

Figure 2. Strategies for improving clinical curative effects of CIK cells. PBMCs are isolated by density gradient centrifugation and expended with IFN-γ, anti-CD3 and IL-2. After 14–21 days, CIK cells are infused into the patient. The anti-tumor activity of CIK cells can be enhanced by adding cytokines like IL-18 or RetroNectin during expansion. DCs have high ability to present tumor antigens and compensate the lack of tumor antigen specificity of CIK cells. Targeted agents such as sunitinib and sorafenib or immune checkpoint inhibitor anti-PD-1 antibodies also have a synergistic effect with CIK cells. CIK cell, cytokine-induced killer cell; PBMC, peripheral blood mononuclear cell; IFN-γ, interferon-γ; IL-2, interleukin-2; IL-18, interleukin-18; VEGFR, vascular endothelial growth factor receptor; PD-1, programmed cell death-1; DC, dendritic cell; RBC, red blood cell.

2. Clinical Studies on CIK Cells for the Treatment of RCC

A total of 15 clinical studies were reviewed here. Six-hundred-and-eight-one patients representing 55.4% of the total with distinct tumor entities were enrolled in CIK cell immunotherapy. Three-hundred-and-eighty-two patients with RCC were treated with CIK cells alone or in combination with DC vaccination, targeted agents sunitinib or sorafenib, and the PD-1 inhibitor pembrolizumab.

2.1. *Clinical Studies on Autologous CIK cells*

Twenty patients with unilateral, locally advanced (TNM stage I or II) RCC who had undergone radical nephrectomy were recruited into a study [19]. The patients were randomly divided into two groups, a CIK cell treatment group and a control group. In the CIK cell group, patients received $1–5 \times 10^9$ autologous CIK cells intravenously per infusion and $2–10 \times 10^9$ CIK cells in total for two consecutive days. Patients were also injected with 20 mg/day thymopentin intramuscularly before CIK cell transfusion and 1 mU rhIL-2 subcutaneously for 10 days after transfusion.

Response Evaluation Criteria in Solid Tumors (RECIST) was used to assess the clinical response every 2 months. In the CIK cell treatment group, a complete response (CR) was achieved in six patients, a partial response (PR) was observed in two patients and stable disease (SD) was remained in two patients. Meanwhile, in the control group, a CR was achieved in five patients, SD remained in three patients, and progressive disease (PD) was observed in two patients. The median progression-free survival (PFS) in the CIK cell group was 32.2 months, which was significantly longer than that of 21.6 months in the control group. However, no statistically significant differences in OS were observed between two groups. All side effects were transient or controllable, including mild arthralgia, laryngeal edema, fatigue, and low-grade fever during lymphocyte infusion or during the early stages of rhIL-2 treatment. Grade 3 or greater adverse events were not observed.

In a retrospective study based on autologous CIK cells, 40 patients with solid tumors were enrolled, including 10 patients with RCC after surgery and chemotherapy [20]. Percentages of CD3+, CD8+ and CD3+CD56+ lymphocyte subsets in patients' peripheral blood were all significantly increased after CIK cell therapy. The 6-month OS rate was 70.0%, 1-year OS rate was 60.0% and 3-year was 57.5%. A favorable safety profile of CIK cells was observed in this study without severe adverse effect. Only two patients had fever and poor appetite and these symptoms could be relieved by simple treatments.

2.2. Clinical Studies on CIK Cells with Improvement of Culture Methods

Liu et al. reported a case applying modified autologous CIK (mCIK) cells for pleural metastasis of collecting duct carcinoma (CDC) [21]. CDC is a rare but highly aggressive RCC arising from the principal cells of the collecting duct. During the generation of mCIK cells, PBMCs were first primed with anti-CD3 antibody, and a mixture of IL-2, IL-18 and IFN-γ was subsequently added after 3 h. This generation method was distinct from the traditional way in which PBMCs are firstly cultured with IFN-γ, followed 24 h later by the addition of anti-CD3 antibody and IL-2. In every cycle, the patient received intrapleural infusion with modified CIK cells at a dose of 10×10^7 once a day for 5 days. After three cycles of therapy, this patient showed relieved cough, dyspnea, chest distress, thoracalgia, and clearer and less pleural fluid. The only adverse reaction was fever after intrapleural infusion and the patient recovered 2 days later.

Another study investigated the efficacy of RetroNectin-activated autologous CIK cells (R-CIK) combined with conventional therapies (chemotherapy and radiotherapy) in patients with metastatic brain tumors [22]. RetroNectin is a 63 kD fragment of recombinant human fibronectin (also called CH-296) that promotes colocalization of virions and target cells to enhance the efficiency of retroviral mediated gene transduction [23]. RetroNectin-activated CIK cells were infused into the participants (1 patient with RCC, 14 patients with non-small cell lung cancer, 4 patients with breast cancer, and 1 patient with thyroid cancer). The OS rate in patients with all tumor entities was 21.4%. The disease control rate was 78.6%. The study also showed that the median PFS of patients receiving R-CIK was 7.7 months and the median OS was 12.6 months. The one patient with RCC achieved a CR without severe toxicities. OS of this patient was 14 months and PFS was 8 months. The results show RetroNectin could be a potential activator to augment the activity of CIK cells.

A study exclusively including patients with metastatic RCC was performed to explore whether the level of the underlying immune inhibitory factor myeloid-derived suppressor cells (MDSCs) was associated with the prognosis of patients receiving CIK cell therapy [24]. Autologous CIK cells were also activated with RetroNectin during generation. Twenty-nine patients received about 5×10^9 CIK cells and 2 million IU IL-2 per day during the following 5 days in one cycle. The treatment schedule for the study consisted of at least 4 and at most 16 cycles in total. Of all evaluable patients, 4 exhibited a PR, 18 remained SD, and 7 showed PD, without CR observed. Moreover, the 1-year survival was 82.8% (24/29). Peripheral blood MDSCs were elevated in almost all RCC patients compared with healthy volunteers and decreased after CIK cell infusion. Also, patients with a relatively low proportion of MDSCs exhibited significantly prolonged survival, which indicated that MDSCs might serve as a potential marker for the prognosis of RCC patients receiving CIK cell treatment.

2.3. Clinical Studies on CIK Cells Combined with Dendritic Cell Vaccination

Dendritic cell (DC)-based vaccines represent a promising therapy that induces anti-tumor immune by initiating an antigen-specific T lymphocyte response [25]. DCs have high ability to present tumor antigens and compensate the lack of tumor antigen specificity of CIK cells. In a randomized controlled trial of 137 patients with postoperative localized and locally advanced RCC, 46 patients were treated with tumor lysate-pulsed DCs and autologous CIK cells, while 45 patients did not receive any postoperative adjuvant therapy [26]. After five intravenous infusions of tumor lysate-pulsed DC-CIK cells (3×10^8 per infusion), an increase of the CD4+/CD8+ ratio and a decrease of CD4+CD25^{high} cells were observed. The metastasis and recurrence rates were significantly decreased, whereas the overall survival rates were significantly increased in the DC-CIK group. The achieved results showed that tumor lysate-pulsed DC-CIK cells could act as a promising postoperative adjuvant immunotherapy by preventing recurrence or metastasis.

In another study involving 121 patients with primary tumors (7 patients with RCC), patients received 1×10^7 DCs for vaccination once a week for 6 weeks and 1×10^9 autologous CIK cells six times within 4 days [27]. The delayed-type hypersensitivity skin tests detected a positive cell-mediated cytotoxicity response with the rate of 76.9%. Most patients achieved improvements in the quality of life (QoL). The treatment was safe and well tolerated and all side effects were mild and controllable.

Wang et al. reported a clinical trial evaluating the efficacy and safety of genetically modified DCs in combination with autologous CIK cells (gmDC-CIK) on patients with RCC [28]. Twenty-eight patients diagnosed with advanced clear cell RCC (ccRCC) (stageIIIB-IV) were enrolled in this study. On day 6 of cell preparation, DCs were pulsed with RNA encoding antigen muc-1 and survivin. In one cycle, patients received four subcutaneous injections of $2–5 \times 10^7$ gmDCs on day 7, 9, 11, and 13 and intravenous infusion of $2–5 \times 10^{10}$ CIK cells on day 11 and 13. The objective response rate (ORR) was 39% and a disease control rate (DCR) was 75%. DCR, but not ORR, was significantly related with cycles of treatment. Only one patient developed grade 1 fever and no other clinically significant side effect was observed.

In another clinical trial, 60 operable RCC patients were randomized to the autologous tumor lysate-pulsed DC-CIK (Ag-DC-CIK) cell treatment group or the control group, and 62 inoperable patients were randomly assigned to the CIK cell treatment group or control group [29]. In operable RCC patients, Ag-DC-CIK cell treatment significantly increased the 3-year disease free survival (DFS) and decreased the recurrence after surgery. Meanwhile, inoperable patients after CIK treatment achieved obviously longer 3-year OS and PFS than patients in the control group. The CD4+/CD8+ T cell ratio in peripheral blood increased after CIK cell treatment, and especially further increased in the autologous tumor lysate-pulsed DC-CIK treatment group. No grade 3 or 4 adverse reaction was observed during the cell transfusion.

Similarly, a study based on DC-CIK cell therapy recruited a total of 410 RCC patients after radical or partial nephrectomy [30]. One-hundred-and-fifty-four patients were included in the DC-CIK cell treatment group, while 256 patients were included in the IFN-α therapy control group. $2–5 \times 10^6$ DCs per day were intradermally injected in the inguinal regions bilaterally and intravenous infusion of $3–6 \times 10^9$ autologous CIK cells were performed once a day. A 6-day treatment was considered as one course, and the second course started after 1-month interval, for a total of three courses. The 3- and 5-year OS rates in the DC-CIK group (96% and 96%, respectively) were significantly more increased than that in the IFN-α group (83% and 74%, respectively). In addition, a statistically higher PFS was also observed in the DC-CIK group. The patients in the DC-CIK group exhibited good tolerance with just transient low-grade fever and fatigue.

A recent study compared the immune response induced by DC-CIK cell treatment and DC activated cytotoxic T cell (DC-ACT) treatment [31]. One-hundred-and-twelve patients with solid tumors (six with RCC) were assigned to the DC-CIK treatment group and 116 patients (six with RCC) were assigned to the DC-ACT group. In every infusion, patients received $(1–3) \times 10^7$ DC cells and $(1–2) \times 10^9$ autologous CIK cells. Each treatment consisted of two DC subcutaneous and three CIK intravenous infusions. Immune cells, such as CD3+ HLA-DR+ T cells and NK cells, and cytokines, like IL-2, IL-6 were significantly increased in DC-CIK group, whereas total CD3+ T cells, CD8+ T cells, CD3+ HLA-DR+ cells and IL-12 were remarkably increased in DC-ACT group. DC-ACT therapy decreased the ratio of IL-4/IFN-γ, IL-4/IL-12 and IL-6/IL-12 when compared with DC-CIK therapy. The results showed DC-ACT therapy promotes immune response towards Th1 cytokine profile, and DC-CIK and DC-ACT therapy may eradicate tumors through different pathways.

2.4. Clinical Studies on CIK Cells Combined with Targeted Agents

Yang et al. reported a case who was a 58-year-old male diagnosed with stage III clear cell RCC without metastasis [32]. After operation, this patient received combinatorial therapy consisting of autologous CIK cells and sorafenib because of the suspicious nodule identified in his left lung. The sorafenib dose was 400 mg twice a day and CIK cell infusion was conducted approximately every 2 weeks. However, adverse side effects, including grade 3 diarrhea, grade 3 fatigue and grade 2 hand-foot syndrome, were apparent and exceeded the patient's tolerance. When sorafenib dose was decreased to 200 mg twice a day with CIK cell immunotherapy continued, the adverse effects became mild and well tolerated.

The nodule remained stable for approximately 6 months and then gradually decreased. Suspect metastases again emerged in the mediastinum and lung 6 months later, but the progress rate of these diseases was very slow. The patient maintained a high quality of life throughout the entire treatment process, with a KPS of 90 and greatly extended OS. These results suggest a potential combinatorial regimen consisting of sorafenib and CIK cells for metastatic RCC patients and indicate the safety of CIK cell-based immunotherapy.

Mai et al. retrospectively analyzed the efficacy of sunitinib/sorafenib in combination with autologous DC-CIK cells in 34 metastatic RCC patients after radical nephrectomy [33]. Fifteen patients in group 1 were treated with sunitinib/sorafenib monotherapy, while 19 patients in group 2 were treated with sunitinib/sorafenib in combination with DC-CIK cells. The median PFS and 3-year OS was significantly higher in group 2 and the cases of PD and deaths were less in group 2 than that in group 1. In addition, the 3-year OS was higher in sunitinib + DC-CIK group than that in sorafenib + DC-CIK group.

2.5. Clinical Studies on CIK Cells Combined with Immune Checkpoint Inhibitors

A phase I study aimed to assess the safety and clinical activity of the PD-1 blockade pembrolizumab in combination with autologous DC-CIK cells [34]. Thirty-seven patients with various solid tumor entities, including 8 with RCC, were enrolled in this study. Patients received more than eight cycles of intravenous infusion of pembrolizumab-activated autologous DC-CIK cells. The median OS and PFS were 270 and 162 days, respectively at the time of report. In RCC patients, objective responses (CR or PR) were observed in two of the eight patients, and the overall disease control rate in RCC patients was 75.0%. Treatment-related adverse reactions were observed in 20/31 patients. Two patients with bladder cancer and hepatocellular carcinoma, respectively, exhibited grade 3 or 4 toxicities, including fever and chills. All adverse reactions were reversible or controllable.

The anti-tumor activity of pembrolizumab-activated DC-CIK cells was then confirmed ex vivo. Autologous renal carcinoma cells were collected from one patient with PR and another with SD after treatment. Expression of PD-L1 was upregulated by DC-CIK cells and after being cocultured with pembrolizumab; the cytotoxicity and IFN-γ secretion level of DC-CIK cells were obviously increased.

Wang et al. reported an RCC case treated with the anti-PD-1 mAb pembrolizumab combined with CIK cell transfer [35]. This patient is an 80-year-old male with multiple metastases after partial nephrectomy. The tumor biopsy from this patient showed moderate CD3+ T cell infiltration, but no PD-1 or PD-L1 expression. After receiving four cycles of pembrolizumab combined with eight cycles of autologous CIK cell transfer, he achieved a CR. This patient developed gingivitis after the first cycle of pembrolizumab and pneumonia after the second cycle of pembrolizumab, for which he received systematic antibiotic treatment. No other severe adverse effects were observed. These findings showed the anti-tumor potency and safety of the PD-1 inhibitor in combination with CIK cell therapy on RCC.

The study design, clinical responses, adverse effects and conclusions of all clinical studies discussed above are outlined in Table 1.

Table 1. Clinical studies applying CIK cells for the treatment of RCC.

Study	Number of Patients	Therapeutic Approach	Clinical Response	Adverse Event	Conclusion
Liu et al. [21]	1 (1 RCC)	Modified auto-CIKs	Symptomatic improvement (relieved cough, dyspnea, chest distress and thoracalgia) and reduction of pleural fluid	Fever (~38 °C) but recovered 2 days later	The patient achieved partial success
Zhan et al. [26]	137 (137 RCC)	Group 1: tumor lysate-pulsed DCs + auto-CIKs Group 2: IFN-α Group 3: no adjuvant therapy	Increased CD4+/CD8+ ratio, decreased CD4+CD25^{high} cells and significantly higher 3- and 5-year OS rates	Controllable fever and fatigue in DC-CIK group	Postoperative immunotherapy with tumor lysate-pulsed DC-CIK cells may prevent recurrence/metastasis and increase OS rates
Zhang et al. [20]	40 (10 RCC)	Auto-CIKs	6-month, 1-year and 3-year OS rates were 70.0, 60.0 and 57.5%, respectively; median OS was 34.9 months; 6 recurrence, 12 metastasis and 15 deaths in all patients (2 recurrence, 5 metastasis and 3 deaths in RCC)	Controllable fever and poor appetite	CIK cell therapy can be an effective adjuvant instrument of the routine anti-tumor treatment
Cui et al. [27]	121 (7 RCC)	Tumor lysate-pulsed DCs + auto-CIKs	Improvements in the physical strength, appetite and sleeping status	Controllable fever, insomnia, anorexia, joint soreness and skin rashes	Tumor lysate-pulsed DC-CIK cells were safe without serious adverse side-effects
Zhang et al. [19]	20 (20 RCC)	Group 1: auto-CIKs Group 2: control	Significantly longer median PFS; 6 CR, 4 SD in CIK group and 5 CR, 3 SD, 2 PD in control group	Mild arthralgia, laryngeal edema, fatigue, and low-grade fever	CIK cell treatment could prolong survival in patients with RCC after radical nephrectomy
Wang et al. [28]	28 (28 RCC)	GmDCs + auto-CIKs	4 CR, 7 PR, 10 SD, 6 PD and 1 death	Flu-like symptoms with fever	DCR was significantly related with cycles of treatment
Wang et al. [24]	29 (29 RCC)	Auto-CIKs + IL-2	4 PR, 18 SD and 7 PD; 1-year survival was 82.8%; median PFS and OS were 7.7 months and 12.6 months, respectively	Grade 1 and 2 fever and grade 2 diarrhea	Auto-CIKs can induce regression of RCC; MDSCs can serve as a potential marker for the prognosis of patients receiving a CIK-based therapy
Li et al. [22]	20 (1 RCC)	RetroNectin-activated auto-CIKs + conventional therapies	1 CR, 5 PR, 9 SD and 5 PD; median PFS and OS were 7.7 months and 12.6 months, respectively (1 CR with an OS of 14 months and PFS of 8 months in RCC)	Fever	RetroNectin-activated CIKs combined with conventional therapies could improve the prognosis of metastatic brain tumor patients
Zheng et al. [30]	410 (410 RCC)	Group 1: tumor lysate-pulsed DCs + auto-CIKs Group 2: IFN-α	Significantly increased 3-, 5-year OS rates and PFS in DC-CIK group	Transient low-grade fever and fatigue	Adjuvant DC-CIK treatment after surgery prolonged PFS and reduced mortality

Table 1. *Cont.*

Study	Number of Patients	Therapeutic Approach	Clinical Response	Adverse Event	Conclusion
Zhao et al. [29]	122 (122 RCC)	In operable patients: Group 1: tumor lysate-pulsed DCs + auto-CIKs Group 2: control in inoperable patients: Group 1: auto-CIKs Group 2: control	Significantly higher 3-year DFS and decreased risk of post-operative disease progression and relapse in operable patients; Significantly higher 3-year OS rate, median OS and PFS in inoperable patients	Flu-like symptoms such as fever and fatigue	DC-CIK cells might be more efficient and personalized for the patients with tumor resection, and CIK cells could improve the prognosis for inoperable patients
Yang et al. [32]	1 (1 RCC)	Auto-CIKs + sorafenib	Metastasis remained stable	No serious adverse reactions	CIK cells combined with sorafenib could result in a synergistic effect
Mai et al. [33]	34 (34 RCC)	Group 1: sunitinib/sorafenib monotherapy Group 2: DCs + auto-CIKs + sunitinib/sorafenib	Significantly higher median PFS and 3-year OS rate; more SD and less PD and death	No serious adverse reactions in group 2; bone marrow suppression, oral ulcer, fatigue, and hand-foot syndrome	Sunitinib/sorafenib combined with CIK cells could significantly prolong the median PFS and 3-year OS
Wang et al. [35]	2 (1 RCC)	Auto-CIKs + pembrolizumab	1 CR (RCC) and 1 near-CR	No serious adverse reactions associated with CIK cells	Pembrolizumab in combination with CIK cells led to potent anti-tumor activity in RCC; CD3+ T cell infiltration in baseline tumor biopsies is a potential predictive biomarker
Chen et al. [34]	37 (8 RCC)	DCs + auto-CIKs + pembrolizumab	2 CR, 5 PR, 13 SD and 11 PD (1 CR, 1 PR, 4 SD, 2 PD in RCC); median OS and PFS were 270 and 162 days	All treatment-related adverse reactions were reversible or controllable; grade 3 or 4 toxicities, including fever and chills, were observed in two patients	Pembrolizumab-activated autologous DC-CIK cells were safe and effective in advanced solid tumors
Li et al. [31]	228 (12 RCC)	Group 1: tumor lysate-pulsed DCs + auto-CIKs Group 2: tumor lysate-pulsed DCs + cytotoxic T cells	Elevated percentage of CD3+ HLA-DR+ T cells, NK cells and cytokines such as IL-2, IL-6 in group 1; Elevated total CD3+ T cells, CD8+ T cells, CD3+ HLA-DR+ cells and IL-12 in group 2	–	DCs combined with cytotoxic T cells have more dominance to induce Th1 cytokine response instead of skewing toward the Th2 cytokine profile

Auto-CIKs: autologous CIK cells; DCs: dendritic cells; IFN-α: interferon-α; OS: overall survival; PFS: progression-free survival; CR: complete response; PR: partial response; SD: stable disease; PD: progressive disease; gmDCs: genetically modified dendritic cells; DFS: disease-free survival; DCR: disease control rate; IL-2: interleukin-2; MDSCs: myeloid-derived suppressor cells.

3. Preclinical Researches to Improve the Anti-Tumoral Activity of CIK Cells

Ever-growing clinical trials have been conducted with CIK cells in cancer patients, owing to the relative easiness of CIK cell preparation ex vivo, low toxicity and GVHD activity, and their encouraging cytolytic activities against various tumor cells [15]. However, the clinical benefits of CIK cells reported in some studies are still limited and fall for inability of exerting a sustained and prolonged anti-tumor response. Researchers are exploring novel methods to modify CIK cell-based immunotherapies for a higher efficacy and more specific recognition against RCC. These preclinical researches conducted with CIK cells are concluded in Table 2.

Genetically modified CIK cells are of potential therapeutic value in the treatment of RCC. IL-7 is a 25kDa cytokine, which induced the proliferation of mature CD4+ and CD8+ T cells and also CIK cells [36]. Finke et al. used the adenovirus-enhanced CD3 receptor-mediated gene transfer for transfection with the IL-7 gene [37]. CIK cells transfected with IL-7 gene showed more IL-7 expression and a higher proliferation rate as compared with non-transfected cells. Expression of IL-7 also increased the production of tumor necrosis factor-α (TNF-α) by CIK cells and improved the cytotoxicity against RCC, malignant melanoma and colon carcinoma cell lines, indicating CIK cells transfected with an IL-7 gene expression construct may be valuable for adoptive immunotherapy on RCC. In another study, DCs were transduced with adenoviruses carrying human CD40L (Ad-hCD40L) to stimulate the anti-tumor activity of CIK cells [38]. CD40L is the ligand of CD40, a member of the tumor necrosis factor receptor family and is essential in antigen-presenting cells (APCs) activation and cytotoxic T lymphocytes (CTLs) generation [39]. DCs transduced with Ad-hCD40L had high expression of soluble CD40L and membrane-bound CD40L and showed a T-helper cell type 1 shift of expressed cytokines/chemokines. In addition, Ad-hCD40L transduction of DCs also significantly stimulated the proliferation of CIK cells and their cytotoxicity against RCC cell lines. This observation shows the immunomodulatory potential of genetically modified DCs for the CIK cell-based immunotherapy.

Telomerase is a ribonucleoprotein enzyme that prevents the end of the chromosome from damage or fusion. Activation of telomerase is detected in nearly all human cancers. Telomerase peptide was added to pulse DCs and induce the tumor-specific lysis of CIK cells [40]. CIK cells had a significant increase in cytotoxic activity against RCC cells after being co-cultured with telomerase peptide pulsed DCs when compared with CIK cells without co-culture, that is 100% versus 41.7% at an effector-to-target (E/T) ratio of 60:1. The activated CIK cells also exerted specific cytotoxicity against autologous, telomerase positive primary cell cultures. Telomerase could, thus, serve as a specific tumor-associated antigen for RCC and allow the generation of antigen specific CIK cells.

T cell Ig and ITIM domain (TIGIT) is a newly identified inhibitory receptor expressed on T and natural killer (NK) cells [44,45]. A study showed that TIGIT was also expressed by CIK cells and interacted with CD155, the human poliovirus receptor expressed in many types of normal and cancer cells [41]. The anti-TIGIT functional antibody blocked TIGIT expression of CIK cells and promoted their proliferation. Cytotoxicity against CD155 positive tumor cells was enhanced with an increased level of cytokines, such as IFN-γ, IL-6, and TNF-α. However, inhibition of DNAX accessory molecule-1 (DNAM-1) reduced the elevated anti-tumor activity and IFN-γ level by TIGIT blockade. The results indicated that TIGIT shared the same ligand, CD155, as DNAM-1 and played an inhibitory role in CIK cell cytotoxicity. This finding provides a new molecular target for the improvement of CIK cell immunotherapy.

Table 2. Summary of preclinical researches conducted with CIK cells on RCC.

Study	Method	Conclusion
Finke et al. [37]	CIK cells transfected with IL-7 gene	Improved proliferation rate and increased TNF-α production of transfected CIK cells; significantly higher cytotoxic activity against the RCC cell line
Hillebrand et al. [38]	DCs transduced with adenoviruses carrying human CD40L (Ad-hCD40L) + CIK cells	Co-culture of Ad-hCD40L DCs with CIK cells led to a significant stimulation of tumor-specific CIK cells, with increased proliferation and cytotoxicity
Sievers et al. [40]	Telomerase peptide pulsed DCs + CIK cells	Significantly increased cytotoxic activity against RCC cell lines and autologous, telomerase positive primary cell cultures
Zhang et al. [41]	An anti-TIGIT functional antibody + CIK cells	CIK cells with TIGIT blocked indicated increased proliferation, higher cytotoxicity against tumor cells expressing CD155 and higher expression of IFN-γ, IL-6, and TNF-α
Setiawan et al. [42]	Peptide P60+ CIK cells	CIK cells combined with P60 resulted in a significant decrease in the viability of renal and pancreatic cancer cell lines
Dehno et al. [43]	CIK cells treated with nivolumab and ipilimumab	CIK cells treated with nivolumab and ipilimumab had no remarkable effect on the viability of RCC cells; the combination of nivolumab and ipilimumab significantly increased the proliferation and IFN-γ secretion of CIK cells

IL-7: interleukin-7; TNF-α: tumor necrosis factor-α; DCs: dendritic cells; TIGIT: T cell Ig and ITIM domain; IFN-γ: interferon-γ; IL-6: interleukin-6.

Peptide P60 has been shown to inhibit the immunosuppressive functions of regulatory T-cells (T-regs) by targeting towards the transcriptional regulator protein forkhead box P3 (FOXP3) [46]. As T-regs was shown to reduce the effectiveness of CIK cells against tumor cells, P60 was added to improve the cytolytic activity against renal and pancreatic cancer cells [12,42]. No increase in IFN-γ secretion and changes in the distribution of major effector cell populations in CIK cells was detected. However, P60 treatment resulted in a significant decrease in the viability of renal and pancreatic cancer cell lines co-cultured with CIK cells.

Recently, the anti-PD-1 mAb nivolumab and anti-CTLA-4 mAb ipilimumab were investigated if the two immune checkpoint inhibitors could stimulate the cytotoxicity of CIK cells against RCC cell lines [43]. Although nivolumab and ipilimumab combined with CIK cells had no remarkable effect on the viability of tumor cells, combination of the two antibodies significantly increased the proliferation and IFN-γ secretion of CIK cells. This finding indicated the possibility of combining immune checkpoint inhibitors with CIK cells as a potential treatment option for RCC.

4. Conclusions

The clinical studies based on CIK cells have shown big promise in the treatment of RCC patients, including those who are in the late stage or refractory to standard therapies. The MHC-unrestricted anti-tumor activity against a wide range of tumor types is one of the most important characteristics of CIK cells. CIK cells are also featured as their relatively low and easily controllable toxicities. In our previous report, the primary side effects of CIK cell therapy were grade 1–2 toxicities like fever, chills, fatigue, headache, and skin rash [47]. Low-grade fever ranged from 37.5 to 40 °C, was the most common adverse event and usually recovered without or with simple treatments [48]. In addition, CIK cells exhibited a reduced risk of GVHD, making CIK cells an ideal candidate for immunotherapy in both matched and mismatched recipients [49].

Many attempts have been made to optimize the treatment modality of CIK cell therapy on RCC. As the clinical studies described above, CIK cells combined with conventional therapies, DC vaccination, targeted drugs or immune checkpoint blockade could achieve better clinical benefits than the standard treatments alone. One of the most successful clinical studies that should be highlighted is reported by Zhao et al. [29]. In 122 patients with different stages of RCC, CIK cell treatment remarkably increased the 3-year survival no matter if it was in operable patients or in inoperable patients. This study suggested personalized CIK cell-based therapy would help to obtain clinical benefits in patients with different stages. Besides sunitinib and sorafenib, which show promising anti-tumor activity combined with CIK cells, other receptor tyrosine kinases, like c-Met, also play an important role in the growth of RCC. Increased expression of c-Met was observed in all RCC subtypes and associated with poor prognosis in RCC [50]. Balan et al. reported that c-Met inhibited immune cell-mediated killing of RCC cells by increasing the expression of PD-L1 [51]. Therefore, c-Met inhibitors may also exert synergistic anti-tumor effect with CIK cells.

Moreover, a variety of preclinical researches have been developed and explored new target molecules and pathways to augment the efficacy of CIK cells' anti-tumor activities. The newly identified inhibitory receptor TIGIT serves as a novel and encouraging target to increase the anti-tumor activity of CIK cells. With the elevated secretion of IFN-γ after TIGIT blockade, expression of PD-1 on CIK cells and PD-L1 on both CIK and tumor cells could also be detected to further develop the cytotoxicity profile of CIK cells by immune checkpoint blockade.

Although there is growing interest in CIK cells as an important cellular anti-tumor therapy on RCC, the heterogeneity in study design, clinical protocol and evaluation criteria of clinical studies all make it difficult to assess and compare the clinical efficacy. In 2010, the first international platform for the registration of clinical trials on CIK cells, IRCC, was established to standardize the clinical data collection [52]. The first update took place in 2015 and the second was published recently [47,53]. Further large-scale studies are required to evaluate the clinical efficacy of CIK cells and more efforts should be performed to identify the optimal CIK cell-based therapeutic combinations on RCC.

Author Contributions: Conceptualization, Y.Z. and I.G.H.S.-W.; writing—original draft preparation, Y.Z.; writing—review and editing, J.E., M.R. and I.G.H.S.-W.; supervision and project administration, I.G.H.S.-W. All authors have read and agreed to the published version of the manuscript.

Acknowledgments: The author Y.Z. would like to acknowledge the support from China Scholarship Council.

References

1. Capitanio, U.; Bensalah, K.; Bex, A.; Boorjian, S.A.; Bray, F.; Coleman, J.; Gore, J.L.; Sun, M.; Wood, C.; Russo, P. Epidemiology of renal cell carcinoma. *Eur. Urol.* **2019**, *75*, 74–84. [CrossRef] [PubMed]
2. Ljungberg, B.; Albiges, L.; Abu-Ghanem, Y.; Bensalah, K.; Dabestani, S.; Fernández-Pello, S.; Giles, R.H.; Hofmann, F.; Hora, M.; Kuczyk, M.A. European association of urology guidelines on renal cell carcinoma: The 2019 update. *Eur. Urol.* **2019**, *75*, 799–810. [CrossRef] [PubMed]
3. Capitanio, U.; Montorsi, F. Renal cancer. *Lancet* **2016**, *387*, 894–906. [CrossRef]
4. Hsieh, J.J.; Purdue, M.P.; Signoretti, S.; Swanton, C.; Albiges, L.; Schmidinger, M.; Heng, D.Y.; Larkin, J.; Ficarra, V. Renal cell carcinoma. *Nat. Rev. Dis. Primers* **2017**, *3*, 17009. [CrossRef]
5. Coppin, C.; Kollmannsberger, C.; Le, L.; Porzsolt, F.; Wilt, T.J. Targeted therapy for advanced renal cell cancer (RCC): A Cochrane systematic review of published randomised trials. *Bju Int.* **2011**, *108*, 1556–1563. [CrossRef]
6. Hudes, G.R. Targeting mTOR in renal cell carcinoma. *Cancer* **2009**, *115*, 2313–2320. [CrossRef]
7. Vuky, J.; Motzer, R.J. Cytokine therapy in renal cell cancer. *Urol. Oncol. Semin. Orig. Investig.* **2000**, *5*, 249–257. [CrossRef]
8. Motzer, R.J.; Tannir, N.M.; McDermott, D.F.; Frontera, O.A.; Melichar, B.; Choueiri, T.K.; Plimack, E.R.; Barthélémy, P.; Porta, C.; George, S. Nivolumab plus ipilimumab versus sunitinib in advanced renal-cell carcinoma. *N. Engl. J. Med.* **2018**, *378*, 1277–1290. [CrossRef]
9. Houot, R.; Schultz, L.M.; Marabelle, A.; Kohrt, H. T-cell–based immunotherapy: Adoptive cell transfer and checkpoint inhibition. *Cancer Immunol. Res.* **2015**, *3*, 1115–1122. [CrossRef]
10. Kim, J.S.; Chung, I.S.; Lim, S.H.; Park, Y.; Park, M.J.; Kim, J.Y.; Kim, Y.G.; Hong, J.T.; Kim, Y.; Han, S.-B. Preclinical and clinical studies on cytokine-induced killer cells for the treatment of renal cell carcinoma. *Arch. Pharm. Res.* **2014**, *37*, 559–566. [CrossRef]
11. Schmidt-Wolf, I.; Finke, S.; Trojaneck, B.; Denkena, A.; Lefterova, P.; Schwella, N.; Heuft, H.; Prange, G.; Korte, M.; Takeya, M. Phase I clinical study applying autologous immunological effector cells transfected with the interleukin-2 gene in patients with metastatic renal cancer, colorectal cancer and lymphoma. *Br. J. Cancer* **1999**, *81*, 1009–1016. [CrossRef] [PubMed]
12. Schmidt-Wolf, I.; Negrin, R.S.; Kiem, H.-P.; Blume, K.G.; Weissman, I.L. Use of a SCID mouse/human lymphoma model to evaluate cytokine-induced killer cells with potent antitumor cell activity. *J. Exp. Med.* **1991**, *174*, 139–149. [CrossRef] [PubMed]
13. Lu, X.; Zhu, A.; Cai, X.; Jia, Z.; Han, W.; Ma, L.; Zhou, M.; Qian, K.; Cen, L.; Chen, B. Role of NKG2D in cytokine-induced killer cells against multiple myeloma cells. *Cancer Biol.* **2012**, *13*, 623–629. [CrossRef] [PubMed]
14. Diefenbach, A.; Jamieson, A.M.; Liu, S.D.; Shastri, N.; Raulet, D.H. Ligands for the murine NKG2D receptor: Expression by tumor cells and activation of NK cells and macrophages. *Nat. Immunol.* **2000**, *1*, 119–126. [CrossRef]
15. Introna, M. CIK as therapeutic agents against tumors. *J. Autoimmun.* **2017**, *85*, 32–44. [CrossRef]
16. Baker, J.; Verneris, M.R.; Ito, M.; Shizuru, J.A.; Negrin, R.S. Expansion of cytolytic CD8+ natural killer T cells with limited capacity for graft-versus-host disease induction due to interferon γ production. *Blood* **2001**, *97*, 2923–2931. [CrossRef]
17. Verneris, M.R.; Ito, M.; Baker, J.; Arshi, A.; Negrin, R.S.; Shizuru, J.A. Engineering hematopoietic grafts: Purified allogeneic hematopoietic stem cells plus expanded CD8+ NK-T cells in the treatment of lymphoma. *Biol. Blood Marrow Transpl.* **2001**, *7*, 532–542. [CrossRef]
18. Jäkel, C.E.; Hauser, S.; Rogenhofer, S.; Müller, S.C.; Brossart, P.; Schmidt-Wolf, I.G. Clinical studies applying cytokine-induced killer cells for the treatment of renal cell carcinoma. *Clin. Dev. Immunol.* **2012**, *2012*, 1–7. [CrossRef]
19. Zhang, Y.; Wang, J.; Wang, Y.; Lu, X.-C.; Fan, H.; Liu, Y.; Zhang, Y.; Feng, K.-C.; Zhang, W.-Y.; Chen, M.-X. Autologous CIK cell immunotherapy in patients with renal cell carcinoma after radical nephrectomy. *Clin. Dev. Immunol.* **2013**, *2013*, 1–12. [CrossRef]

20. Zhang, J.; Zhu, L.; Wei, J.; Liu, L.; Yin, Y.; Gu, Y.; Shu, Y. The effects of cytokine-induced killer cells for the treatment of patients with solid tumors: A clinical retrospective study. *J. Cancer Res. Clin. Oncol.* **2012**, *138*, 1057–1062. [CrossRef]
21. Liu, J.; Sui, J.; Zhang, Z.; Ren, X.; Luan, L.; Yang, Q.; Gu, S.; Wank, R.; Laumbacher, B.; Song, X. Inhibition of pleural metastasis of collecting duct carcinoma of the kidney by modified cytokine-induced killer cells: A case report and review of the literature. *Oncol. Lett.* **2010**, *1*, 955–958. [CrossRef] [PubMed]
22. Li, W.; Wang, Y.; Zhao, L.; Xu, L.; Zhang, Y.; Mai, L.; Gao, Q. Efficacy of RetroNectin-activated cytokine-induced killer cell therapy in metastatic brain tumor patients. *Oncol. Res. Treat.* **2015**, *38*, 160–165. [CrossRef] [PubMed]
23. Kimizuku, F.; Taguchi, Y.; Ohdate, Y.; Kawase, Y.; Shimojo, T.; Hashino, K.; Kato, I.; Sekiguchi, K.; Titani, K. Production and characterization of functional domains of human fibronectin expressed in Escherichia coli. *J. Biochem.* **1991**, *110*, 284–291. [CrossRef] [PubMed]
24. Wang, Z.; Zhang, Y.; Liu, Y.; Wang, L.; Zhao, L.; Yang, T.; He, C.; Song, Y.; Gao, Q. Association of myeloid-derived suppressor cells and efficacy of cytokine-induced killer cell immunotherapy in metastatic renal cell carcinoma patients. *J. Immunother.* **2014**, *37*, 43–50. [CrossRef]
25. Santos, P.M.; Butterfield, L.H. Dendritic cell–based cancer vaccines. *J. Immunol.* **2018**, *200*, 443–449. [CrossRef]
26. Zhan, H.; Xin, G.; Pu, X.; Li, W.; Li, Z.; Zhou, X.; Qiu, J. A randomized controlled trial of postoperative tumor lysate-pulsed dendritic cells and cytokine-induced killer cells immunotherapy in patients with localized and locally advanced renal cell carcinoma. *Chin. Med. J.* **2012**, *125*, 3771–3777.
27. Cui, Y.; Yang, X.; Zhu, W.; Li, J.; Wu, X.; Pang, Y. Immune response, clinical outcome and safety of dendritic cell vaccine in combination with cytokine-induced killer cell therapy in cancer patients. *Oncol. Lett.* **2013**, *6*, 537–541. [CrossRef]
28. Wang, D.; Zhang, B.; Gao, H.; Ding, G.; Wu, Q.; Zhang, J.; Liao, L.; Chen, H. Clinical research of genetically modified dendritic cells in combination with cytokine-induced killer cell treatment in advanced renal cancer. *BMC Cancer* **2014**, *14*, 251. [CrossRef]
29. Zhao, X.; Zhang, Z.; Li, H.; Huang, J.; Yang, S.; Xie, T.; Huang, L.; Yue, D.; Xu, L.; Wang, L. Cytokine induced killer cell-based immunotherapies in patients with different stages of renal cell carcinoma. *Cancer Lett.* **2015**, *362*, 192–198. [CrossRef]
30. Zheng, K.; Tan, J.-M.; Wu, W.-Z.; Qiu, Y.-M.; Zhang, H.; Xu, T.-Z.; Sun, X.-H.; Zhuo, W.-L.; Wang, D.; Zhang, J.-P. Adjuvant dendritic cells vaccine combined with cytokine-induced-killer cell therapy after renal cell carcinoma surgery. *J. BUON* **2015**, *20*, 505–513.
31. Li, C.; Zhu, D.; Zhao, Y.; Guo, Q.; Sun, W.; Li, L.; Gao, D.; Zhao, P. Dendritic Cells Therapy with Cytokine-Induced Killer Cells and Activated Cytotoxic T Cells Attenuated Th2 Bias Immune Response. *Immunol. Investig.* **2019**, *49*, 522–534. [CrossRef] [PubMed]
32. Yang, Y.; Lin, H.; Zhao, L.; Song, Y.; Gao, Q. Combination of sorafenib and cytokine-induced killer cells in metastatic renal cell carcinoma: A potential regimen. *Immunotherapy* **2017**, *9*, 629–635. [CrossRef] [PubMed]
33. Mai, H.-X.; Mei, G.-H.; Zhao, F.-L.; Li, B.-T.; Tang, Y.-Y.; Zhang, B.; Xu, X.-J.; Chen, L.-J. Retrospective analysis on the efficacy of sunitinib/sorafenib in combination with dendritic cells-cytokine-induced killer in metastasis renal cell carcinoma after radical nephrectomy. *J. Cancer Res.* **2018**, *14*, 427.
34. Chen, C.-L.; Pan, Q.-Z.; Weng, D.-S.; Xie, C.-M.; Zhao, J.-J.; Chen, M.-S.; Peng, R.-Q.; Li, D.-D.; Wang, Y.; Tang, Y. Safety and activity of PD-1 blockade-activated DC-CIK cells in patients with advanced solid tumors. *Oncoimmunology* **2018**, *7*, e1417721. [CrossRef]
35. Wang, Z.; Liu, X.; Till, B.; Sun, M.; Li, X.; Gao, Q. Combination of cytokine-induced killer cells and programmed cell death-1 blockade works synergistically to enhance therapeutic efficacy in metastatic renal cell carcinoma and non-small cell lung cancer. *Front. Immunol.* **2018**, *9*, 1513. [CrossRef]
36. Zoll, B.; Lefterova, P.; Csipai, M.; Finke, S.; Trojaneck, B.; Ebert, O.; Micka, B.; Roigk, K.; Fehlinger, M.; Schmidt-Wolf, G.D. Generation of cytokine-induced killer cells using exogenous interleukin-2,-7 or-12. *Cancer Immunol. Immunother.* **1998**, *47*, 221–226. [CrossRef] [PubMed]
37. Finke, S.; Trojaneck, B.; Lefterova, P.; Csipai, M.; Wagner, E.; Kircheis, R.; Neubauer, A.; Huhn, D.; Wittig, B.; Schmidt-Wolf, I. Increase of proliferation rate and enhancement of antitumor cytotoxicity of expanded human CD3+ CD56+ immunologic effector cells by receptor-mediated transfection with the interleukin-7 gene. *Gene Ther.* **1998**, *5*, 31–39. [CrossRef] [PubMed]

38. Hillebrand, R.M.; Vogt, A.; Strassburg, C.P.; Gonzalez-Carmona, M.A.; Schmidt-Wolf, I.G. Immune Check Point CD40–CD40L Activates Dendritic and Effector Cells Against Human Renal Carcinoma Cells. *Anticancer Res.* **2019**, *39*, 4643–4652. [CrossRef] [PubMed]
39. French, R.R.; Chan, H.C.; Tutt, A.L.; Glennie, M.J. CD40 antibody evokes a cytotoxic T-cell response that eradicates lymphoma and bypasses T-cell help. *Nat. Med.* **1999**, *5*, 548–553. [CrossRef]
40. Sievers, E.; Albers, P.; Schmidt-Wolf, I.G.; MÄRTEN, A. Telomerase pulsed dendritic cells for immunotherapy for renal cell carcinoma. *J. Urol.* **2004**, *171*, 114–119. [CrossRef]
41. Zhang, B.; Zhao, W.; Li, H.; Chen, Y.; Tian, H.; Li, L.; Zhang, L.; Gao, C.; Zheng, J. Immunoreceptor TIGIT inhibits the cytotoxicity of human cytokine-induced killer cells by interacting with CD155. *Cancer Immunol. Immunother.* **2016**, *65*, 305–314. [CrossRef] [PubMed]
42. Setiawan, M.F.; Rudan, O.; Vogt, A.; Gonzalez-Carmona, M.A.; Langhans, B.; Schmidt-Wolf, R.; Garofano, F.; Strassburg, C.P.; Lasarte, J.J.; Casares, N. FOXP3 Inhibitory Peptide P60 Increases Efficacy of Cytokine-induced Killer Cells Against Renal and Pancreatic Cancer Cells. *Anticancer Res.* **2019**, *39*, 5369–5374. [CrossRef] [PubMed]
43. Dehno, M.N.; Li, Y.; Weiher, H.; Schmidt-Wolf, I.G. Increase in Efficacy of Checkpoint Inhibition by Cytokine-Induced-Killer Cells as a Combination Immunotherapy for Renal Cancer. *Int. J. Mol. Sci.* **2020**, *21*, 3078. [CrossRef] [PubMed]
44. Yu, X.; Harden, K.; Gonzalez, L.C.; Francesco, M.; Chiang, E.; Irving, B.; Tom, I.; Ivelja, S.; Refino, C.J.; Clark, H. The surface protein TIGIT suppresses T cell activation by promoting the generation of mature immunoregulatory dendritic cells. *Nat. Immunol.* **2009**, *10*, 48. [CrossRef] [PubMed]
45. Stanietsky, N.; Simic, H.; Arapovic, J.; Toporik, A.; Levy, O.; Novik, A.; Levine, Z.; Beiman, M.; Dassa, L.; Achdout, H. The interaction of TIGIT with PVR and PVRL2 inhibits human NK cell cytotoxicity. *Proc. Natl. Acad. Sci. USA* **2009**, *106*, 17858–17863. [CrossRef]
46. Casares, N.; Rudilla, F.; Arribillaga, L.; Llopiz, D.; Riezu-Boj, J.I.; Lozano, T.; López-Sagaseta, J.; Guembe, L.; Sarobe, P.; Prieto, J. A peptide inhibitor of FOXP3 impairs regulatory T cell activity and improves vaccine efficacy in mice. *J. Immunol.* **2010**, *185*, 5150–5159. [CrossRef]
47. Zhang, Y.; Schmidt-Wolf, I.G. Ten-year update of the international registry on cytokine-induced killer cells in cancer immunotherapy. *J. Cell. Physiol.* **2020**. [CrossRef]
48. Zhang, Y.; Xia, L.; Zhang, Y.; Wang, Y.; Lu, X.; Shi, F.; Liu, Y.; Chen, M.; Feng, K.; Zhang, W. Analysis of adverse events following the treatment of autologous cytokine-induced killer cells for adoptive immunotherapy in malignant tumour sufferers. *Expert Opin. Biol.* **2015**, *15*, 481–493. [CrossRef]
49. Introna, M.; Lussana, F.; Algarotti, A.; Gotti, E.; Valgardsdottir, R.; Micò, C.; Grassi, A.; Pavoni, C.; Ferrari, M.L.; Delaini, F. Phase II study of sequential infusion of donor lymphocyte infusion and cytokine-induced killer cells for patients relapsed after allogeneic hematopoietic stem cell transplantation. *Biol. Blood Marrow Transpl.* **2017**, *23*, 2070–2078. [CrossRef]
50. Gibney, G.; Aziz, S.; Camp, R.; Conrad, P.; Schwartz, B.; Chen, C.; Kelly, W.; Kluger, H. c-Met is a prognostic marker and potential therapeutic target in clear cell renal cell carcinoma. *Ann. Oncol.* **2013**, *24*, 343–349. [CrossRef]
51. Balan, M.; Teran, E.M.Y.; Waaga-Gasser, A.M.; Gasser, M.; Choueiri, T.K.; Freeman, G.; Pal, S. Novel roles of c-Met in the survival of renal cancer cells through the regulation of HO-1 and PD-L1 expression. *J. Biol. Chem.* **2015**, *290*, 8110–8120. [CrossRef] [PubMed]
52. Hontscha, C.; Borck, Y.; Zhou, H.; Messmer, D.; Schmidt-Wolf, I. Clinical trials on CIK cells: First report of the international registry on CIK cells (IRCC). *J. Cancer Res. Clin. Oncol.* **2011**, *137*, 305–310. [CrossRef] [PubMed]
53. Schmeel, L.C.; Schmeel, F.C.; Coch, C.; Schmidt-Wolf, I.G. Cytokine-induced killer (CIK) cells in cancer immunotherapy: Report of the international registry on CIK cells (IRCC). *J. Cancer Res. Clin. Oncol.* **2015**, *141*, 839–849. [CrossRef] [PubMed]

5

Individualizing Systemic Therapies in First Line Treatment and beyond for Advanced Renal Cell Carcinoma

Yasir Khan, Timothy D. Slattery and Lisa M. Pickering *

The Royal Marsden Hospital NHS Foundation Trust, Fulham Road, London SW3 6JJ, UK; yasir.khan@rmh.nhs.uk (Y.K.); tim.slattery@rmh.nhs.uk (T.D.S.)

* Correspondence: lisa.pickering@rmh.nhs.uk

Simple Summary: In recent years, a number of new, effective treatments have become available for advanced renal (kidney) cancer. However, with more drugs available it has become more difficult to decide which drugs to choose for particular patients, and in which order to use them. In addition, the new treatments do not work for all patients and they can have troublesome side effects. At the moment, these choices are made according to factors including the type of renal carcinoma from a biopsy, the extent of cancer for that patient, their previous health and their current fitness. The options are summarized in guidelines although these do not make recommendations for individual patients. It is hoped that ongoing research will uncover new tests that allow these decisions to be made more accurately in a "personalized" manner. This article describes how the process is undertaken at present and how it may change in the future.

Abstract: Therapeutic options for treating advanced renal cell cancer (RCC) are rapidly evolving. Vascular endothelial growth factor (VEGF)-directed therapy, predominantly VEGF receptor (VEGFr) tyrosine kinase inhibitors (TKIs) had been the most effective first line treatment since 2005 irrespective of International Metastatic RCC Database Consortium (IMDC) risk stratification. However, immune checkpoint inhibitors (ICI) have recently changed the treatment paradigm for advanced RCC particularly as the first-line systemic treatment modality. The combination of Ipilimumab and Nivolumab provides better disease control and long-term outcomes compared with the anti-VEGFr TKI Sunitinib for IMDC intermediate- to poor-risk patients and we now have the option of using ICI with TKI upfront for all IMDC risk groups. This poses a challenge for physicians, both to select the most suitable first line regimen and the most suitable subsequent therapy given the lack of data about sequencing in this setting. This treatment landscape is expected to become more complex with the emerging treatment options. Moreover, these therapeutic options cannot be generalized as significant variability exists between individual's disease biologies and their physiologies for handling treatment adverse effects. Notable efforts are being made to identify promising predictive biomarkers ranging from neo-antigen load to gene expression profiling. These biomarkers need prospective validation to justify their utility in clinical practice and in treatment decision making. This review article discusses various clinicopathological characteristics that should be carefully evaluated to help select appropriate treatment and discusses the current status of biomarker-based selection.

Keywords: renal cell cancer; immune checkpoint inhibitors; tyrosine kinase inhibitors; biomarkers; individualization

1. Introduction

Renal cell carcinoma (RCC) is the most common type of kidney cancer with increasing incidence worldwide in recent years [1]. The subtypes of RCC differ in their morphological and histological features as well as in the biology and molecular pathways that drive cancer growth. The most common subtype of RCC is clear cell RCC (ccRCC) which accounts for 75–85% of cases [2]. Other sub-types are sometimes collectively termed "non-clear cell" for convenience but are biologically and genetically distinct. These include papillary (15–20%), chromophobe (5%), collecting duct, medullary and translocation RCC [3,4]. Papillary RCC (PRCC) is further subdivided into type 1 and 2 PRCC based on certain genetic alterations.

RCC is one of the few solid organ malignancies in which it has long been recognized that the immune system plays a significant role. RCC does not carry a high mutation burden but nevertheless is responsive to immune modulation. Spontaneous regression is a well observed phenomenon in RCC and therefore, immune modulating agents like Interferon (IFN) and Interleukin-2 (IL-2) were commonly used treatments before the advent of TKIs [5–7]. Although durable, complete responses were seen with IL-2 in particular, that was achieved in fewer than 10% of patients and the effectiveness was further limited by a high rate of treatment-related toxicity.

Vascular endothelial growth factor (VEGF)-directed therapies, including anti-VEGF receptor (anti-VEGFr) TKIs became the new standard of care in 2005 following enhanced understanding of RCC biology. Their effectiveness is well established in ccRCC on the basis of randomized phase III registration studies [8–11]. These agents are also widely used in non-ccRCC on the basis of open label phase two trials, and reported off trial experience, but lack level one evidence. Over the last five years, immune checkpoint inhibitors (ICI) have further transformed the treatment of advanced RCC. These drugs work particularly well for cancers with increased mutational load and highly expressed neo-antigens. Nivolumab was the first anti-Programmed cell death (anti-PD-1) drug approved in the second line setting for advanced RCC in 2015 based on the results of the Checkmate 025 phase III trial [12]. Since then, ICI have been trialed in the first line setting and we now have a plethora of first line treatment options for individual IMDC risk categories ranging from ICI-based combinations and new generation TKIs which add to and now have largely superseded earlier generation TKIs. The updated treatment algorithms of European Society for Medical Oncology (ESMO) as well as National Comprehensive Cancer Network (NCCN) have incorporated all but the most recently presented of these data [13,14].

2. Selection of Treatment

As the number of approved systemic options to treat advanced RCC patients continues to increase, it has become increasingly challenging to select between them. Treatment algorithms provide general guidance (Figure 1) but data that clearly guide selection and sequencing at a personalized level in the first line setting and beyond are lacking. In this review article we will discuss how demographic, prognostic, clinical, and increasingly biomarker information can be used to individualize the treatment for the advanced RCC patients.

2.1. IMDC Risk-Based Treatment Selection

It has been recognized for some time that patients with advanced RCC can be categorized by clinical criteria into differing risk groups that have variable prognostic outcomes. The most commonly used model for risk assessment in current use is the International Metastatic RCC Database Consortium (IMDC) classification. In this model, patients are grouped as favorable (score 0), intermediate (score 1–2), and poor risk (score 3–6) based on their Karnofsky performance status, time from the diagnosis to initiate systemic treatment, hemoglobin level, neutrophil and platelet count and serum calcium level. Some reported clinical trials have utilized these risk criteria in defining the eligible trial population, and almost all current trials report efficacy outcomes stratified by IMDC risk category. Furthermore, the approvals of some treatments are restricted by risk category (Figure 1). Thus, the risk category of individual patients can help guide therapy choices.

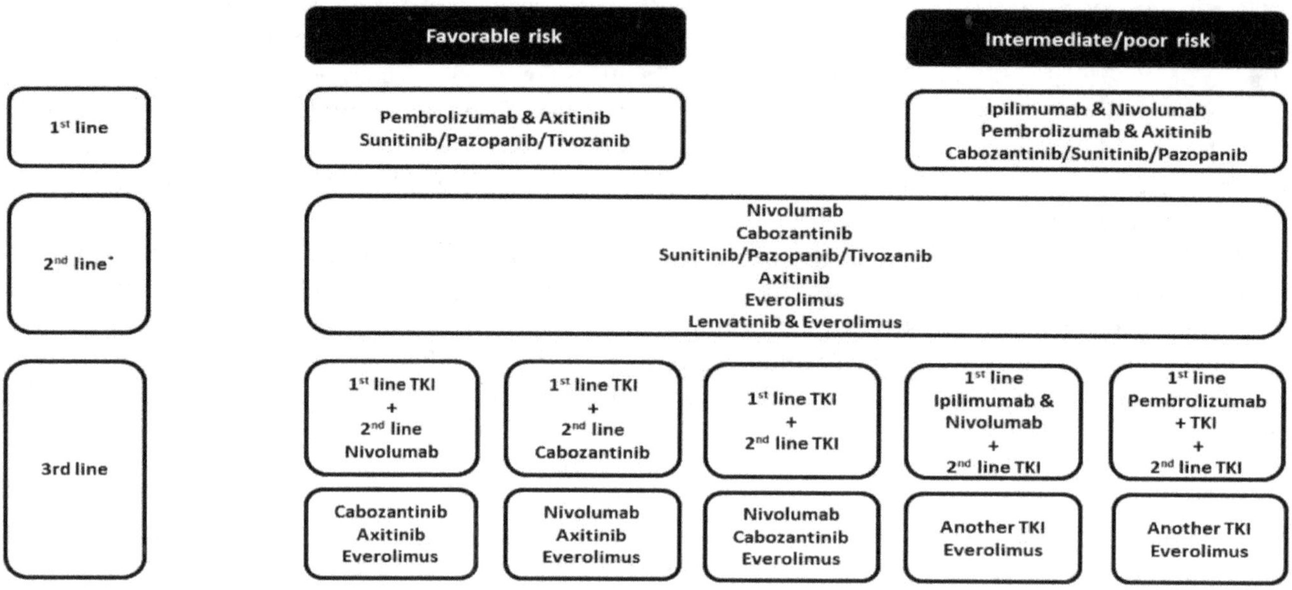

Figure 1. Treatment algorithm for International Metastatic Renal Cell Cancer Database Consortium (IMDC) risk categories [13]. * Based on 1st line treatment. TKI: Tyrosine kinase inhibitors.

There are now various management options to treat favorable risk patients including active surveillance, single agent TKI, or most recently the option of using ICI upfront in combination with a TKI. Anti-VEGFr TKI monotherapy has been the treatment of choice for treating advanced RCC patients with IMDC favorable risk disease since the mid 2000s. Both Sunitinib and Pazopanib are first generation multi-targeted TKIs and the efficacy benefits of each were seen across risk groups, including the favorable risk cohort. Tivozanib is a second generation TKI that was compared against Sorafenib as initial or second-line therapy for patients with advanced RCC in the TIVO-1 open label, randomized phase III trial. The majority of patients had favorable or intermediate risk disease. This trial showed a statistically significant PFS benefit for Tivozanib overall, with PFS of 16.7 months for Tivozanib versus 10.8 months for Sorafenib favorable risk patients (HR 0.59; CI 0.37–0.92; $p = 0.018$) [15]. Despite positive results for TIVO-1, Tivozanib has, as yet, failed to get regulatory approval from the Food and Drug Administration (FDA) but is being used in Europe and United Kingdom (UK) since its approval by the European Medical Agency (EMA) in 2017 [15].

The combinations of Pembrolizumab with Axitinib, and Avelumab with Axitinib, have recently been added to the list of FDA and EMA-approved first line treatment options. Both combinations are approved for all IMDC risk groups. The Pembrolizumab and Axitinib combination demonstrated significant improvement for OS at 12 months versus Sunitinib (89.9% vs. 78.3%) as well as longer median progression free survival (PFS), (15.1 months vs. 11.1 months, HR 0.69; 95% CI, 0.57– 0.84; $p < 0.001$). Similarly, in JAVELIN Renal 101, the Avelumab and Axitinib combination showed better PFS than Sunitinib although no OS advantage has been observed to date [16]. Both trials included more IMDC intermediate- and poor-risk than favorable-risk patients, however sub-group analysis demonstrated clinical benefit across all IMDC risk groups, specifically including the favorable risk cohort. CheckMate 9ER also looked at ICI/TKI combination for all IMDC risk groups and initial results presented at ESMO 2020 favored combination of Nivolumab and Cabozantinib over Sunitinib with manageable toxicities. Median PFS was doubled with combination Nivolumab and Cabozantinib (16.6 months) versus Sunitinib (8.3 months), (HR 0.51; 95% CI, 0.41–0.64; $p < 0.0001$) and OS also favored the Nivolumab/Cabozantinib combination (HR 0.60; 98.89 CI 0.40–0.89); $p = 0.0010$) [17]. There are two other options that have recently been approved for intermediate and poor risk patients;

the combination of Nivolumab and Ipilimumab, and single agent Cabozantinib. However, neither has demonstrated efficacy advantages over Sunitinib for favorable risk patients and as such are not considered appropriate options at this time.

Active surveillance is also considered to be an appropriate option for some favorable risk patients if they have asymptomatic low volume disease and the trajectory of the progression is relatively slow [18,19]. Rini et al. performed a prospective phase II trial evaluating active surveillance for advanced RCC and reported PFS of 17.0% and 11.0% for the entire cohort at 24 and 36 months respectively [18]. In this trial, the number of involved organs and IMDC risk factors were independently associated with shorter PFS. This approach is certainly feasible for patients with indolent disease where it can help to preserve quality of life for a longer period of time seemingly without compromising future outcomes. Although with increasing numbers of increasingly effective options, its use is becoming more selective.

In summary, for patients with favorable risk disease who have met a threshold for requiring active systemic anti-cancer therapy, a combination of ICI and TKI is now considered the standard first line regimen where available, given the demonstrated superior efficacy of these combinations over Sunitinib. However single agent TKIs have long-proven efficacy and are still appropriate in a subset of patients, particularly when the risk ICI-induced toxicity is a concern.

ICI have a prominent role to play in the treatment of intermediate- and poor-risk patients based on the published data. Historically, Sunitinib and Pazopanib were widely used in these patients, as was Temsirolimus particularly in the mid 2000s, on the basis of data showing a survival advantage for Temsirolimus over IFN-a in poor risk patients as defined in the trial criteria [20]. However, in the last couple of years those options have been superseded. Current recommended options to treat these subgroups are combinations of Ipilimumab/Nivolumab, Pembrolizumab/Axitinib and Avelumab/Axitinib, or single agent Cabozantinib.

The Ipilimumab and Nivolumab combination had statistically superior efficacy compared to Sunitinib in intermediate- and poor-risk subgroups, most notably for the primary end point of OS. In CheckMate 214, Ipilimumab and Nivolumab produced an objective response rate (ORR) of 42.0% and a striking complete response rate (CR) of 11.0% in intermediate- and poor-risk patients (Table 1) [20–26]. Updated data presented at ASCO GU 2020 reported median OS of 47 months with Ipilimumab and Nivolumab versus 26.6 months with Sunitinib (HR 0.66; 95% CI 0.55–0.90; $p < 0.0001$) with median follow up of 42.0 months. The durability of benefit was confirmed in this update as median duration of response (DOR) was still not reached for the responders. The Pembrolizumab and Axitinib combination demonstrated a CR rate of 5.8% in Keynote 426. Subgroup analyses showed 12-month OS and PFS of 91.4% and 70.3% in Pembrolizumab and Axitinib arm for intermediate- and poor-risk patients versus 76.7% and 45.2% with Sunitinib respectively.

Table 1. Summary of studies evaluating individualized treatment based on clinicopathological characteristics.

Study	Study Type	Treatment Individualization	Treatment	Treatment Setting	Outcomes
Hudes et al. [20]	Prospective, randomized phase III	Clinical risk category based (Trial protocol defined poor risk group RCC)	Temsirolimus vs. IFN-a vs. Temsirolimus + IFN-a	First line	OS 10.9 vs. 7.3 vs. 8.4 months ($p = 0.008$)
Checkmate 214 [21]	Prospective, randomized phase III	Clinical risk category based (IMDC intermediate- and poor-risk groups RCC)	Nivolumab + Ipilimumab vs. Sunitinib	First line	OS of 47.0 vs. 26.6 months ($p < 0.0001$)
CABOSUN [22]	Prospective, randomized phase II	Clinical risk category based (IMDC intermediate- and poor-risk groups RCC)	Cabozantinib vs. Sunitinib	First line	PFS of 8.6 vs. 5.3 months ($p = 0.0008$)

Table 1. *Cont.*

Study	Study Type	Treatment Individualization	Treatment	Treatment Setting	Outcomes
RESTORE [23]	Prospective, randomized phase II	Toxicity based	Standard Sunitinib schedule (4/2) vs. altered Sunitinib schedule (2/1)	First line TKI	6-month FFS 44.0% vs. 63.0% ($p = 0.029$)
Bjarnason et al. [24]	Prospective phase II	Toxicity based	Individualized Sunitinib dose and scheduled	First line	PFS 12.5 months ($p < 0.001$)
PISCES [25]	Prospective, randomized phase II	Patient preference based	Pazopanib vs. Sunitinib	First line	70% of patients favoured Pazopanib
Gravis et al. [26]	Retrospective	Disease distribution based (Glandular metastasis vs. Non-glandular metastasis at first presentation)	Any systemic treatment	First line and beyond	OS 61.5 vs. 37.4 months ($p < 0.001$)

Abbreviations: IMDC, International Metastatic RCC Database Consortium; OS, overall survival; PFS, progression free survival.

Cabozantinib is a second generation multi-targeted TKI which was granted accelerated approval by the FDA for the first line therapy for IMDC intermediate- and poor-risk RCC patients based on the CABOSUN trial; a randomized phase II trial compared with Sunitinib [22]. An update of the trial was published in 2018 which confirmed the preliminary results [27]. This trial reported median PFS of 8.6 months with Cabozantinib compared with 5.3 months with Sunitinib (HR 0.48; 95% CI 0.31–0.74; $p = 0.0008$) with one patient achieving CR.

There are no available direct comparisons of the above-mentioned treatment options and trial populations differ between the studies although of note each used the same standard comparator of Sunitinib. The benefits of these newer regimens over Sunitinib, based on the data described, are now reflected in current international guidelines with the exception of the very recently presented data for Nivolumab/Cabozantanib which has not yet been evaluated for approval [13,14]. At present the combination of Ipilimumab and Nivolumab has the longest follow-up and therefore the most mature data for durability of response at this time. In addition, a recent update showed that anti-VEGFr TKIs in the second-line setting post Ipilimumab and Nivolumab do seem to retain their efficacy [28]. The data for Keynote 426 and JAVELIN Renal 101 are not yet as mature; time will demonstrate their effectiveness for long term disease control. Cabozantinib monotherapy does have good efficacy in this setting, however this was a randomized phase II rather than a phase III trial, evidence of durable benefit is lacking, and as such its use should be restricted to situations where ICI-containing regimens are not appropriate or unavailable.

2.2. *Histology-Based Treatment Selection*

Knowledge of the histological sub-type of mRCC can be used to guide treatment. At a patient level, it is determined by sampling the original nephrectomy specimen if available, or from a biopsy taken at the time of relapse or of diagnosis of metastatic disease. ccRCC accounts for over 80.0% of all cases of RCC [2], meaning that the vast majority of data arise from clinical trials conducted in this histological sub-type. Non-ccRCC is recognized as a collection of separate entities, with clinical and morphological characteristics that differ from ccRCC and from each other. This is important because RCCs with differing histologies are associated with distinct genomic alterations, clinical features, and manifestations. It is therefore to be expected that these histologies confer differing responses to and outcomes with available regimens.

Systemic anticancer agents approved for treatment of ccRCC are often used in patients with non-ccRCC. However, the described ORR, durations of response, and OS in patients with non-ccRCC are typically inferior in the literature. However, the non-ccRCC histological sub-types are frequently excluded from larger randomized phase III trials thus most existing data in these groups are derived from fairly small prospective phase II trials or subgroup analyses. In fact, despite collectively representing up to a quarter of all RCC histological subtypes, there are currently no specific FDA and EMA approved treatment options for non-ccRCC alone [29]. This section will focus on the benefit of determining histology to guide treatment, particularly in the non-ccRCC histology subtypes in which appropriate choices are less apparent from guidelines due to their relative rarity and consequent lack of robust randomized trial data.

One trial that did allow inclusion of differing histological sub-types of mRCC was the randomized phase II RECORD-3 trial. This trial compared first-line Sunitinib followed by Everolimus at progression, with first-line Everolimus followed by Sunitinib at progression in patients with metastatic RCC of whom 86% had ccRCC and 14% had non-ccRCC [30]. In the trial as a whole, the results favored use of Sunitinib over Everolimus first-line (PFS of 10.7 vs. 7.9 months; HR 1.43; 95% CI 1.15–1.77). When the ccRCC group was sub-analyzed, although there was no statistical difference in OS between the two arms there was a notable numerical difference. Median OS was 23.9 months for Everolimus followed by Sunitinib ($n = 207$) and 30.2 months for Sunitinib followed by Everolimus ($n = 197$) (HR 1.1; 95% CI 0.9–1.4). Thus, the results favored selecting anti-VEGFr TKIs in preference to mTOR inhibitors in the first line setting in ccRCC. This is reflected in guidelines for treatment of metastatic RCC worldwide. In contrast, the differences in PFS and OS seen in the two different sequences were not replicated in the non-ccRCC cohort. Median OS in the non-ccRCC subgroup was 16.2 months for sequential Everolimus and Sunitinib ($n = 29$) and 16.8 months for sequential Sunitinib and Everolimus ($n = 35$) (HR 1.0; 95% CI 0.6–1.8). Clearly, the OS from both agents was lower in the non-ccRCC cohort but not noticeably different from each other. This lack of observed difference could be in part due to the smaller numbers in this cohort, or it could indicate a much lower responsiveness to Sunitinib and/or that Everolimus does have some activity against non-ccRCC.

The use of anti-VEGFr-TKIs in non-ccRCC has also been investigated in a number of dedicated trials. One small retrospective phase II study of 53 patients did show a benefit for Sunitinib over Sorafenib in PRCC, with an increased PFS (11.9 vs. 5.1 months, $p < 0.001$) (Table 2) [31–37]. The same study did not show any statistically significant difference in the PFS between Sunitinib and Sorafenib in a small number ($n = 11$) of chromophobe RCC (ChRCC). Similarly, mTOR inhibitors were first studied over a decade ago across all RCC subtypes; the subgroup analysis in the phase III ARCC trial supported the use of Temsirolimus over IFN-α in non-ccRCC, with an improved OS (8.2 vs. 4.3 months; HR 0.49; 95% CI 0.29–0.85). Although this was a retrospective analysis, it led to the option of using mTOR inhibitors in the treatment of non-ccRCC, and subsequently its use as one of the arms in later non-ccRCC trials. Subsequently two notable trials in non-ccRCC were developed that compared Sunitinib and Everolimus. Both showed activity for these drugs, although the efficacy seemed less than that previously seen in ccRCC [38,39]. In the ASPEN Trial, Sunitinib improved PFS compared with Everolimus across the whole cohort of 108 patients Sunitinib (8.3 months 80% CI 5.8–11.4 versus 5.6 months 80% CI 5.5–6.0; HR 1.41 80% CI 1.03–1.92; $p = 0.16$). However, this was not consistent and in the small number of patients ($n = 16$) with ChRCC the PFS numerically favored Everolimus [39]. However, the number of ChRCC patients were too low to reach statistical significance. The randomized phase II ESPN trial similarly demonstrated that both agents had modest efficacy with a small numerical but non-statistically superior efficacy advantage for Sunitinib [38].

The efficacy of immunotherapy-based regimens is also being investigated in non-ccRCC subtypes in both retrospective and prospective studies. One retrospective multicenter analysis of 43 patients with metastatic non-ccRCC who had had a variety of PD-1- or PD-L-1-targeting agents found that ORR, the primary endpoint of the study, was 19.0% in this heterogenous group. This included responses in patients with papillary non-ccRCC and those whose cancers had sarcomatoid differentiation [34].

Two prospective studies have also shown efficacy of immunotherapy in treating non-ccRCC. In the phase IIIb/IV CheckMate 374 study, the ORR in 44 patients treated with Nivolumab was 13.6% at a median follow-up of 11 months [40]. Most subtypes of non-ccRCC were all fairly well-represented in this study, with one patient with ChRCC showing a complete response to Nivolumab. In the single-arm phase II Keynote 427 study which looked at Pembrolizumab as a first-line treatment option, the preliminary data show an ORR of 25.0% for PRCC, 9.5% for ChRCC, and 35.0% for unclassified RCC, with a median follow-up of 11 months [35]. There have been several studies looking at immunotherapy in combination with other agents, such as MET inhibitors, other immunotherapy agents, and VEGF inhibitors. For example, the combination of Durvalumab and Savolitinib was looked at in 42 patients with PRCC, with an ORR of 29.0% [41]. The combination of Nivolumab and Ipilimumab showed an ORR of 28.0% when studied in 18 patients with various types of non-ccRCC [36]. Atezolizumab and Bevacizumab was also studied in 60 patients with various types of RCC, with an ORR of 26.0% across the cohort of non-ccRCC [42].

Table 2. Select list of studies for non-clear cell renal cell cancer (non-ccRCC) histologies.

Study	Study Type	Histology	Treatment	Outcomes
Choueiri et al [31]	Retrospective analysis	PRCC	Sunitinib vs. Sorafenib	PFS of 11.9 vs. 5.1 months ($p < 0.001$)
Dutcher et al. [32]	Retrospective analysis	Non-ccRCC	Temsirolimus vs. IFN-a	OS of 11.6 vs. 4.3 months (HR 0.49; 95% CI 0.29–0.85)
KEYNOTE 426 [33]	Prospective, randomized phase III (sub-group analysis)	RCC with sarcomatoid differentiation	Pembrolizumab + Axitinib vs. Sunitinib	PFS not reached vs. 8.4 months (HR 0.54; 95% CI 0.29–1.00)
McKay et al. [34]	Retrospective analysis	Non-ccRCC	Monotherapy or combination PD-1/PD-L1 inhibitor	ORR 28% for PRCC 33% for translocation 43% for sarcomatoid/rhabdoid differentiation
KEYNOTE 427 [35]	Prospective, open-label phase II	Non-ccRCC	Pembrolizumab	ORR 25.4% for PRCC 9.5% for ChRCC 34.6% for unclassified RCC
CheckMate 214 [36]	Prospective, randomized phase III (post-hoc analyses)	RCC with sarcomatoid differentiation	Ipilimumab + Nivolumab vs. Sunitinib	ORR of 56.7% vs. 19.2%
Oudard et al. [37]	Prospective, open-label phase II	CDCs	Cisplatin and Gemcitabine	ORR 26.0% OS of 11.0 months

Abbreviations: CDCs, collecting duct carcinomas; ChRCC, chromophobe renal cell cancers; non-ccRCC, non-clear cell renal cell cancer; ORR, objective response rate; OS, overall survival; PFS, progression free survival; PRCC, papillary renal cell cancer; RCC, renal cell cancer.

Renal cell cancers with sarcomatoid differentiation are not recognized as a separate entity (as per the 2016 WHO criteria) but deserve recognition as they are generally associated with a poorer outcome [43]. Immunotherapy has been a treatment of interest in RCC with sarcomatoid differentiation. Research has suggested that sarcomatoid tumors have a high degree of inflammation, and often have poor-risk features, and so may be sensitive to ICI as indicated in the retrospective analysis described above [34]. This has been further supported by three recent prospective trials looking at immunotherapy to treat RCC in ccRCC with sub-analyses focusing on tumors that including sarcomatoid differentiation. The Keynote 426 trial which compared Axitinib/Pembrolizumab to Sunitinib included 105 patients with sarcomatoid features [33]. The results heavily favored the combination treatment arm with PFS not reached, against 8.4 months in the Sunitinib arm (HR 0.54; 95% CI 0.29–1.00), and with an ORR of 58.8%. Similarly, in the ImMotion 151 trial which compared Atezolizumab/Bevacizumab with Sunitinib, there were 142 patients analysed that had tumors with sarcomatoid differentiation [44]. Although this combination is not currently being further developed in RCC, the findings are relevant regarding the efficacy in the sarcomatoid subgroup. There was strong evidence favoring the combination arm, with improved PFS in the intention to treat (ITT) population (HR 0.56; 95% CI 0.38–0.83). An update from the CheckMate 214 study was recently published, looking specifically at subgroup analyses including tumors with sarcomatoid differentiation [45]. The PFS achieved with Ipilimumab/Nivolumab was superior to Sunitinib with HR 0.61 (95% CI 0.38–0.97), further demonstrating the efficacy of immunotherapy combinations in RCC with sarcomatoid differentiation.

Translocation renal cell carcinoma (TRCC) constitutes only 1–4% of adult RCCs and typically responds poorly to conventional ccRCC therapies. It is associated with TFE3, TFEB, or MITF gene fusions, with various associated targetable signaling pathways. An example is the presence of an *SFPQ-TFE* fusion [t(X;1) (p11.2; p34)] resulting in "Xp11.2 translocation carcinoma", in which TFE3 chromatin immunoprecipitation followed by deep sequencing analysis indicated a strong enrichment for the PI3K/AKT/mTOR pathway [46]. This led to the concept of targeting both the PI3K/AKT and mTOR pathways simultaneously, and while no agent has yet made it to a large-scale clinical trial, there have been some promising results in smaller studies. The novel inhibitor SN202, a dual inhibitor of PI3K and mTOR pathways, has been studied in vitro and in mice, with a decrease in the phosphorylation of PI3K downstream signaling molecules AKT and S6K in renal cancer cells seen [47]. Similarly, miR-205-5p is a negative regulator of both PI3K/AKT and mTOR pathways which has also been shown to decrease the production of renal cancer cells in vitro and in mice, through both direct targeting of vascular endothelial growth factor A and promotion of apoptosis and inhibition of epithelial to mesenchymal transition in renal cancer cells, leading to reduced cell proliferation, invasion and migration of ccRCC [48]. Although at present these tumors are treated according to algorithms for ccRCC or for other non-ccRCC sub-types, it is hoped these results will yield other approaches for possible future therapies for TRCC.

Renal medullary carcinoma (RMC) is an aggressive subtype of RCC, with up to 94% of patients presenting with stage IV disease [49]. RMC makes up <0.5% of all RCCs, and frequently affects young adults with haemoglobinopathies such as sickle cell trait [50]. For many years, the mainstay of treatment has been cytotoxic chemotherapy, most commonly with platinum-containing doublet regimens [51]. However durable benefit is rare and the search for more effective therapeutic strategies is ongoing. Case reports have described responses to ICIs in RMC with one reporting a CR in one of three patients with RMC treated with Nivolumab [51]. Three clinical trials of ICIs alone or in combination are now recruiting in RMC.

Chemotherapy has a place in the treatment of a small group of non-ccRCC, despite a relative paucity of evidence. Oudard et al. conducted an open-label phase II trial of 23 patients with collecting duct RCC where ORR of 26.0% were achieved Cisplatin and Gemcitabine with median OS of approximately 11 months [37]. Conventional RCC-type approaches also lead to responses in some patients with collecting duct RCC. Combining these approaches, it was found that the addition of Bevacizumab to chemotherapy produced improved PFS and OS in collecting duct carcinomas (CDCs) (15.1 and 27.8 months, respectively) [52]. Although this was a small study, the results suggested Bevacizumab plus chemotherapy may be a feasible treatment option in this otherwise morbid tumor subtype.

2.3. *Toxicity-Driven Treatment Selection and Modification*

All delivered treatments confer toxicities that differ both between regimens and patients. Their presence or absence, and severity, can be usefully employed to individualize treatment regimens for patients. There is considerable research effort to identify and utilize biomarkers for toxicity but none are in routine practice in RCC at this time; toxicities are more often used to adjust treatment than to select it. Strategies used to modify treatment in response to toxicity are dose reduction, dose interruption, schedule modification, and regimen change and in all cases should be accompanied by supportive therapies for toxicity management.

Based on considerable experience with Sunitinib in particular, there is now evidence that modified dosing and scheduling of TKIs can be effectively used for treatment individualization. All phase III trials of Sunitinib used the standard, licensed dosing schedule of four weeks on treatment followed by a two week break from treatment (4/2). However, we know that there is inter-patient variability in tolerating the standard schedule (SS). A number of studies have been conducted to compare the standard dosing schedule with altered schedules (AS) to evaluate whether AS could deliver improved tolerability whilst retaining drug efficacy. RESTORE was a prospective phase II randomized trial which compared 4/2 schedule with two weeks on, one week off (2/1) schedule. In this trial, failure free survival (FFS) was defined as treatment discontinuation due to disease progression or treatment toxicities. The alternate "two weeks on, one week off" (2/1) Sunitinib schedule was associated with 63.0% FFS at 6 months as compared to 44.0% with the standard 4/2 schedule. Median time to treatment failure (TTF) was also statistically better with 7.6 months for the 2/1 schedule versus 6.0 months for 4/2 schedule ($p = 0.029$) [23]. Another prospective phase II trial evaluated the efficacy and safety of Sunitinib in the first line setting utilizing an individualized approach. Patients had the dose of Sunitinib, and the number of days on treatment, adjusted according to reported rates of toxicity with an aim that toxicities remained ≤ grade II intensity. This trial reported PFS of 12.5 months ($p < 0.001$) and clinical benefit rate of 84.6% with the individualized approached [24]. A number of retrospective analyses have also shown that alternate dosing schedules, particularly the 2/1 schedule, can deliver good efficacy with acceptable tolerability [53,54]. Whilst the design of these studies varies, and they were not powered to demonstrate superiority of AS for efficacy, collectively they suggest that Sunitinib schedule and the dose can be personalized according to adverse effects without losing its efficacy.

The earlier generation VEGFr-TKIs differ slightly in their side effect profiles but have broadly similar and overlapping toxicities. However interestingly, individual patients can develop different side effects to each of these TKIs therefore switching between TKIs to another can improve tolerability whilst retaining efficacy and cancer control. PISCES was a phase IIIb randomized, double blind, cross-over trial evaluating patients' preference for Pazopanib versus Sunitinib. Patient preference was assessed by questionnaire at the end of the two treatment periods and the results overall favored Pazopanib but not in all patents (Table 1) [25]. Therefore, adjusting on an individual patient basis and being prepared to switch regimen is an important principle that remains relevant despite these treatments themselves now being largely superseded.

While the data for the altered dosing of Sunitinib comes from phase II trials and retrospective studies, Axitinib dose escalation and de-escalation strategies have been evaluated prospectively in phase III trials. In a pharmacokinetic and pharmacodynamic study of Axitinib, a clear association was found between circulating drug levels and efficacy of Axitinib; higher ORR was seen with higher drug exposure [55]. The same study demonstrated that the presence of Axitinib-induced hypertension, an "on-target" toxicity, could be used to guide Axitinib dose in order to optimize efficacy. It showed that amongst patients who developed diastolic blood pressure (dBP) of ≥90 mmHg in response to Axitinib median PFS was 14.6 months as compared to 7.8 months in the cohort in whom dBP remained <90 mmHg whilst on Axitinib.

Patients develop specific toxicities from ICI known as immune-related adverse events. However, there is overlap with those toxicities caused by TKIs, e.g., diarrhea, elevated liver enzymes, and skin rashes. The emergence of ICI and TKI in combination as a treatment strategy, poses a new challenge to identify the cause of emergent toxicities and to adjust treatment accordingly. The consensus statement from The Society for Immunotherapy of Cancer, described differing possible approaches for overlapping toxicities. The majority of the committee recommended stopping the TKI for 2–3 days as a first step given the shorter half-life of TKIs, particularly Axitinib, which is used as a backbone in two of these regimens. Others recommended holding both drugs with or without steroids, or continuing Axitinib but holding ICI and treat with steroids [56]. Ultimately the choice depends on the specific toxicity, its grade and physician judgement.

2.4. Consideration of Comorbidities in Treatment Selection

As with any disease, patients with more significant comorbidities and worse performance status may have a poorer outcome than those with fewer comorbidities and good performance status.

The effect of comorbidities (including age) were studied in a retrospective analysis, with data coming from the Surveillance Epidemiology and End Results (SEER) database in the United States [57]. The Charlson Comorbidity Index (CCI) was used, with a higher score indicating the presence of more severe comorbidities. It was found that patients with a higher CCI had decreasing probabilities of receiving systemic treatment versus no treatment, when all patients with RCC were studied (OR 0.86; 95% CI 0.77–0.96). For all patients who were alive at the landmark six month point of analysis, there was a statistically non-significant swing towards those who had received some form of systemic treatment (OR 1.04; 95% CI 0.87–1.23). This could be explained by the fact that those who are alive at six months were more likely to have a better performance status and/or higher pre-treatment estimate of longer OS, thus were more suitable for active therapy. Also, a study looking at comorbidities as prognostic markers showed that while the investigated co-morbidities could induce pathophysiological changes that predisposed to tumor progression, none were independent prognostic factors in patients with RCC [58].

It is often appropriate for severely comorbid patients with advanced RCC not to receive any systemic anti-cancer therapy, with more of a focus on symptomatic relief and improved quality of life. However active, treatment should be considered in stage IV RCC and can be deliverable to many patients by adapting choices with knowledge of their specific comorbidities. This is especially relevant in the present paradigm, given the range of systemic treatment options with manageable tolerability [59]. One example is selecting immunotherapy or mTOR inhibitors in patients with advanced RCC who have existing significant circulatory disease, to avoid VEGFr-TKI-driven increase in the risk of vascular events. Conversely, patients who have inflammatory-driven pathologies (e.g., inflammatory bowel disease, autoimmune diseases) are at higher risk of adverse effects from immunotherapy and according to the severity, may be more suited to a targeted therapy option. Although there are few situations where individual therapies are absolutely contraindicated, the knowledge of comorbidities and expected toxicities can guide preferences to limit the risk of exacerbating established comorbidities.

2.5. *Assessment of Disease Distribution to Guide Treatment*

Consideration of the sites and extent of RCC metastases can also be helpful in driving treatment selection. For example, it has long been standard practice to utilize local treatment modalities for patients with a limited metastatic burden. In such cases, surgical resection (metastasectomy) and/or stereotactic radiosurgery can lead to excellent disease control whilst avoiding the duration of exposure to, and toxicities from, systemic anticancer treatments [60,61]. In addition, the location of metastases and overall tumor burden, can also have relevance for individualizing treatment.

One example is the choice of initial surveillance for a subset of RCC patients with low metastatic burden that is not amenable to a local therapy option [18]. A real-world study showed that stage IV RCC patients with lung (HR 1.27; 95% CI 1.06–1.53), liver (HR 1.42; 95% CI 1.10–1.84), and bone (HR 1.37; 95% CI 1.13–1.66) metastases respectively had shorter OS than those without these sites of disease [62]. Other studies have analyzed the effectiveness of treatment regimens according to locations of metastases. A sub-analysis of the METEOR trial focused on outcomes in patients with bone metastases. This showed that for patients with bone metastases at baseline, treatment with Cabozantinib versus Everolimus, led to a significant improvement in PFS (7.4 months vs. 2.7 months; HR 0.33, 95% CI 0.21–0.51), OS (20.1 months v 12.1 months; HR 0.54, 95% CI 0.34–0.84) and ORR (17.0% vs. 0%), as well as improved response on bone scan (20.0% vs. 10.0%) [63]. The CABOSUN trial also demonstrated that the degree of benefit for Cabozantinib over Sunitinib was greater for patients with metastatic bone disease. The median PFS in patients with bone disease was almost double with 6.1 months for Cabozantinib as compared to 3.3 months for Sunitinib with an impressive HR of 0.54 [22]. Cabozantinib has become widely recognized as an appropriate TKI for RCC patients with bone metastases.

A further example is the observation that the presence of metastases to endocrine (or "glandular") organs is associated with relatively favorable outcomes in patients with advanced ccRCC [26]. At first presentation of metastatic RCC, patients with at least one glandular metastasis compared to those without glandular metastases were more likely to have favorable risk disease (37.2% vs. 18.0%), less likely to have poor-risk disease (10.7% vs. 27.0%), and had considerably longer OS (61.5 months vs. 37.4 months, HR 1.70; 95% CI 1.30–2.20, $p < 0.001$) (Table 1). Interestingly, these findings were irrespective of the presence or absence of bone or liver metastases, suggesting that the potential for improved OS must be recognized when determining management of patients with advanced ccRCC and glandular metastases. This is relevant, as it may affect treatment choice in this subgroup, particularly in those with limited sites of metastatic disease in whom a radical treatment approach should be adopted where possible. If a radical approach is not deemed possible, it is reasonable to adopt a period of initial surveillance to avoid the toxicities of systemic therapy, as the disease may remain indolent for a long period of time and potentially for a number of years.

Conversely, brain metastases confer a relatively poor prognosis, which is often less than 12 months from the time of diagnosis [64]. While this is frequently still the case, patients are receiving more aggressive intervention for brain metastases such as the increased use of stereotactic brain radiosurgery. This has led to improved local control of intracranial metastases particularly for those with a solitary brain deposits. For example, Suarez-Sarmiento Jr et al. showed that relapse free survival (RFS) in RCC patients with brain metastases was correlated with the number of brain lesions; RFS was 27.5 months for those with only one lesion, but 12 months for those with more than one lesion ($p = 0.0026$) [64]. This supports a more aggressive approach to limited brain metastases in patients with RCC.

A further factor that may influence treatment selection is whether there is any clinical benefit in achieving tumor shrinkage, as opposed to stability, in order to improve cancer-related symptoms. This is particularly relevant in anatomical sites where tumor growth may lead to adverse consequences, such as metastases affecting the spinal canal, and mediastinum disease. In such cases, the likelihood of inducing meaningful disease response, and the time to achieve response can be relevant in guiding therapy choice. Regimens that have achieved relatively short time to treatment response (TTR), in addition to meeting their survival endpoints, include Nivolumab plus Ipilimumab in CheckMate 214, Pembrolizumab plus Axitinib in KEYNOTE 426 and most recently Nivolumab plus Cabozantanib in Checkmate 9-ER. In these trials, ORR with Nivolumab plus Ipilimumab was 42%, and was 56% with both Pembrolizumab plus Axitinib and Nivolumab plus Cabozantanib. It is also worth noting that the progressive disease rate was higher with Nivolumab plus Ipilimumab at 27%, compared to 14.6% for Pembrolizumab plus Axitinib and 13.7% with Nivolumab plus Cabozantanib. Acknowledging the limitations of cross trial comparisons, this suggests that in cases where a rapid response is desirable, a reasonable strategy is to select a TKI–containing regimen, ideally as a TKI + ICI combination.

2.6. *Role of Genomic Markers and Biomarkers in Treatment Selection*

Potential benefits of comprehensive genomic analyses of renal cancers include the identification of biomarkers for prognosis and/or prediction of treatment benefit, and in identifying pathways suitable for targeted therapies. Each subtype of RCC has a unique pathophysiology that may be appropriate for separate therapeutic development [29,65]. Furthermore, many genetic/familial syndromes are strongly associated with specific gene mutations and the presence of RCC subtypes. Numerous active therapeutic trials have been designed in utilizing this paradigm, evaluating treatments in both ccRCC and non-ccRCC.

ccRCC is characterized by the inactivation of Von Hippel-Lindau (VHL) tumor suppressor protein and subsequent VHL mutation in essentially all cases, which results in the accumulation of hypoxia-inducible factor (HIF) and subsequent downstream activation of pathways involved in cell metabolism, proliferation and angiogenesis. Several ongoing studies are addressing the development of HIF-targeted therapeutic approaches. The CXC-chemokine receptor-4 (CXCR4) inhibitor X4P-001, which has been shown to downregulate HIF-2α, is being studied in combination with Axitinib, with the intent of overcoming or delaying resistance to VEGFr TKIs (Table 3) [66–79]. PT2385 is a direct HIF-2α antagonist that is being evaluated in patients with ccRCC in a world-first study [67], with the preliminary results showing a favorable safety profile and activity in patients with heavily pre-treated ccRCC. Recently the HIF-2α antagonist MK-6482 was studied in a small group of patients with ccRCC, with PFS at 12 months of 98% (95% CI 89–100%), and DOR) in confirmed responders not reached (range 12–62 weeks) [68].

Table 3. Summary of studies using mutations and biomarkers to individualize treatment.

Study	Tumour Subtype	Study Type	Marker	Results, Comments
Atkins et al. [66]	ccRCC	Phase I/II study	HIF2α	CXCR4 + Axitinib delaying ± overcoming resistance to VEGFr inhibitors.
Courtney et al. [67]	ccRCC	Phase I/II study	HIF-2α	PT2385 shows favourable safety profile and activity in patients with heavily pre-treated ccRCC.
Srinivasan et al. [68]	ccRCC	Phase II study	HIF-2α	Improved PFS (98% at 12 months); DOR in confirmed responses NR (range 12–62 months).
Hakimi et al. [69]	ccRCC	Single institution cohort study	PBRM1, SETD2, BAP1, KDM5C	Mutations in all genes are asssociated with advanced stage, grade, and possibly worse CSS
Voss et al. [70]	Advanced/ metastatic RCC	Retrospective cohort study (COMPARZ and RECORD-3)	PBRM1, BAP1, TP53	Loss of PBRM1, gain of BAP1 and/or TP53 associated with improved PFS and OS in stage IV setting
Hsieh et al. [71]	ccRCC	Retrospective analysis (RECORD-3)	PBRM1, BAP1, KDM5C	PBRM1 and BAP1 mutations associated with longer and shorter PFS with 1L Everolimus in stage IV setting; KDM5C mutation assocaited with longer PFS with 1L Sunitinib.
IMmotion 150 [72]	Treatment-naïve stage IV RCC	Randomized, phase II study	TMB, angiogenic gene signature	TMB and neoantigen burden not associated with PFS; angiogenesis and T-effector response strongly associated with PFS
CREATE [73]	Type 1 PRCC	Multicentre, non-randomized, open-label phase II study	MET	Crizotinib improved PFS in MET positive/ amplified arm compared to MET negative/ non-amplified arm (80% v 22%); OS similar in both arms.
Voss et al. [74]	Advanced/ metastatic RCC	Randomized, phase II study	PTEN	Loss of PTEN IHC expression had improved PFS when treated with Everolimus, compared to retained PTEN IHC expression (10.5 months v 5.3 months).
Iacovelli et al. [75] Thompson et al. [76]	Advanced/ metastatic RCC	Systematic review/ meta-analysis	PD-L1	Limited utility of PD-L1 as a predictive biomarker due to the lack of negative predictive value.
Choueiri et al. [77]	Metastatic ccRCC	Randomized, phase III study (COMPARZ)	PD-L1	Increased PD-L1 was associated with shorter survival in patients with metastatic RCC receiving VEGFr inhibitor agents.
IMmotion 151 [78]	Treatment-naïve stage IV RCC	Randomized, phase III study	Angiogenic gene signature, T-effector gene signature	Confirmation of angiogenesis and T-effector response strongly associating with PFS; also finding associations between angiogenesis and T-effector response, tissue subtypes, and treatment options.
Pal et al. [79]	Stage IV RCC	Retrospective analysis	ctDNA: TP53, VHL, NF1, EGFR, PIK3CA, ARID1A	Disparity in genomic alteration frequencies in post first-line vs. first-line were in *TP53* (49% vs. 24%), *VHL* (29% vs. 18%), *NF1* (20% vs. 3%), *EGFR* (15% vs. 8%), and *PIK3CA* (17% vs. 8%)

Abbreviations: 1L, first line; ctDNA, circulating tumor DNA; ccRCC, clear cell renal cell cancer; CSS, cancer specific survival; CXCR4, CXC-chemokine receptor-4; DOR, duration of response; HIF-2a, hypoxia-inducible factor-2a; NR, not reported; OS, overall survival; PFS, progression free survival; PD-L1, programmed death-ligand 1; TMB, tumor mutational burden; VEGFr, vascular endothelial growth factor receptor.

In patients with ccRCC, PBRM1 is the second most commonly altered gene, with up to 40% of these cancers having somatic loss-of-function mutations [50]. In the localized disease setting, loss of PBRM1 is associated with unfavorable clinical outcomes, with these patients more likely to have stage III disease at presentation, as well as more aggressive pathology, and a higher likelihood of developing stage IV disease in the future [69]. There have been other histone modifying and chromatin remodeling genes in ccRCC studied (SETD2, BAP1, KDM5C), all of which are associated with advanced stage, grade, and possibly worse cancer-specific survival [69]. In the metastatic setting, however, loss of PBRM1 is associated with both improved PFS and OS [70], and may be explained by tumors harboring PBRM1 mutations being strongly angiogenic, resulting in the upregulation of targets of VEGF-directed therapies (e.g., HIF) [80]. The favorable outcome associated with loss of PBRM1 is also found in the RECORD-3 and ImMotion150 trials, irrespective of treatment choice in each trial [71,72].

PRCC has a long list of associated genetic mutations [81]. Type 1 PRCC has been associated with both alterations in the MET gene and a gain in chromosome 7 (where the MET gene is located). There have been some promising results in recent studies looking at treatment of type 1 PRCC with MET inhibitors. Crizotinib is a small-molecule TKI that inhibits MET as well as anaplastic lymphoma kinase (ALK) and ROS proto-oncogene 1 receptor tyrosine kinase (ROS1), which has been shown to be effective in Type 1 PRCC. The effect of Crizotinib in type 1 PRCC patients was studied in tumors with MET-positivity and/or MET-amplification, against those that were MET-negative and not MET-amplified [73]. PFS at one year was 80.0% (95% CI 20.4–96.9) in the MET-positive/amplified arm, against 22.0% (95% CI 5.4–45.6) in the MET-negative/non-amplified arm. The OS was relatively similar in each arm, and the numbers in this study were quite small (23 evaluable subjects), but nevertheless it may provide us with a potential treatment option for type 1 PRCC and is currently being trialed in larger studies. Furthermore, two respective phase II trials looking at Foretinib and Savolitinib, both multi-kinase inhibitors targeting MET, demonstrated significant response rates in patients with MET-driven papillary RCC's [82,83]. Foretinib had a 50.0% response rate among patients with a germline MET mutation, and Savolitinib had a 18.0% ORR in MET-driven tumors (compared to 0% ORR in non-MET driven tumors) with a median PFS of 6.2 months against 1.4 months in the respective arms (HR 0.33, 95% CI 0.20–0.52). There is an ongoing phase II randomized controlled trial which was designed to compare Crizotinib, Savolitinib, Cabozantinib, and Sunitinib in patients with PRCC [84]. The Crizotinib and Savolitinib arms were closed in mid-2018 for futility after an interim analysis, leaving the efficacy of Cabozantinib and Sunitinib to be studied in both MET mutated and MET expressing tumors. However, none of the trials has yet yielded results that translate into mutation-driven selection in clinical practice. At present, appropriate first line choices for MET-positive non-ccRCC on a biological basis could be Sunitinib or Cabozantinib. Cabozantinib has activity against MET as well as other signaling pathways but lacks clinical trial evidence in phase III clinical trials in non-ccRCC. Sunitinib, conversely, is listed as the default option in many clinical guidelines, based on the trial results described previously. Type 2 PRCC has been linked to mutations in CDKN2A, SETD2, BAP1, PBRM1, TERT, NF2, FH, and NRF2-ARE pathway genes (among others), as well as a CpG island methylator phenotype [85]. Various mutations in CDK2NA have also been seen frequently in CDCs although it is unclear whether and how this knowledge may be harnessed in future therapy selection [86].

The chromophobic and oncocytic subtypes have a correlation with Birt-Hogg-Dubé syndrome. Various types of non-ccRCC have been associated with Tuberous Sclerosis Complex (TSC) with one study showing a high incidence of both papillary and chromophobe/oncocytic subtypes [87]. Apart from MET-mutated PRCC, there is no strong evidence for other mutations due to a lack of adequately sized cohorts, although the trials are ongoing. As an example, given the known association, the presence of FH may lead to the use of treatment regimens efficacious in patients with hereditary leiomyomata and renal cell cancer (HLRCC) or PRCC [50].

An association between mutation status for TSC1/TSC2/mTOR and therapeutic outcome with Everolimus was tested, but not confirmed. Clinically meaningful differences in PFS, however, were seen based on PTEN expression by IHC, which was lost in >50% of patients [74]. A loss of PTEN IHC expression led to favorable outcomes in patients treated with Everolimus when compared to retained PTEN IHC expression (median PFS 10.5 vs. 5.3 months, HR 2.5, $p < 0.001$). Such differences were not seen with Sunitinib, suggesting that TKIs may be a preferred therapeutic option in those with retained PTEN IHC expression.

For ICI across all tumor types as well as in RCC, PD-L1 expression is the most thoroughly researched biomarker. Its expression has an association with aggressive disease biology in RCC, including high nuclear grade, lymph node involvement, and distant metastases; however, its utility as a predictive biomarker is limited as it lacks negative predictive value [75,76]. Though treatment efficacy is greater in PD-L1 positive patients, it has been repeatedly demonstrated that ICI also provide clinical benefit to PD-L1 negative patients [16,33,44]. Hence, PD-L1 expression does not help segregate responders from non-responders. The proposed explanations of this inconsistency as a biomarker are variable expression of PD-L1 on fresh versus archival tissue, intra-tumoral heterogeneity, and heterogenous expression of PD-L1 on primary versus metastatic sites, as well as lack of using a uniform assay [88]. Interestingly however, an association with high PD-L1 and poor outcome when treated with VEGFr inhibitors has been shown [77].

Tumor mutational burden (TMB) is perhaps the most promising biomarker for ICI in recent times for tumor types with high mutational loads such as melanoma and urothelial cancer. However, the mutational load in RCC is usually very low and as yet, it is not in routine clinical use as a predictive biomarker in any setting. The generation of tumor neoantigens may come from higher frequencies of frameshift insertion and deletion mutations [89], and the ongoing TRACERx Renal study has shown secondary mutations and chromosomal changes involved in tumor evolution, outlining their clinical relevance [90]. In the IMmotion 150 trial, exploratory biomarker analysis was conducted evaluating TMB and neo-antigen burden but found no association with PFS [72]. Strongly angiogenic tumors are more responsive to anti-VEGF TKI as compared to ICI. Gene expression profiling can identify RCC into high and low angiogenic tumors. As mentioned previously, tumors harboring PBRM1 mutations tend to be strongly angiogenic while BAP1 mutation is associated with poorly angiogenic tumors. These genetic signatures were integrated prospectively in phase III study (IMmotion 151), with the data recently validating both angiogenesis and T-effector gene signatures as predictors of outcome [44,90]. Patients with favorable risk RCC are characterized by an angiogenesis^{High} gene signature. In renal tumors with T-effector^{High} and angiogenesis^{Low} signatures, Atezolizumab/Bevacizumab improved PFS compared to Sunitinib. Patients with an angiogenesis^{High} gene signature had improved PFS compared to angiogenesis^{Low} group in the Sunitinib arm. Supporting the data mentioned previously on tumors with sarcomatoid differentiation, sarcomatoid RCCs were shown to be characterized by angiogenesis^{Low} and T-effector^{High} gene signatures, with higher PD-L1 expression, and hence greater benefit with immunotherapy [78]. This may be a significant step in the understanding of the biology of RCC, and the subsequent information obtained to direct therapy.

Circulating tumor DNA (ctDNA) is the most widely used blood-based test for assessment of cancer biomarkers. It is a means of assessing for tumor-based material less invasively, and its use as a predictive and prognostic biomarker has been validated across multiple solid tumor types [91,92]. The use of ctDNA in RCC is still under investigation, although the rationale is very much justified. Multiple genomic alterations including those in VHL, TP53, EGFR, and NF1 have been identified in ctDNA, with the same report showing genomic alterations in any gene detected in 78.6% of patients with metastatic RCC [79]. The ctDNA count to assess tumor response to treatment has been studied since, with a positive correlation between detectable ctDNA and radiographic burden of disease found [93]. Although the limitations of many studies include a lack of power (due to small sample sizes), more specific genomic analyses would likely benefit further from ctDNA analysis in terms of prognostication, an example being MET-deficient RCC [94].

A new area of focus these days is gut microbiota where pre-clinical studies have shown that certain micro-organisms may predict positive or negative responses from ICI [95]. Exposure to antibiotics and dietary habits impact our gut microbiome and further research is being carried out to segregate the groups of micro-organisms which are consistent with ICI related outcomes.

The available published data for predictive biomarkers is not sufficiently strong to change current clinical practice. Most of the literature is based on retrospective analysis on archival tissues but there are many ongoing studies which are prospectively evaluating various biomarkers. The current evidence to use biomarkers in treatment decision is lacking and needs validation before it can be used for clinical decision making.

3. Selection of Second-Line Treatment and beyond

The treatment landscape beyond the first line setting has changed considerably in the last few years, and has been further complicated since several agents previously used in the second and third line settings are now indicated first line, either alone or in combination. In fact, only five years ago the standard of care for second-line treatment was limited to Axitinib or Everolimus for patients who had received a TKI as their first-line treatment for metastatic RCC [96].

The same principles apply in choosing subsequent lines of treatment in advanced RCC to those adopted in choosing initial therapy. There is evidence that patients exposed to ICI upfront can respond well to VEGF-targeting TKIs on progression [28]. This was reported in a follow-on observational study in 33 patients who had progressed on upfront ICI therapy in the Checkmate 214 trial and who subsequently received a VEGFr-TKI. The reported ORR was 36.0% with a median PFS of 7.0–8.0 months achieved with the VEGFr-TKIs Sunitinib, Pazopanib, Cabozantinib, and Axitinib. This was particularly respectable given that the trial population had predominantly intermediate and poor risk disease. These four VEGFr-TKIs together with Tivozanib, and Sorafenib can all be appropriately considered after first-line VEGFr-TKIs on the basis of randomized trial data [97–109].

There is continuing research into the benefit of immunotherapy in advanced RCC in second and later lines of therapy after a variety of initial treatments. The phase III CheckMate 025 study evaluated efficacy outcomes from Nivolumab and Everolimus in patients who had progressed after one or two prior TKIs. It demonstrated a statistically significant improvement in ORR, PFS, and OS with Nivolumab, compared to Everolimus [12]. No other checkpoint inhibitor therapy agent is yet indicated for use in second-line treatment and beyond in advanced ccRCC although other trials are recruiting including using different ICI-containing regimens in those exposed to upfront ICI therapy.

It has long been known that mTOR inhibitors are also beneficial in treating advanced RCC beyond first-line therapy. Everolimus showed an improved PFS when compared to placebo [110]. With the advance of TKI treatment options, and subsequent randomized trial data showing superiority of both Nivolumab and Cabozantinib over Everolimus, mTOR inhibitors are less-frequently used as monotherapy if other options are available [12,101]. However, the use of Everolimus in combination with the VEGFr-TKI Lenvatinib is approved and in routine use. In a randomized phase II study of 150 patients, the combination of Lenvatinib and Everolimus showed PFS and OS benefit over Everolimus monotherapy [111].

Therapy with IL-2 is now uncommon for treatment of ccRCC. It is FDA-approved for treatment of metastatic RCC but is only available at select institutions world-wide for patients with low-volume disease. ORR are 14.0–20.0%, but patients who have a complete response may enter a long-term remission [6,112]. Toxicity may be profound, and treatment-associated deaths have been reported. Its use has largely been superseded by the advent of the plethora of ICI-based and other treatment regimens.

Selecting the most suitable treatment option for second-line and beyond in advanced RCC is heavily dependent on the regimen given in the first-line setting, in addition to consideration of those factors used to select first line treatment such as efficacy data, local availability, comorbidities, physician/patient preference, and, to a lesser extent, histological subtype. Despite the many therapeutic advancements made in the last few years, there is a lack of well-validated prognostic and predictive biomarkers to further personalize the management of advanced RCC, although this means a very active research field. Based on the efficacy and strength of data, the most widely recommended second-line treatment options for advanced ccRCC are Cabozantinib and Nivolumab although Lenvatinib with Everolimus of merit and is increasingly used [12,100,101]. Beyond this, the options include any of the other approved treatments and of course recruitment to clinical trials is to be encouraged where available.

4. Conclusions

Over the last decade, there has been a major shift in the treatment of advanced RCC. The progress of medicine has led to improved survival, making the management of complex disease processes as important as ever. The evolution of both immunotherapy and targeted therapy treatment options, along with the significant advances in research into personalized medicine, have led to greatly improved survival and quality of life in this previously morbid tumor group. Treatment choice is primarily selected utilizing internationally-recognized, evidence-based consensus guidelines. However, choice between treatments that are regarded to have broadly equivalent efficacy is often required and, to date, has been driven by clinico-pathological features including RCC risk category, histological sub-type, patient fitness, and comorbidities. However, the development of these treatment options has been accompanied by enormous advances in understanding of the molecular and genomic basis of RCC. It is therefore hoped that the continuing development of validated tumor genomic markers and biomarkers, together with new ways of predicting and prognosticating outcome, will eventually allow for more educated, accurate and tailored treatment individualization.

Author Contributions: Y.K., T.D.S., and L.M.P. outlined and wrote this manuscript. L.M.P. provided objective critique and revisions to the subsequent drafts of this manuscript. All authors have read and agreed to the published version of the manuscript.

Abbreviations

ALK	anaplastic lymphoma kinase
CCI	Charlson comorbidity index
ccRCC	clear cell renal cell cancer
CDCs	collecting duct carcinomas
ChRCC	chromophobe renal cell cancer
CR	complete response
ctDNA	circulating tumor DNA
CXCR4	CXC-chemokine receptor-4
dBP	diastolic blood pressure
DOR	duration of response
EMA	European medical agency
ESMO	European society for medical oncology
FDA	food and drug administration
FFS	failure free survival
HIF	hypoxia-inducible factor
HLRCC	hereditary leiomyomata and renal cell cancer
ICI	immune checkpoint inhibitors
IFN	interferon
IL-2	interleukin-2
IMDC	International Metastatic RCC Database Consortium
ITT	intention to treat
NCCN	national comprehensive cancer network

ORR	objective response rate
OS	overall survival
PD-1	programmed cell death-1
PD-L1	programmed cell death-ligand 1
PFS	progression free survival
PRCC	papillary renal cell cancer
RCC	renal cell cancer
RFS	relapse free survival;
RMC	renal medullary carcinoma
ROS1, ROS	proto-oncogene 1 receptor tyrosine kinase
SEER	surveillance epidemiology and end results
TKIs	tyrosine kinase inhibitors
TMB	tumor mutational burden
TRCC	translocation renal cell carcinoma
TSC	tuberous sclerosis complex
TTF	time to treatment failure
TTR	time to treatment response
VEGFr	vascular endothelial growth factor receptor
VHL	Von Hippel-Lindau

References

1. Saad, A.M.; Gad, M.M.; Al-Husseini, M.J.; Ruhban, I.A.; Sonbol, M.B.; Ho, T.H. Trends in Renal-Cell Carcinoma Incidence and Mortality in the United States in the Last 2 Decades: A SEER-Based Study. *Clin. Genitourin. Cancer* **2019**, *17*, 46–57.e5. [CrossRef] [PubMed]
2. Adashek, J.J.; Salgia, M.M.; Posadas, E.M.; Figlin, R.A.; Gong, J. Role of Biomarkers in Prediction of Response to Therapeutics in Metastatic Renal-Cell Carcinoma. *Clin. Genitourin. Cancer* **2019**, *17*, e454–e460. [CrossRef] [PubMed]
3. Smith, K.E.R.; Bilen, M.A. A Review of Papillary Renal Cell Carcinoma and MET Inhibitors. *Kidney Cancer* **2019**, *3*, 151–161. [CrossRef] [PubMed]
4. Mitchell, T.J.; Rossi, S.H.; Klatte, T.; Stewart, G.D. Genomics and clinical correlates of renal cell carcinoma. *World J. Urol.* **2018**, *36*, 1899–1911. [CrossRef]
5. Dekernion, J.; Sarna, G.; Figlin, R.; Lindner, A.; Smith, R.B. The Treatment of Renal Cell Carcinoma with Human Leukocyte Alpha-Interferon. *J. Urol.* **1983**, *130*, 1063–1066. [CrossRef]
6. Fyfe, G.; Fisher, R.I.; Rosenberg, S.A.; Sznol, M.; Parkinson, D.R.; Louie, A.C. Results of treatment of 255 patients with metastatic renal cell carcinoma who received high-dose recombinant interleukin-2 therapy. *J. Clin. Oncol.* **1995**, *13*, 688–696. [CrossRef]
7. Yamamoto, T.; Kitamura, H.; Masumori, N. Complete response to interferon-alpha in a patient with metastatic renal cell carcinoma after unsuccessful molecular-targeted therapies. *Int. J. Urol.* **2014**, *21*, 839–840. [CrossRef]
8. Motzer, R.J.; Hutson, T.E.; Tomczak, P.; Michaelson, M.D.; Bukowski, R.M.; Rixe, O.; Oudard, S.; Negrier, S.; Szczylik, C.; Kim, S.T.; et al. Sunitinib versus Interferon Alfa in Metastatic Renal-Cell Carcinoma. *N. Engl. J. Med.* **2007**, *356*, 115–124. [CrossRef]
9. Sternberg, C.N.; Davis, I.D.; Mardiak, J.; Szczylik, C.; Lee, E.; Wagstaff, J.; Barrios, C.H.; Salman, P.; Gladkov, O.A.; Kavina, A.; et al. Pazopanib in Locally Advanced or Metastatic Renal Cell Carcinoma: Results of a Randomized Phase III Trial. *J. Clin. Oncol.* **2010**, *28*, 1061–1068. [CrossRef]
10. Escudier, B.; Pluzanska, A.; Koralewski, P.; Ravaud, A.; Bracarda, S.; Szczylik, C.; Chevreau, C.; Filipek, M.; Melichar, B.; Bajetta, E.; et al. Bevacizumab plus interferon alfa-2a for treatment of metastatic renal cell carcinoma: A randomised, double-blind phase III trial. *Lancet* **2007**, *370*, 2103–2111. [CrossRef]
11. Rini, B.; Halabi, S.; Rosenberg, J.E.; Stadler, W.M.; Vaena, D.A.; Archer, L.; Atkins, J.N.; Picus, J.; Czaykowski, P.; Dutcher, J.; et al. Phase III Trial of Bevacizumab Plus Interferon Alfa Versus Interferon Alfa Monotherapy

in Patients with Metastatic Renal Cell Carcinoma: Final Results of CALGB 90206. *J. Clin. Oncol.* **2010**, *28*, 2137–2143. [CrossRef] [PubMed]

12. Motzer, R.J.; Escudier, B.; McDermott, D.F.; George, S.; Hammers, H.J.; Srinivas, S.; Tykodi, S.S.; Sosman, J.A.; Procopio, G.; Plimack, E.R.; et al. Nivolumab versus Everolimus in Advanced Renal-Cell Carcinoma. *N. Engl. J. Med.* **2015**, *373*, 1803–1813. [CrossRef] [PubMed]
13. Escudier, B.; Porta, C.; Schmidinger, M.; Rioux-Leclercq, N.; Bex, A.; Khoo, V.; Grünwald, V.; Gillessen, S.; Horwich, A. Renal cell carcinoma: ESMO Clinical Practice Guidelines for diagnosis, treatment and follow-up. *Ann. Oncol.* **2019**, *30*, 706–720. [CrossRef] [PubMed]
14. NCCN. Clinical Practice Guidelines in Oncology (NCCN Guidelines): Kidney Cancer. Available online: https://www.nccn.org/professionals/physician_gls/pdf/kidney.pdf (accessed on 20 October 2020).
15. Motzer, R.J.; Nosov, D.; Eisen, T.; Bondarenko, I.; Lesovoy, V.; Lipatov, O.; Tomczak, P.; Lyulko, O.; Alyasova, A.; Harza, M.; et al. Tivozanib Versus Sorafenib As Initial Targeted Therapy for Patients with Metastatic Renal Cell Carcinoma: Results from a Phase III Trial. *J. Clin. Oncol.* **2013**, *31*, 3791–3799. [CrossRef]
16. Motzer, R.J.; Penkov, K.; Haanen, J.; Rini, B.; Albiges, L.; Campbell, M.T.; Venugopal, B.; Kollmannsberger, C.; Negrier, S.; Uemura, M.; et al. Avelumab plus Axitinib versus Sunitinib for Advanced Renal-Cell Carcinoma. *N. Engl. J. Med.* **2019**, *380*, 1103–1115. [CrossRef]
17. Choueiri, T.; Powles, T.; Burotto, M.; Bourlon, M.; Zurawski, B.; Juárez, V.O.; Hsieh, J.; Basso, U.; Shah, A.; Suarez, C.; et al. 696O_PR Nivolumab + cabozantinib vs. sunitinib in first-line treatment for advanced renal cell carcinoma: First results from the randomized phase III CheckMate 9ER trial. *Ann. Oncol.* **2020**, *31*, S1159. [CrossRef]
18. Rini, B.I.; Dorff, T.B.; Elson, P.; Rodriguez, C.S.; Shepard, D.; Wood, L.; Humbert, J.; Pyle, L.; Wong, Y.-N.; Finke, J.H.; et al. Active surveillance in metastatic renal-cell carcinoma: A prospective, phase 2 trial. *Lancet Oncol.* **2016**, *17*, 1317–1324. [CrossRef]
19. Park, I.; Lee, J.-L.; Ahn, J.-H.; Lee, D.-H.; Lee, K.-H.; Jeong, I.G.; Song, C.; Hong, B.; Hong, J.H.; Ahn, H. Active surveillance for metastatic or recurrent renal cell carcinoma. *J. Cancer Res. Clin. Oncol.* **2014**, *140*, 1421–1428. [CrossRef]
20. Hudes, G.; Carducci, M.; Tomczak, P.; Dutcher, J.; Figlin, R.; Kapoor, A.; Staroslawska, E.; Sosman, J.; McDermott, D.; Bodrogi, I.; et al. Temsirolimus, Interferon Alfa, or Both for Advanced Renal-Cell Carcinoma. *N. Engl. J. Med.* **2007**, *356*, 2271–2281. [CrossRef]
21. Motzer, R.J.; Tannir, N.M.; McDermott, D.F.; Frontera, O.A.; Melichar, B.; Choueiri, T.K.; Plimack, E.R.; Barthélémy, P.; Porta, C.; George, S.; et al. Nivolumab plus Ipilimumab versus Sunitinib in Advanced Renal-Cell Carcinoma. *N. Engl. J. Med.* **2018**, *378*, 1277–1290. [CrossRef]
22. Choueiri, T.K.; Halabi, S.; Sanford, B.L.; Hahn, O.; Michaelson, M.D.; Walsh, M.K.; Feldman, D.R.; Olencki, T.; Picus, J.; Small, E.J.; et al. Cabozantinib Versus Sunitinib As Initial Targeted Therapy for Patients with Metastatic Renal Cell Carcinoma of Poor or Intermediate Risk: The Alliance A031203 CABOSUN Trial. *J. Clin. Oncol.* **2017**, *35*, 591–597. [CrossRef] [PubMed]
23. Lee, J.-L.; Kim, M.K.; Park, I.; Ahn, J.-H.; Lee, D.H.; Ryoo, H.M.; Song, C.; Hong, B.; Hong, J.H.; Ahn, H. RandomizEd phase II trial of Sunitinib four weeks on and two weeks off versus Two weeks on and One week off in metastatic clear-cell type REnal cell carcinoma: RESTORE trial. *Ann. Oncol.* **2015**, *26*, 2300–2305. [CrossRef] [PubMed]
24. Bjarnason, G.A.; Knox, J.J.; Kollmannsberger, C.K.; Soulieres, D.; Ernst, D.S.; Zalewski, P.; Canil, C.M.; Winquist, E.; Hotte, S.J.; North, S.; et al. The efficacy and safety of sunitinib given on an individualised schedule as first-line therapy for metastatic renal cell carcinoma: A phase 2 clinical trial. *Eur. J. Cancer* **2019**, *108*, 69–77. [CrossRef] [PubMed]
25. Escudier, B.; Porta, C.; Bono, P.; Powles, T.; Eisen, T.; Sternberg, C.N.; Gschwend, J.E.; De Giorgi, U.; Parikh, O.; Hawkins, R.; et al. Randomized, Controlled, Double-Blind, Cross-Over Trial Assessing Treatment Preference for Pazopanib Versus Sunitinib in Patients with Metastatic Renal Cell Carcinoma: PISCES Study. *J. Clin. Oncol.* **2014**, *32*, 1412–1418. [CrossRef] [PubMed]
26. Gravis, G.; Chanez, B.; DeRosa, L.; Beuselinck, B.; Barthélémy, P.; Laguerre, B.; Brachet, P.-E.; Joly, F.; Escudier, B.; Harrison, D.; et al. Effect of glandular metastases on overall survival of patients with metastatic clear cell renal cell carcinoma in the antiangiogenic therapy era. *Urol. Oncol. Semin. Orig. Investig.* **2016**, *34*, 167.e17–167.e23. [CrossRef] [PubMed]

27. Choueiri, T.K.; Hessel, C.; Halabi, S.; Sanford, B.; Michaelson, M.D.; Hahn, O.; Walsh, M.; Olencki, T.; Picus, J.; Small, E.J.; et al. Cabozantinib versus sunitinib as initial therapy for metastatic renal cell carcinoma of intermediate or poor risk (Alliance A031203 CABOSUN randomised trial): Progression-free survival by independent review and overall survival update. *Eur. J. Cancer* **2018**, *94*, 115–125. [CrossRef]
28. Auvray, M.; Auclin, E.; Barthelemy, P.; Bono, P.; Kellokumpu-Lehtinen, P.; Gross-Goupil, M.; De Velasco, G.; Powles, T.; Mouillet, G.; Vano, Y.-A.; et al. Second-line targeted therapies after nivolumab-ipilimumab failure in metastatic renal cell carcinoma. *Eur. J. Cancer* **2019**, *108*, 33–40. [CrossRef]
29. Vaishampayan, U. Evolving Treatment Paradigms in Non-clear Cell Kidney Cancer. *Curr. Treat. Options Oncol.* **2018**, *19*, 5. [CrossRef]
30. Knox, J.J.; Barrios, C.H.; Kim, T.M.; Cosgriff, T.; Srimuninnimit, V.; Pittman, K.; Sabbatini, R.; Rha, S.Y.; Flaig, T.W.; Page, R.D.; et al. Final overall survival analysis for the phase II RECORD-3 study of first-line everolimus followed by sunitinib versus first-line sunitinib followed by everolimus in metastatic RCC. *Ann. Oncol.* **2017**, *28*, 1339–1345. [CrossRef]
31. Choueiri, T.K.; Plantade, A.; Elson, P.; Negrier, S.; Ravaud, A.; Oudard, S.; Zhou, M.; Rini, B.I.; Bukowski, R.M.; Escudier, B. Efficacy of Sunitinib and Sorafenib in Metastatic Papillary and Chromophobe Renal Cell Carcinoma. *J. Clin. Oncol.* **2008**, *26*, 127–131. [CrossRef]
32. Dutcher, J.P.; De Souza, P.; McDermott, D.; Figlin, R.A.; Berkenblit, A.; Thiele, A.; Krygowski, M.; Strahs, A.; Feingold, J.; Hudes, G. Effect of temsirolimus versus interferon-α on outcome of patients with advanced renal cell carcinoma of different tumor histologies. *Med. Oncol.* **2009**, *26*, 202–209. [CrossRef] [PubMed]
33. Rini, B.I.; Plimack, E.R.; Stus, V.; Gafanov, R.; Hawkins, R.; Nosov, D.; Pouliot, F.; Alekseev, B.; Soulières, D.; Melichar, B.; et al. Pembrolizumab plus Axitinib versus Sunitinib for Advanced Renal-Cell Carcinoma. *N. Engl. J. Med.* **2019**, *380*, 1116–1127. [CrossRef] [PubMed]
34. McKay, R.R.; Bossé, D.; Xie, W.; Wankowicz, S.A.; Flaifel, A.; Brandao, R.; Lalani, A.-K.A.; Martini, D.J.; Wei, X.X.; Braun, D.A.; et al. The Clinical Activity of PD-1/PD-L1 Inhibitors in Metastatic Non–Clear Cell Renal Cell Carcinoma. *Cancer Immunol. Res.* **2018**, *6*, 758–765. [CrossRef] [PubMed]
35. McDermott, D.F.; Lee, J.-L.; Ziobro, M.; Gafanov, R.A.; Matveev, V.B.; Suárez, C.; Donskov, F.; Pouliot, F.; Alekseev, B.Y.; Wiechno, P.; et al. First-line pembrolizumab (pembro) monotherapy for advanced non-clear cell renal cell carcinoma (nccRCC): Results from KEYNOTE-427 cohort B. *J. Clin. Oncol.* **2019**, *37*, 546. [CrossRef]
36. Gupta, R.; Ornstein, M.C.; Gul, A.; Allman, K.D.; Ball, J.; Wood, L.S.; Garcia, J.A.; VonMerveldt, D.; Hammers, H.; Rini, B.I. Clinical activity of ipilimumab plus nivolumab (Ipi/Nivo) in patients (pts) with metastatic non-clear cell renal cell carcinoma (nccRCC). *J. Clin. Oncol.* **2019**, *37* (Suppl. 15), e16084. [CrossRef]
37. Oudard, S.; Banu, E.; Vieillefond, A.; Fournier, L.; Priou, F.; Medioni, J.; Banu, A.; Duclos, B.; Rolland, F.; Escudier, B.; et al. Prospective Multicenter Phase II Study of Gemcitabine Plus Platinum Salt for Metastatic Collecting Duct Carcinoma: Results of a GETUG (Groupe d'Etudes des Tumeurs Uro-Génitales) Study. *J. Urol.* **2007**, *177*, 1698–1702. [CrossRef]
38. Tannir, N.M.; Jonasch, E.; Albiges, L.; Altinmakas, E.; Ng, C.S.; Matin, S.F.; Wang, X.; Qiao, W.; Lim, Z.D.; Tamboli, P.; et al. Everolimus Versus Sunitinib Prospective Evaluation in Metastatic Non–Clear Cell Renal Cell Carcinoma (ESPN): A Randomized Multicenter Phase 2 Trial. *Eur. Urol.* **2016**, *69*, 866–874. [CrossRef]
39. Armstrong, A.J.; Halabi, S.; Eisen, T.; Broderick, S.; Stadler, W.M.; Jones, R.J.; Garcia, J.A.; Vaishampayan, U.N.; Picus, J.; Hawkins, R.E.; et al. Everolimus versus sunitinib for patients with metastatic non-clear cell renal cell carcinoma (ASPEN): A multicentre, open-label, randomised phase 2 trial. *Lancet Oncol.* **2016**, *17*, 378–388. [CrossRef]
40. Vogelzang, N.J.; Olsen, M.R.; McFarlane, J.J.; Arrowsmith, E.; Bauer, T.M.; Jain, R.K.; Somer, B.; Lam, E.T.; Kochenderfer, M.D.; Molina, A. Safety and Efficacy of Nivolumab in Patients with Advanced Non-Clear Cell Renal Cell Carcinoma: Results from the Phase IIIb/IV CheckMate 374 Study. *Clin. Genitourin. Cancer* **2020**. [CrossRef]
41. Powles, T.; Larkin, J.M.G.; Patel, P.; Pérez-Valderrama, B.; Rodriguez-Vida, A.; Glen, H.; Thistlethwaite, F.; Ralph, C.; Srinivasan, G.; Mendez-Vidal, M.J.; et al. A phase II study investigating the safety and efficacy of savolitinib and durvalumab in metastatic papillary renal cancer (CALYPSO). *J. Clin. Oncol.* **2019**, *37*, 545. [CrossRef]

42. McGregor, B.A.; McKay, R.R.; Braun, D.A.; Werner, L.; Gray, K.; Flaifel, A.; Signoretti, S.; Hirsch, M.S.; Steinharter, J.A.; Bakouny, Z.; et al. Results of a Multicenter Phase II Study of Atezolizumab and Bevacizumab for Patients with Metastatic Renal Cell Carcinoma with Variant Histology and/or Sarcomatoid Features. *J. Clin. Oncol.* **2020**, *38*, 63–70. [CrossRef] [PubMed]
43. Keskin, S.K.; Msaouel, P.; Hess, K.R.; Yu, K.-J.; Matin, S.F.; Sircar, K.; Tamboli, P.; Jonasch, E.; Wood, C.G.; Karam, J.A.; et al. Outcomes of Patients with Renal Cell Carcinoma and Sarcomatoid Dedifferentiation Treated with Nephrectomy and Systemic Therapies: Comparison between the Cytokine and Targeted Therapy Eras. *J. Urol.* **2017**, *198*, 530–537. [CrossRef] [PubMed]
44. Rini, B.I.; Powles, T.; Atkins, M.B.; Escudier, B.; McDermott, D.F.; Suarez, C.; Bracarda, S.; Stadler, W.M.; Donskov, F.; Lee, J.L.; et al. Atezolizumab plus bevacizumab versus sunitinib in patients with previously untreated metastatic renal cell carcinoma (IMmotion151): A multicentre, open-label, phase 3, randomised controlled trial. *Lancet* **2019**, *393*, 2404–2415. [CrossRef]
45. McDermott, D.F.; Choueiri, T.K.; Motzer, R.J.; Aren, O.R.; George, S.; Powles, T.; Donskov, F.; Harrison, M.R.; Cid, J.R.R.R.; Ishii, Y.; et al. CheckMate 214 post-hoc analyses of nivolumab plus ipilimumab or sunitinib in IMDC intermediate/poor-risk patients with previously untreated advanced renal cell carcinoma with sarcomatoid features. *J. Clin. Oncol.* **2019**, *37*, 4513. [CrossRef]
46. Damayanti, N.P.; Budka, J.A.; Khella, H.W.Z.; Ferris, M.W.; Ku, S.Y.; Kauffman, E.; Wood, A.C.; Ahmed, K.; Chintala, V.N.; Adelaiye-Ogala, R.; et al. Therapeutic Targeting of TFE3/IRS-1/PI3K/mTOR Axis in Translocation Renal Cell Carcinoma. *Clin. Cancer Res.* **2018**, *24*, 5977–5989. [CrossRef]
47. Wang, W.; Liao, L.; Wang, Y.; Li, H.; Suo, Z.; Long, K.; Tang, P. Preclinical evaluation of novel PI3K/mTOR dual inhibitor SN202 as potential anti-renal cancer agent. *Cancer Biol. Ther.* **2018**, *19*, 1015–1022. [CrossRef]
48. Huang, J.; Wang, X.; Wen, G.; Ren, Y. miRNA-205-5p functions as a tumor suppressor by negatively regulating VEGFA and PI3K/Akt/mTOR signaling in renal carcinoma cells. *Oncol. Rep.* **2019**, *42*, 1677–1688. [CrossRef]
49. Shah, A.Y.; Karam, J.A.; Malouf, G.G.; Rao, P.; Lim, Z.D.; Jonasch, E.; Xiao, L.; Gao, J.; Vaishampayan, U.N.; Heng, D.Y.; et al. Management and outcomes of patients with renal medullary carcinoma: A multicentre collaborative study. *BJU Int.* **2016**, *120*, 782–792. [CrossRef]
50. Kotecha, R.R.; Motzer, R.J.; Voss, M.H. Towards individualized therapy for metastatic renal cell carcinoma. *Nat. Rev. Clin. Oncol.* **2019**, *16*, 621–633. [CrossRef]
51. Msaouel, P.; Hong, A.L.; Mullen, E.A.; Atkins, M.B.; Walker, C.L.; Lee, C.-H.; Carden, M.A.; Genovese, G.; Linehan, W.M.; Rao, P.; et al. Updated Recommendations on the Diagnosis, Management, and Clinical Trial Eligibility Criteria for Patients with Renal Medullary Carcinoma. *Clin. Genitourin. Cancer* **2019**, *17*, 1–6. [CrossRef]
52. Pécuchet, N.; Bigot, F.; Gachet, J.; Massard, C.; Albiges, L.; Teghom, C.; Allory, Y.; Méjean, A.; Escudier, B.; Oudard, S. Triple combination of bevacizumab, gemcitabine and platinum salt in metastatic collecting duct carcinoma. *Ann. Oncol.* **2013**, *24*, 2963–2967. [CrossRef] [PubMed]
53. Atkinson, B.J.; Kalra, S.; Wang, X.; Bathala, T.; Corn, P.; Tannir, N.M.; Jonasch, E. Clinical outcomes in patients with metastatic renal cell carcinoma treated with alternative sunitinib schedules. *J. Urol.* **2014**, *19*, 611–618. [CrossRef] [PubMed]
54. Bjarnason, G.A.; Khalil, B.; Hudson, J.M.; Williams, R.; Milot, L.M.; Atri, M.; Kiss, A.; Burns, P.N. Outcomes in patients with metastatic renal cell cancer treated with individualized sunitinib therapy: Correlation with dynamic microbubble ultrasound data and review of the literature. *Urol. Oncol. Semin. Orig. Investig.* **2014**, *32*, 480–487. [CrossRef] [PubMed]
55. Rini, B.I.; Garrett, M.; Poland, B.; Dutcher, J.P.; Rixe, O.; Wilding, G.; Stadler, W.M.; Pithavala, Y.K.; Kim, S.; Tarazi, J.; et al. Axitinib in Metastatic Renal Cell Carcinoma: Results of a Pharmacokinetic and Pharmacodynamic Analysis. *J. Clin. Pharmacol.* **2013**, *53*, 491–504. [CrossRef] [PubMed]
56. Rini, B.I.; Battle, D.; Figlin, R.A.; George, D.J.; Hammers, H.; Hutson, T.; Jonasch, E.; Joseph, R.W.; McDermott, D.F.; Motzer, R.J.; et al. The society for immunotherapy of cancer consensus statement on immunotherapy for the treatment of advanced renal cell carcinoma (RCC). *J. Immunother. Cancer* **2019**, *7*, 354. [CrossRef] [PubMed]
57. Hollenbeak, C.S.; Schaefer, E.W.; Doan, J.; Raman, J.D. Determinants of treatment in patients with stage IV renal cell carcinoma. *BMC Urol.* **2019**, *19*, 123. [CrossRef]

58. Heide, J.; Ribback, S.; Klatte, T.; Shariat, S.; Burchardt, M.; Dombrowski, F.; Belldegrun, A.S.; Drakaki, A.; Pantuck, A.J.; Kröger, N. Evaluation of the prognostic role of co-morbidities on disease outcome in renal cell carcinoma patients. *World J. Urol.* **2020**, *38*, 1525–1533. [CrossRef]
59. Hansen, C.R.; Grimm, D.; Bauer, J.; Wehland, M.; Magnusson, N.E. Effects and Side Effects of Using Sorafenib and Sunitinib in the Treatment of Metastatic Renal Cell Carcinoma. *Int. J. Mol. Sci.* **2017**, *18*, 461. [CrossRef]
60. Ljungberg, B. The Role of Metastasectomy in Renal Cell Carcinoma in the Era of Targeted Therapy. *Curr. Urol. Rep.* **2012**, *14*, 19–25. [CrossRef]
61. Ouzaid, I.; Capitanio, U.; Staehler, M.; Wood, C.G.; Leibovich, B.C.; Ljungberg, B.; Van Poppel, H.; Bensalah, K. Young Academic Urologists Kidney Cancer Working Group of the European Association of Urology. Surgical Metastasectomy in Renal Cell Carcinoma: A Systematic Review. *Eur. Urol. Oncol.* **2019**, *2*, 141–149. [CrossRef]
62. Pal, S.K.; Ghate, S.R.; Li, N.; Swallow, E.; Peeples, M.; Zichlin, M.L.; Perez, J.R.; Agarwal, N.; Vogelzang, N.J. Real-World Survival Outcomes and Prognostic Factors Among Patients Receiving First Targeted Therapy for Advanced Renal Cell Carcinoma: A SEER–Medicare Database Analysis. *Clin. Genitourin. Cancer* **2017**, *15*, e573–e582. [CrossRef] [PubMed]
63. Escudier, B.; Powles, T.; Motzer, R.J.; Olencki, T.; Frontera, O.A.; Oudard, S.; Rolland, F.; Tomczak, P.; Castellano, D.; Appleman, L.J.; et al. Cabozantinib, a New Standard of Care for Patients with Advanced Renal Cell Carcinoma and Bone Metastases? Subgroup Analysis of the METEOR Trial. *J. Clin. Oncol.* **2018**, *36*, 765–772. [CrossRef] [PubMed]
64. Suarez-Sarmiento, A.; Nguyen, K.A.; Syed, J.S.; Nolte, A.; Ghabili, K.; Cheng, M.; Liu, S.T.; Chiang, V.; Kluger, H.; Hurwitz, M.E.; et al. Brain Metastasis from Renal-Cell Carcinoma: An Institutional Study. *Clin. Genitourin. Cancer* **2019**, *17*, e1163–e1170. [CrossRef] [PubMed]
65. Linehan, W.M. Genetic basis of kidney cancer: Role of genomics for the development of disease-based therapeutics. *Genome Res.* **2012**, *22*, 2089–2100. [CrossRef] [PubMed]
66. Atkins, M.; Joseph, R.; Ho, T.; Vaishampayan, U.; Ali, S.; Matrana, M.; Alter, R.; Edenfield, J.; Wang, Y.; Blanchette, S.; et al. A phase 1 dose-finding study of X4P-001 (an oral CXCR4 inhibitor) and axitinib in patients with advanced renal cell carcinoma (RCC). *Mol. Cancer Ther* **2018**, *17* (Suppl. 1), B201.
67. Courtney, K.D.; Infante, J.R.; Lam, E.T.; Figlin, R.A.; Rini, B.I.; Brugarolas, J.; Zojwalla, N.J.; Lowe, A.M.; Wang, K.; Wallace, E.M.; et al. Phase I Dose-Escalation Trial of PT2385, a First-in-Class Hypoxia-Inducible Factor-2α Antagonist in Patients with Previously Treated Advanced Clear Cell Renal Cell Carcinoma. *J. Clin. Oncol.* **2018**, *36*, 867–874. [CrossRef]
68. Srinivasan, R.; Donskov, F.; Iliopoulos, O.; Rathmell, W.; Narayan, V.; Maughan, B.; Oudard, S.; Else, T.; Maranchie, J.; Welsh, S.; et al. LBA26 Phase II study of the oral HIF-2α inhibitor MK-6482 for Von Hippel-Lindau (VHL) disease-associated clear cell renal cell carcinoma (ccRCC): Update on RCC and non-RCC disease. *Ann. Oncol.* **2020**, *31*, S1158. [CrossRef]
69. Hakimi, A.A.; Chen, Y.-B.; Wren, J.; Gonen, M.; Abdel-Wahab, O.; Heguy, A.; Liu, H.; Takeda, S.; Tickoo, S.K.; Reuter, V.E.; et al. Clinical and Pathologic Impact of Select Chromatin-modulating Tumor Suppressors in Clear Cell Renal Cell Carcinoma. *Eur. Urol.* **2013**, *63*, 848–854. [CrossRef]
70. Voss, M.H.; Reising, A.; Cheng, Y.; Patel, P.; Marker, M.; Kuo, F.; Chan, T.A.; Choueiri, T.K.; Hsieh, J.J.; Hakimi, A.A.; et al. Genomically annotated risk model for advanced renal-cell carcinoma: A retrospective cohort study. *Lancet Oncol.* **2018**, *19*, 1688–1698. [CrossRef]
71. Hsieh, J.J.; Chen, D.; Wang, P.I.; Marker, M.; Redzematovic, A.; Chen, Y.-B.; Selcuklu, S.D.; Weinhold, N.; Bouvier, N.; Huberman, K.H.; et al. Genomic Biomarkers of a Randomized Trial Comparing First-line Everolimus and Sunitinib in Patients with Metastatic Renal Cell Carcinoma. *Eur. Urol.* **2017**, *71*, 405–414. [CrossRef]
72. McDermott, D.F.; Huseni, M.A.; Atkins, M.B.; Motzer, R.J.; Rini, B.I.; Escudier, B.; Fong, L.; Joseph, R.W.; Pal, S.K.; Reeves, J.A.; et al. Clinical activity and molecular correlates of response to atezolizumab alone or in combination with bevacizumab versus sunitinib in renal cell carcinoma. *Nat. Med.* **2018**, *24*, 749–757. [CrossRef] [PubMed]
73. Schöffski, P.; Wozniak, A.; Escudier, B.; Rutkowski, P.; Anthoney, A.; Bauer, S.; Sufliarsky, J.; Van Herpen, C.; Lindner, L.H.; Grünwald, V.; et al. Crizotinib achieves long-lasting disease control in advanced papillary renal-cell carcinoma type 1 patients with MET mutations or amplification. EORTC 90101 CREATE trial. *Eur. J. Cancer* **2017**, *87*, 147–163. [CrossRef] [PubMed]

74. Voss, M.H.; Chen, D.; Reising, A.; Marker, M.; Shi, J.; Xu, J.; Ostrovnaya, I.; Seshan, V.; Redzematovic, A.; Chen, Y.B.; et al. PTEN Expression, Not Mutation Status in TSC1, TSC2, or mTOR, Correlates with the Outcome on Everolimus in Patients with Renal Cell Carcinoma Treated on the Randomized RECORD-3 Trial. *Clin. Cancer Res.* **2019**, *25*, 506–514. [CrossRef] [PubMed]
75. Iacovelli, R.; Nolè, F.; Verri, E.; Renne, G.; Paglino, C.; Santoni, M.; Rocca, M.C.; Giglione, P.; Aurilio, G.; Cullurà, D.; et al. Prognostic Role of PD-L1 Expression in Renal Cell Carcinoma. A Systematic Review and Meta-Analysis. *Target. Oncol.* **2016**, *11*, 143–148. [CrossRef] [PubMed]
76. Thompson, R.H.; Dong, H.; Kwon, E.D. Implications of B7-H1 Expression in Clear Cell Carcinoma of the Kidney for Prognostication and Therapy. *Clin. Cancer Res.* **2007**, *13*, 709s–715s. [CrossRef] [PubMed]
77. Choueiri, T.K.; Figueroa, D.J.; Fay, A.P.; Signoretti, S.; Liu, Y.; Gagnon, R.; Deen, K.; Carpenter, C.; Benson, P.; Ho, T.H.; et al. Correlation of PD-L1 Tumor Expression and Treatment Outcomes in Patients with Renal Cell Carcinoma Receiving Sunitinib or Pazopanib: Results from COMPARZ, a Randomized Controlled Trial. *Clin. Cancer Res.* **2015**, *21*, 1071–1077. [CrossRef]
78. Rini, B.; Huseni, M.; Atkins, M.; McDermott, D.; Powles, T.; Escudier, B.; Banchereau, R.; Liu, L.-F.; Leng, N.; Fan, J.; et al. Molecular correlates differentiate response to atezolizumab (atezo) + bevacizumab (bev) vs. sunitinib (sun): Results from a phase III study (IMmotion151) in untreated metastatic renal cell carcinoma (mRCC). *Ann. Oncol.* **2018**, *29*, viii724–viii725. [CrossRef]
79. Pal, S.K.; Sonpavde, G.; Agarwal, N.; Vogelzang, N.J.; Srinivas, S.; Haas, N.B.; Signoretti, S.; McGregor, B.A.; Jones, J.; Lanman, R.B.; et al. Evolution of Circulating Tumor DNA Profile from First-line to Subsequent Therapy in Metastatic Renal Cell Carcinoma. *Eur. Urol.* **2017**, *72*, 557–564. [CrossRef]
80. Gao, W.; Li, W.; Xiao, T.; Liu, X.S.; Kaelin, W.G., Jr. Inactivation of the PBRM1 tumor suppressor gene amplifies the HIF-response in VHL−/− clear cell renal carcinoma. *Proc. Natl. Acad. Sci. USA* **2017**, *114*, 1027–1032. [CrossRef]
81. Massari, F.; Di Nunno, V.; Santoni, M.; Gatto, L.; Caserta, C.; Morelli, F.; Zafarana, E.; Carrozza, F.; Mosca, A.; Mollica, V.; et al. Toward a genome-based treatment landscape for renal cell carcinoma. *Crit. Rev. Oncol.* **2019**, *142*, 141–152. [CrossRef]
82. Choueiri, T.K.; Vaishampayan, U.; Rosenberg, J.E.; Logan, T.F.; Harzstark, A.L.; Bukowski, R.M.; Rini, B.I.; Srinivas, S.; Stein, M.N.; Adams, L.M.; et al. Phase II and Biomarker Study of the Dual MET/VEGFR2 Inhibitor Foretinib in Patients with Papillary Renal Cell Carcinoma. *J. Clin. Oncol.* **2013**, *31*, 181–186. [CrossRef] [PubMed]
83. Choueiri, T.K.; Plimack, E.; Arkenau, H.-T.; Jonasch, E.; Heng, D.Y.C.; Powles, T.; Frigault, M.M.; Clark, E.A.; Handzel, A.A.; Gardner, H.; et al. Biomarker-Based Phase II Trial of Savolitinib in Patients with Advanced Papillary Renal Cell Cancer. *J. Clin. Oncol.* **2017**, *35*, 2993–3001. [CrossRef] [PubMed]
84. Cabozantinib S-Malate, Crizotinib, Savolitinib, or Sunitinib Malate in Treating Patients with Locally Advanced or Metastatic Kidney Cancer—Full Text View ClinicalTrials.gov. Available online: https://clinicaltrials.gov/ct2/show/NCT02761057 (accessed on 20 October 2020).
85. Haas, N.B.; Nathanson, K.L. Hereditary Kidney Cancer Syndromes. *Adv. Chronic Kidney Dis.* **2014**, *21*, 81–90. [CrossRef] [PubMed]
86. Wang, J.; Papanicolau-Sengos, A.; Chintala, S.; Wei, L.; Liu, B.; Hu, Q.; Miles, K.M.; Conroy, J.M.; Glenn, S.T.; Costantini, M.; et al. Collecting duct carcinoma of the kidney is associated with CDKN2A deletion and SLC family gene up-regulation. *Oncotarget* **2016**, *7*, 29901–29915. [CrossRef]
87. Yang, P.; Cornejo, K.M.; Sadow, P.M.; Cheng, L.; Wang, M.; Xiao, Y.; Jiang, Z.; Oliva, E.; Jozwiak, S.; Nussbaum, R.L.; et al. Renal Cell Carcinoma in Tuberous Sclerosis Complex. *Am. J. Surg. Pathol.* **2014**, *38*, 895–909. [CrossRef]
88. Callea, M.; Albiges, L.; Gupta, M.; Cheng, S.-C.; Genega, E.M.; Fay, A.P.; Song, J.; Carvo, I.; Bhatt, R.S.; Atkins, M.B.; et al. Differential Expression of PD-L1 between Primary and Metastatic Sites in Clear-Cell Renal Cell Carcinoma. *Cancer Immunol. Res.* **2015**, *3*, 1158–1164. [CrossRef]
89. Turajlic, S.; Litchfield, K.; Xu, H.; Rosenthal, R.; McGranahan, N.; Reading, J.L.; Wong, Y.N.S.; Rowan, A.; Kanu, N.; Al Bakir, M.; et al. Insertion-and-deletion-derived tumour-specific neoantigens and the immunogenic phenotype: A pan-cancer analysis. *Lancet Oncol.* **2017**, *18*, 1009–1021. [CrossRef]
90. Turajlic, S.; Xu, H.; Litchfield, K.; Rowan, A.; Horswell, S.; Chambers, T.; O'Brien, T.; Lopez, J.I.; Watkins, T.B.; Nicol, D.; et al. Deterministic Evolutionary Trajectories Influence Primary Tumor Growth: TRACERx Renal. *Cell* **2018**, *173*, 595–610.e11. [CrossRef]

91. Oxnard, G.R.; Thress, K.S.; Alden, R.S.; Lawrance, R.; Paweletz, C.P.; Cantarini, M.; Yang, J.C.-H.; Barrett, J.C.; Jänne, P.A. Association Between Plasma Genotyping and Outcomes of Treatment with Osimertinib (AZD9291) in Advanced Non–Small-Cell Lung Cancer. *J. Clin. Oncol.* **2016**, *34*, 3375–3382. [CrossRef]
92. Thierry, A.R.; Mouliere, F.; El Messaoudi, S.; Mollevi, C.; Lopez-Crapez, E.; Rolet, F.; Gillet, B.; Gongora, C.; Dechelotte, P.; Robert, B.; et al. Clinical validation of the detection of KRAS and BRAF mutations from circulating tumor DNA. *Nat. Med.* **2014**, *20*, 430–435. [CrossRef]
93. Maia, M.C.; Bergerot, P.G.; Dizman, N.; Hsu, J.; Jones, J.; Choueiri, T.K.; Sonpavde, G.; Lanman, R.B.; Banks, K.; Pal, S. Association of Circulating Tumor DNA (ctDNA) Detection in Metastatic Renal Cell Carcinoma (mRCC) with Tumor Burden. *Kidney Cancer* **2017**, *1*, 65–70. [CrossRef] [PubMed]
94. Ikeda, S.; Schwaederle, M.; Mohindra, M.; Jardim, D.L.; Kurzrock, R. MET alterations detected in blood-derived circulating tumor DNA correlate with bone metastases and poor prognosis. *J. Hematol. Oncol.* **2018**, *11*, 76. [CrossRef] [PubMed]
95. Routy, B.; Le Chatelier, E.; DeRosa, L.; Duong, C.P.M.; Alou, M.T.; Daillère, R.; Fluckiger, A.; Messaoudene, M.; Rauber, C.; Roberti, M.P.; et al. Gut microbiome influences efficacy of PD-1–based immunotherapy against epithelial tumors. *Science* **2018**, *359*, 91–97. [CrossRef] [PubMed]
96. Fischer, S.; Gillessen, P.D.S.; Rothermundt, C. Sequence of treatment in locally advanced and metastatic renal cell carcinoma. *Transl. Androl. Urol.* **2015**, *4*, 310–325.
97. Rini, B.I.; Escudier, B.; Tomczak, P.; Kaprin, A.; Szczylik, C.; Hutson, T.E.; Michaelson, M.D.; Gorbunova, V.A.; Gore, M.E.; Rusakov, I.G.; et al. Comparative effectiveness of axitinib versus sorafenib in advanced renal cell carcinoma (AXIS): A randomised phase 3 trial. *Lancet* **2011**, *378*, 1931–1939. [CrossRef]
98. Motzer, R.J.; Escudier, B.; Tomczak, P.; Hutson, T.X.; Michaelson, M.D.; Négrier, S.; Oudard, S.; Gore, M.; Tarazi, J.; Hariharan, S.; et al. Axitinib versus sorafenib as second-line treatment for advanced renal cell carcinoma: Overall survival analysis and updated results from a randomised phase 3 trial. *Lancet Oncol.* **2013**, *14*, 552–562. [CrossRef]
99. Cella, D.; Escudier, B.; Rini, B.; Chen, C.; Bhattacharyya, H.; Tarazi, J.; Rosbrook, B.; Kim, S.; Motzer, R.J. Patient-reported outcomes for axitinib vs. sorafenib in metastatic renal cell carcinoma: Phase III (AXIS) trial. *Br. J. Cancer* **2013**, *108*, 1571–1578. [CrossRef]
100. Choueiri, T.K.; Escudier, B.; Powles, T.; Mainwaring, P.N.; Rini, B.I.; Donskov, F.; Hammers, H.; Hutson, T.E.; Lee, J.L.; Peltola, K. Cabozantinib versus everolimus in advanced renal-cell carcinoma. *N. Engl. J. Med.* **2015**, *373*, 1814–1823. [CrossRef]
101. Choueiri, T.K.; Escudier, B.; Powles, T.; Tannir, N.M.; Mainwaring, P.N.; Rini, B.I.; Hammers, H.J.; Donskov, F.; Roth, B.J.; Peltola, K.; et al. Cabozantinib versus everolimus in advanced renal cell carcinoma (METEOR): Final results from a randomised, open-label, phase 3 trial. *Lancet Oncol.* **2016**, *17*, 917–927. [CrossRef]
102. Motzer, R.; Hutson, T.; Cella, D.; Reeves, J.; Hawkins, R.; Guo, J.; Nathan, P.; Staehler, M.; de Souza, P.; Merchan, J.R. Pazopanib versus sunitinib in metastatic renal-cell carcinoma. *N. Engl. J. Med.* **2013**, *369*, 722–731. [CrossRef]
103. Motzer, R.J.; Hutson, T.X.; McCann, L.; Deen, K.; Choueiri, T.K. Overall Survival in Renal-Cell Carcinoma with Pazopanib versus Sunitinib. *N. Engl. J. Med.* **2014**, *370*, 1769–1770. [CrossRef] [PubMed]
104. Escudier, B.; Eisen, T.; Stadler, W.M.; Szczylik, C.; Oudard, S.; Siebels, M.; Negrier, S.; Chevreau, C.; Solska, E.; Desai, A.A.; et al. Sorafenib in Advanced Clear-Cell Renal-Cell Carcinoma. *N. Engl. J. Med.* **2007**, *356*, 125–134. [CrossRef] [PubMed]
105. Hutson, T.E.; Escudier, B.; Esteban, E.; Bjarnason, G.A.; Lim, H.Y.; Pittman, K.B.; Senico, P.; Niethammer, A.; Lu, D.R.; Hariharan, S.; et al. Randomized Phase III Trial of Temsirolimus Versus Sorafenib As Second-Line Therapy After Sunitinib in Patients with Metastatic Renal Cell Carcinoma. *J. Clin. Oncol.* **2014**, *32*, 760–767. [CrossRef] [PubMed]
106. Escudier, B.; Eisen, T.; Stadler, W.M.; Szczylik, C.; Oudard, S.; Staehler, M.; Negrier, S.; Chevreau, C.; Desai, A.A.; Rolland, F.; et al. Sorafenib for Treatment of Renal Cell Carcinoma: Final Efficacy and Safety Results of the Phase III Treatment Approaches in Renal Cancer Global Evaluation Trial. *J. Clin. Oncol.* **2009**, *27*, 3312–3331. [CrossRef] [PubMed]
107. Motzer, R.J.; Hutson, T.E.; Tomczak, P.; Michaelson, M.D.; Bukowski, R.M.; Oudard, S.; Negrier, S.; Szczylik, C.; Pili, R.; Bjarnason, G.A.; et al. Overall Survival and Updated Results for Sunitinib Compared with Interferon Alfa in Patients with Metastatic Renal Cell Carcinoma. *J. Clin. Oncol.* **2009**, *27*, 3584–3590. [CrossRef] [PubMed]

108. Cella, D.; Li, J.Z.; Cappelleri, J.C.; Bushmakin, A.; Charbonneau, C.; Kim, S.T.; Chen, I.; Motzer, R.J. Quality of Life in Patients with Metastatic Renal Cell Carcinoma Treated with Sunitinib or Interferon Alfa: Results from a Phase III Randomized Trial. *J. Clin. Oncol.* **2008**, *26*, 3763–3769. [CrossRef]
109. Rini, B.I.; Pal, S.K.; Escudier, B.J.; Atkins, M.B.; Hutson, T.E.; Porta, C.; Verzoni, E.; Needle, M.N.; McDermott, D.F. Tivozanib versus sorafenib in patients with advanced renal cell carcinoma (TIVO-3): A phase 3, multicentre, randomised, controlled, open-label study. *Lancet Oncol.* **2020**, *21*, 95–104. [CrossRef]
110. Motzer, R.J.; Escudier, B.; Oudard, S.; Hutson, T.E.; Porta, C.; Bracarda, S.; Grünwald, V.; Thompson, J.A.; Figlin, R.A.; Hollaender, N.; et al. Efficacy of everolimus in advanced renal cell carcinoma: A double-blind, randomised, placebo-controlled phase III trial. *Lancet* **2008**, *372*, 449–456. [CrossRef]
111. Motzer, R.J.; Hutson, T.X.; Glen, H.; Michaelson, M.D.; Molina, A.; Eisen, T.; Jassem, J.; Zolnierek, J.; Maroto, J.P.; Mellado, B.; et al. Lenvatinib, everolimus, and the combination in patients with metastatic renal cell carcinoma: A randomised, phase 2, open-label, multicentre trial. *Lancet Oncol.* **2015**, *16*, 1473–1482. [CrossRef]
112. Klapper, J.A.; Downey, S.G.; Smith, F.O.; Yang, J.C.; Hughes, M.S.; Kammula, U.S.; Sherry, R.M.; Royal, R.E.; Steinbrg, S.M.; Rosenberg, S. High-dose interleukin-2 for the treatment of metastatic renal cell carcinoma: A retrospective analysis of response and survival in patients treated in the surgery branch at the National Cancer Institute between 1986 and 2006. *Cancer* **2008**, *113*, 293–301. [CrossRef]

Comparative Efficacy of First-Line Immune-Based Combination Therapies in Metastatic Renal Cell Carcinoma

Reza Elaidi [1,*,†], Letuan Phan [1,†], Delphine Borchiellini [2], Philippe Barthelemy [3], Alain Ravaud [4], Stéphane Oudard [5] and Yann Vano [5]

1 ARTIC (Association pour la Recherche sur les Thérapeutiques Innovantes en Cancérologie), Hôpital Européen Georges Pompidou, 75015 Paris, France; letuanp@gmail.com
2 Department of Medical Oncology, Centre Antoine-Lacassagne, 06100 Nice, France; delphine.borchiellini@nice.unicancer.fr
3 Department of Medical Oncology, Hôpital civil, 67091 Strasbourg, France; p.barthelemy@icans.eu
4 Department of Medical Oncology, Hôpital St Andre, 33000 Bordeaux, France; alain.ravaud@chu-bordeaux.fr
5 Department of Medical Oncology, Hôpital Européen Georges Pompidou, 75015 Paris, France; stephane.oudard@aphp.fr (S.O.); yann.vano@aphp.fr (Y.V.)
* Correspondence: reza-thierry.elaidi-ext@aphp.fr
† These two authors contributed equally to this work.

Abstract: Three drug combinations, ipilimumab-nivolumab (Ipi-Nivo), pembrolizumab-axitinib (Pembro-Axi), and avelumab-axitinib (Ave-Axi), have received regulatory approval in the USA and Europe for the treatment of metastatic renal cell carcinoma with clear cell component (mRCC). However, no head-to-head comparison data are available to identify the best option. Therefore, we aimed to compare these new treatments in a first-line setting. We conducted a systematic search in PubMed, the Cochrane Library, and clinicaltrials.gov for any randomized controlled trials of treatment-naïve patients with mRCC, from January 2015 to October 2019. The process was performed according to PRISMA guidelines. We performed a Bayesian network meta-analysis with two different approaches, a contrast-based model comparing HRs and ORs between studies and arm-based using parametric modeling. The outcomes for the analysis were overall survival, progression-free survival (PFS), and objective response rate. Our search identified 3 published phase 3 randomized clinical trials (2835 patients). In the contrast-based model, Ave-Axi (SUCRA = 83%) and Pembro-Axi (SUCRA = 80%) exhibited the best ranking probabilities for PFS. For overall survival (OS), Pembro-Axi (SUCRA = 96%) was the most preferable option against Ave-Axi and Ipi-Nivo. Objective response rate analysis showed Ave-Axi as the best (SUCRA: 94%) and Pembro-Axi as the second best option. In the parametric models, the risk of progression was comparable for Ave-Axi and Ipi-Nivo, whereas Pembro-Axi exhibited a lower risk during the first 6 months of treatment and a higher risk afterwards. Furthermore, Pembro-Axi exhibited a net advantage in terms of OS over the two other regimens, while Ave-Axi was the least preferable option. Overall evidence suggests that pembrolizumab plus axitinib seems to have a slight advantage over the other two combinations.

Keywords: metastatic renal cell carcinoma; immune-based combination therapies; network meta-analysis

1. Background

Over the past few years, the treatment for metastatic renal cell carcinoma with clear cell component (mRCC) has drastically changed with the introduction of targeted therapy, immunotherapy, and a better understanding of RCC biology [1–4]. So far, the first-line and second-line systematic therapies for mRCC have been mainly composed of agents targeting the vascular endothelial growth factor receptor (VEGFR) and inhibiting the mammalian target of rapamycin (mTOR), with the last in class being axitinib and cabozantinib [5,6]. Currently, drug development in mRCC focuses on immune checkpoint inhibitors (ICIs), targeting programmed cell death 1 (PD-1), programmed cell death-ligand 1 (PD-L1) pathway, or cytotoxic T-lymphocyte-associated protein 4 (CTLA-4) [4,7]. Four combinations have demonstrated either progression-free survival (PFS) or overall survival (OS) improvements over the VEGFR tyrosine kinase inhibitor (TKI) standard of care (SOC) sunitinib in the first-line setting for advanced or metastatic RCC with clear cell component: nivolumab (anti-PD-1) plus ipilimumab (anti-CTLA-4) [8], pembrolizumab (anti-PD-1) plus axitinib (VEGFR-TKI) [9], avelumab (anti-PD-L1) plus axitinib [10], and atezolizumab (anti-PD-L 1) plus bevacizumab (anti-VEGF) [11].

The shift in systemic therapy of mRCC has just begun, and phase 3 results with these new available combinations raise many questions that need to be addressed in order to make better use of them in clinical practice. In addition, we still lack predictive biomarkers and prognostic characteristics in patients or the disease to guide treatment allocation. Results of these phase 3 trials should be interpreted in the context of the International Metastatic RCC Database Consortium (IMDC) risk classification, which has proven its utility since the targeted therapy era [12,13].

Comparison between these therapeutic options is one of the main concerns for clinicians and patients [14]. However, since no clinical trial has provided any head-to-head comparison data of these combinations, we conducted a network meta-analysis (NMA) to indirectly compare their efficacies in terms of progression-free survival (PFS), overall survival (OS), and objective response rate (ORR) in the first-line setting for patients with mRCC.

2. Methods

2.1. Search Strategy and Selection Criteria

We specifically focused on randomized controlled trials (RCTs), including naïve-treatment patients with mRCC with clear cell component who received one of the combinations involving ICIs in the first-line setting, with no patient restrictions on PD-L1 or the IMDC subgroup. The study was conducted based on PRISMA extended guidelines for network meta-analysis [15]. We performed a systematic literature search for articles or abstracts in PubMed, the Cochrane Library, clinicaltrials.gov, and ESMO or ASCO congress, from January 2015 to August 2019 (full search strategy detailed in File S1). References of relevant articles were checked to ensure that no combinations with ICIs were missed. If several data reports were available from the same trial, we retained the latest updated source. The outcomes were PFS, OS, and ORR in the intention-to-treat (ITT) population, and per IMDC subgroup if available. For PFS and OS, hazard ratios (HRs) with 95% confidence intervals (CIs), and their corresponding Kaplan–Meier curves (when available) were retained for our study.

The whole process of trial selection, full-text screening, and data extraction was performed by two investigators (R-E, L-P) independently; if disagreement occurred, it was resolved by discussion with other investigators. For all selected studies, risk of bias was assessed with the Cochrane Handbook tool [16].

2.2. Statistical Analysis

We used two different approaches: a contrast-based method comparing the relative treatment effect in the intention-to-treat population as well as in the IMDC subgroups, and an arm-based method using Kaplan–Meier curves to estimate the parametric survival model (in the ITT population only). We performed both fixed-effect and random-effect models for the contrast-based approach.

To assess which treatment was likely to be the best option, we used rank probabilities and the surface under the cumulative ranking curve (SUCRA) [17] in the contrast-based NMA model and assessed time-dependent HRs derived from the arm-based NMA approach. Additionally, an exploratory analysis of the PFS of sarcomatoid carcinoma patients was performed to investigate the recently observed benefit of these combinations in this subpopulation.

2.2.1. Contrast-Based Approach

This approach focused on relative effects using HR on a log scale to run an NMA model as described in Dias 2013 [18].

2.2.2. Arm-Based Approach

To circumvent the apparent violation of the proportional hazard assumption of the Cox model in the published PFS Kaplan–Meier curves of the CheckMate 214 study [4], we also considered a method relying on time-dependent HRs. We used fractional polynomials to estimate parametric functions from the Kaplan–Meier curves in a Bayesian hierarchical model [19,20].

Statistical analyses were all performed within a Bayesian framework. Credible intervals were all reported at the 95% level. The contrast-based analysis was performed using R (version 3·6·0) (Core Team 2019, Vienna, Austria) and JAGS (version 4·3·0) with the package "getmtc" (version 0·8·2) [21] and Openbugs (version 3·2·3). Kaplan–Meier curves were reconstructed using GetData Graph Digitizer (version 2·26).

2.3. *Role of the Funding Source*

There was no funding source for this study. The corresponding author had full access to all the data in the study and had final responsibility for the decision to submit for publication.

3. Results

Our search identified 72 results. Of these, three published phase 3 randomized clinical trials matched our selection criteria (2843 patients, Figure 1): CheckMate 209–214 [4], Keynote 426 [8], and Javelin Renal 101 [9]. These evaluated three different combinations: nivolumab plus ipilimumab (Ipi-Nivo), pembrolizumab plus axitinib (Pembro-Axi), and avelumab plus axitinib (Ave-Axi), respectively (detailed search in File S1). The Immotion 151 trial investigating atezolizumab plus bevacizumab (Atezo-Beva) was excluded due to the non-superiority of OS compared to sunitinib in the intention-to-treat population. Therefore, it is unlikely that this combination will be recommended as a treatment in a near future. In the three retained trials, the combinations were compared to sunitinib (star-shaped network), which was the common comparator (trial characteristics are provided in Table 1). Risk of bias for each trial was considered acceptable in view of the Cochrane assessment grid (Table S1). Data sources for all the analyses are provided in Table S2.

Table 1. Outcomes reported in each trial of the network. Ave: avelumab; Axi: axitinib; Ipi: ipilimumab; Nivo: nivolumab; NR: not reached; ORR: objective response rate; OS: overall survival; Pembro: pembrolizumab; PFS: progression-free survival.

Study	Treatment	Number of Patients	ORR (95% CI)	Median OS (Months)	Median PFS (Months)	HR OS (95% CI)	HR PFS (95% CI)
CheckMate 214	Sunitinib	546	32% (28–36)	37.9	12.3	-	-
	Nivo + Ipi	550	39% (35–43)	NR	12.4	0.71 (0.59–0.86)	0.85 (0.73–0.98)
Keynote 426	Sunitinib	429	35.7% (31–40)	NR	11.1	-	-
	Pembro + Axi	432	59% (54–64)	NR	15.1	0.53 (0.38–0.74)	0.69 (0.57–0.84)
Javelin Renal 101	Sunitinib	444	25% (22–30)	NR	8.4	-	-
	Ave + Axi	442	51% (47–56)	NR	13.8	0.78 (0.55–1.08)	0.69 (0.56–0.84)

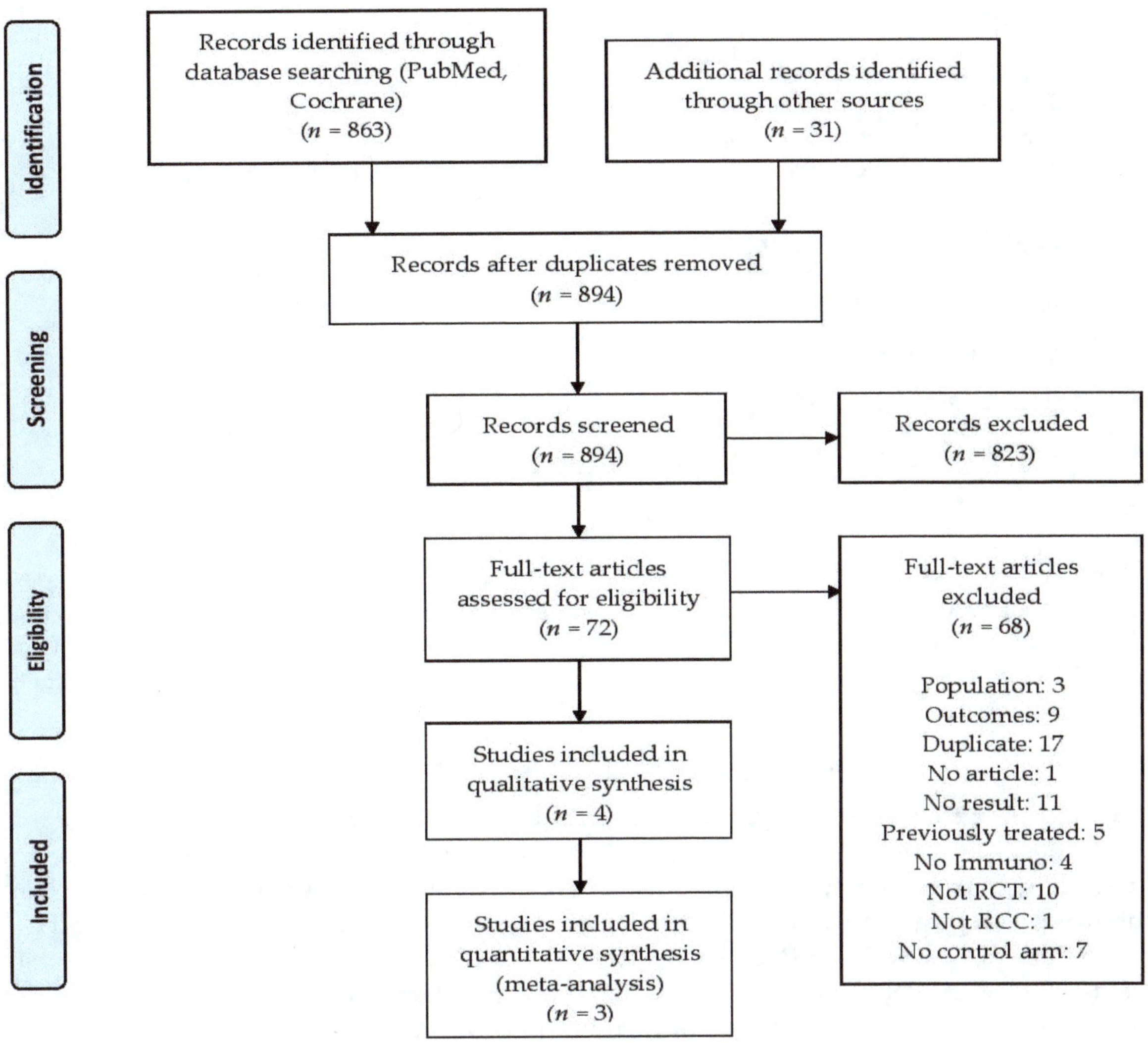

Figure 1. Flowchart of the systematic search. PRISMA flow diagram.

3.1. Contrast-Based Approach in Intention-to-Treat Population

Both Pembro-Axi and Ave-Axi showed similar efficacy for PFS (HR: 1.00 (0.68–1.50)). However, the Ipi-Nivo combination was less efficient (HR: 0.81 (0.57–1.20)) compared to Ave-Axi or Pembro-Axi (HR: 0.82 (0.58–1.20)). Ranking suggested Ave-Axi as the best option (SUCRA = 83%) and Pembro-Axi as the second best (SUCRA = 80%), but the difference was not clinically relevant (Table S3). For OS, NMA suggested Pembro-Axi (SUCRA = 96%) had better efficacy than Ave-Axi or Ipi-Nivo (HR: 0.68 (0.35–1.30), HR: 0.75 (0.44–1.30), respectively). Similarly, for ORR, NMA suggested that Ave-Axi (SUCRA = 94%) was the most preferable option compared to Pembro-Axi or Ipi-Nivo (odds ratio (OR) 0.81 (0.46–1.40), OR: 0.44 (0.27–0.72) respectively). These results are summarized in the form of forest plots for indirect comparisons (Figure 2) and direct comparisons (Figure S1) for the ITT population.

Fixed-effect and random-effect models yielded similar results, with larger credibility intervals for the random-effect model (Figure S2 and Table S3). Sensitivity analysis, either adding the fourth combination atezolizumab plus bevacizumab or using slightly informative priors, provided very close results with an unchanged rank order for the three combinations of the main analysis (Figure S3).

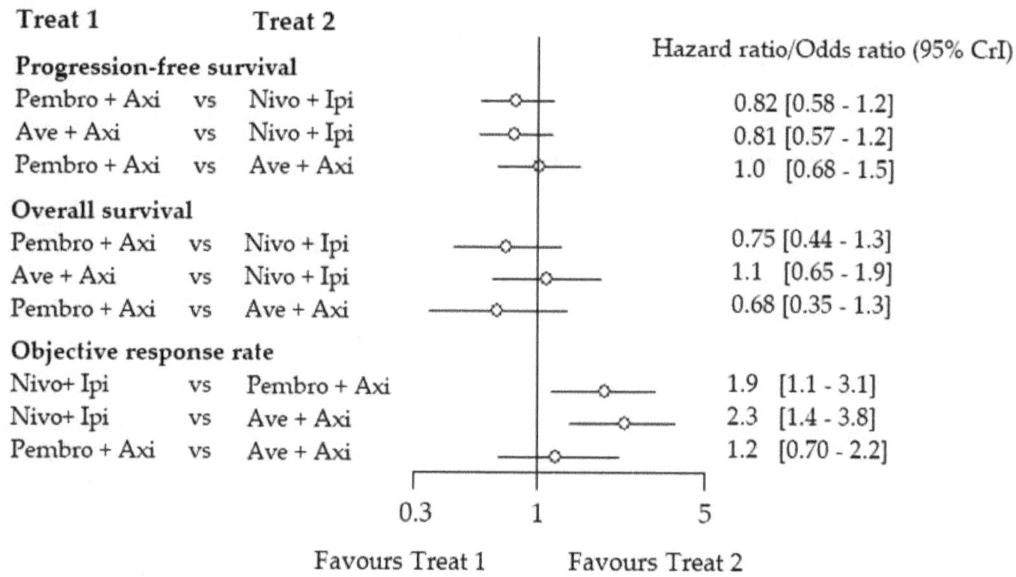

Figure 2. Indirect comparison of the contrast-based network meta-analysis (NMA) (fixed effect) in the ITT) population. Forest plot of the indirect comparison between each combination for the 3 outcomes in the ITT population. For the ORR, the odds ratio favoring treatment 1 Treat 1, means that treatment 1 had a lower response rate than treatment 2 (Treat 2).

3.2. Contrast-Based Approach per IMDC Subgroup

The IMDC subgroup analysis was performed for PFS and ORR only, since OS data were immature with many censored patients from the Javelin Renal 101 trial. We pooled the intermediate and poor IMDC risk subgroups to match the CheckMate 214 results with the other trials. Patient proportion in each subgroup is reported in Table 2. In the IMDC favorable risk group, Ave-Axi turned out to be superior to Pembro-Axi (HR for PFS: 0.67 (0.26–1.70), ORR: 1.8 (0.69–4.60)) and to Ipi-Nivo (HR for PFS: 0.44 (0.19–1.00), ORR: 5.6 (2.40–13.00)). In the intermediate and poor risk groups, Pembro-Axi and Ave-Axi were the two best options and compared favorably to Ipi-Nivo (Pembro-Axi HR for PFS: 0.87 (0.58–1.30), OR: 1.1 (0.76–1.70), Ave-Axi HR for PFS: 0.91 (0.58–1.40), OR: 1.7 (1.10–2.70)). The three combinations exhibited striking differences in the favorable risk group compared to the ITT analysis in terms of treatment effect, despite enlarged credibility intervals (Figure 3). Fixed-effect and random-effect models yielded similar results (ranking Table S4).

Table 2. Summary data in each IMDC subgroup.

Trial	Treatment	Favorable Prognosis			Intermediate and Poor Prognosis		
		N (%)	HR IC 95%	ORR IC 95%	N (%)	HR IC 95%	ORR IC 95%
CheckMate 214	Sunitinib	124 (23)		50%	424 (77)		29%
	Nivo + Ipi	125 (23)	1.23 (0.90–1.69)	39%	423 (77)	0.77 (0.65–0.90)	42%
Keynote 426	Sunitinib	131 (31)		49.6%	298 (69)		29.5%
	Pembro + Axi	138 (32)	0.81 (0.53–1.24)	66.7%	294 (68)	0.67 (0.53–0.85)	55.8%
Javelin Renal 101	Sunitinib	96 (22)		37%	347 (78)		22.5%
	Ave + Axi	94 (22)	0.54 (0.32–0.91)	68.1%	343 (78)	0.70 (0.53–0.94)	46.9%

Note: the sum of patients in the (reported) subgroup analysis was different from the overall number of patients reported in the articles.

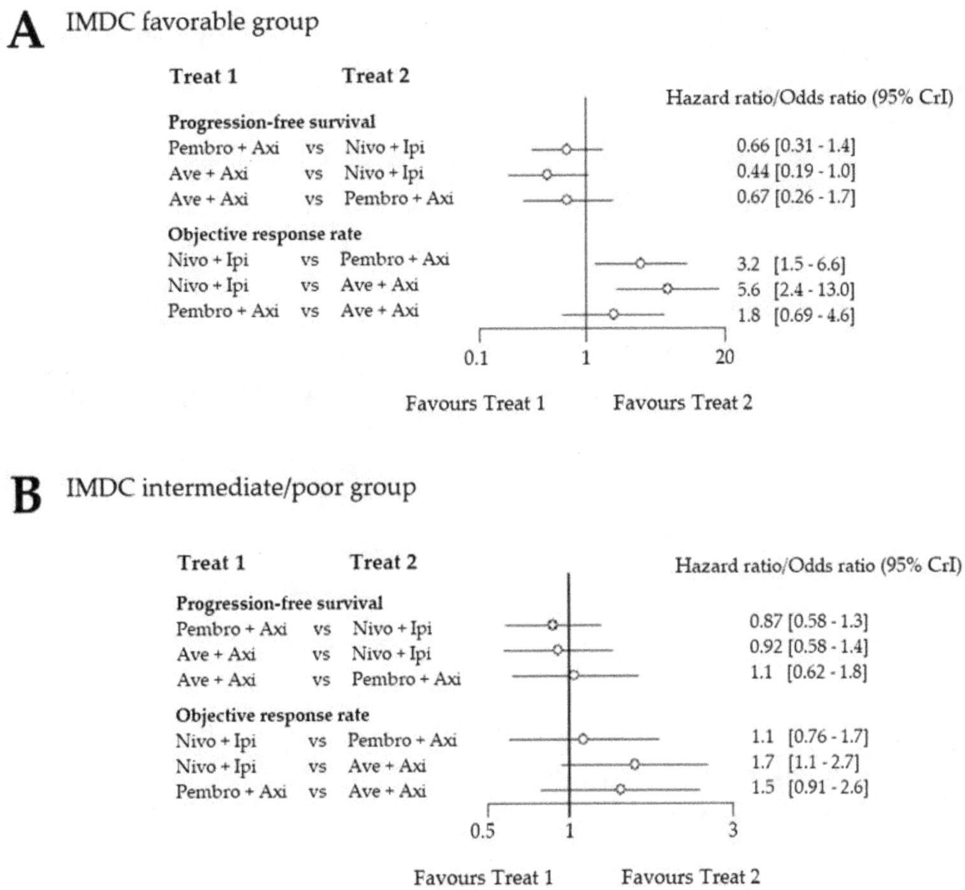

Figure 3. Forest plot of the indirect comparison between each combination. (**A**) results in the IMDC favorable risk group; (**B**) results in the IMDC intermediate and poor (pooled) risk group. For the For ORR, the odds ratio favouring treatment 1 (Treat 1) means that treatment 1 had a lower response rate than treatment 2 (Treat 2).

3.3. Arm-Based Approach

Among the different models tested, a Weibull model offered the best compromise between fit and complexity.

3.4. Progression-Free Survival in Intention-to-Treat Population

The time-dependent HR of the drug combinations vs. sunitinib clearly suggest a violation of the main assumption of proportional hazards in the three trials, primarily for OS, and especially in the CheckMate 214 trial for both OS and PFS (Figure 4A). Risk of progression was higher with Ipi-Nivo compared to other combinations during the first 15 months; this difference vanished past this time period. Pembro-Axi and Ave-Axi exhibited close HR over the follow-up period; we considered that the seemingly different curves of time-dependent HR (increasing Pembro-Axi vs. decreasing Ave-Axi) were more a consequence of the models' parameters than a real difference in the combinations' effects (see parameter estimations, Table S5).

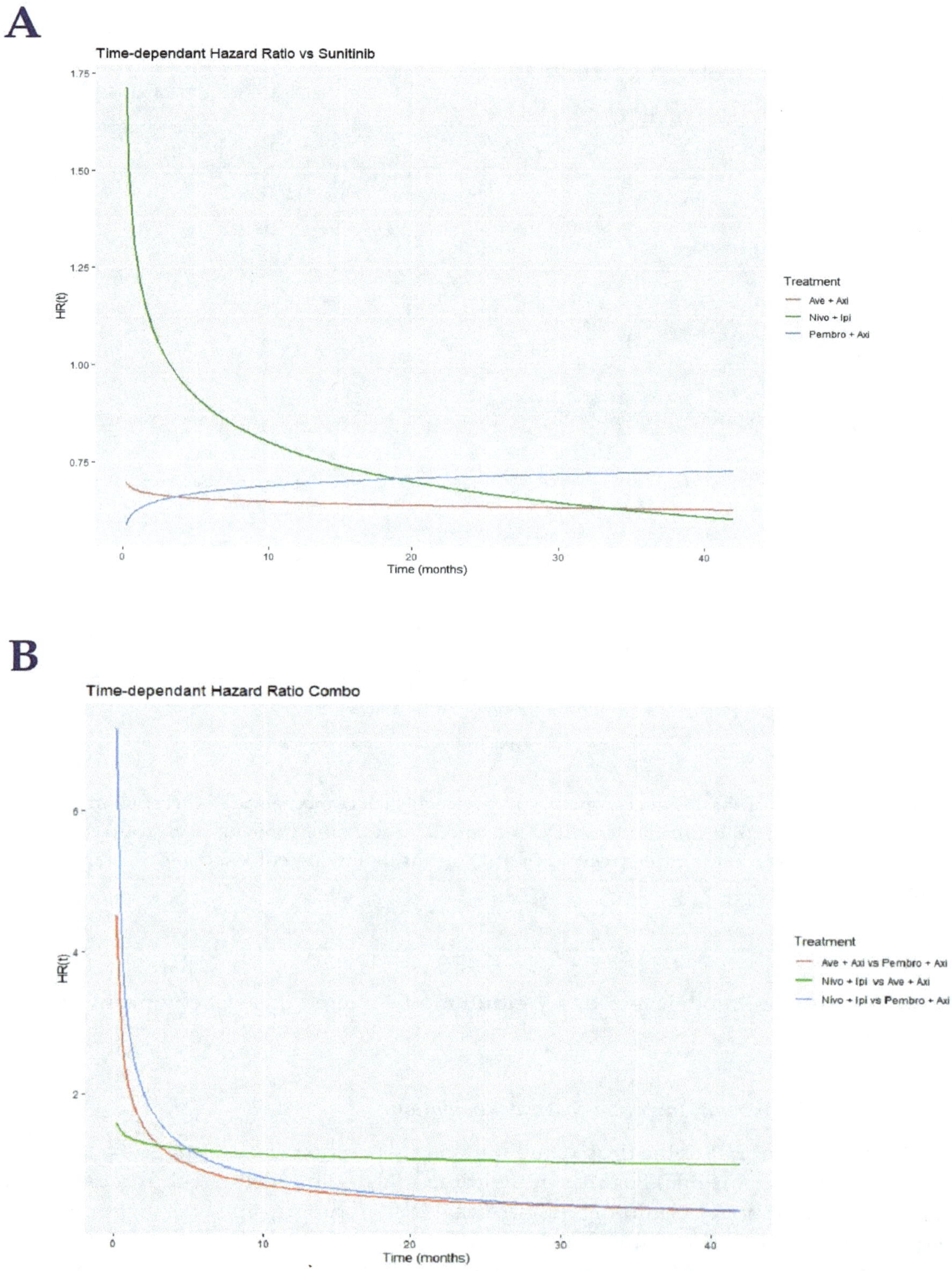

Figure 4. Time-dependent HRs for PFS of combinations. (**A**) Time-dependent hazard ratio vs. sunitinib. (**B**) Time-dependent hazard ratio between combinations.

The aim of this study was to provide an indirect comparison between the three combinations. We allowed sunitinib's effect to be different across each study instead of arbitrarily taking a mean effect, accounting for the variability of sunitinib's effect, as observed in the different control arms. Benefit was in favor of Pembro-Axi over Ave-Axi and Ipi-Nivo during the first 5–7 months of treatment, which reversed afterwards. Ipi-Nivo and Ave-Axi displayed a comparable benefit with a higher risk of progression for Ipi-Nivo at the beginning of the treatment period, as in Figure 4B.

3.5. Overall Survival in Intention-to-Treat Population

The time-dependent HR curves for OS suggested that all three drug combinations have comparable time effects on OS (Figure 5A). We also showed that for each trial, the computed mean HR across the follow-up period exhibited fairly similar estimates, as in the contrast-based approach, and close to published HRs, which established the coherence between the two methods and conferred robustness to our results.

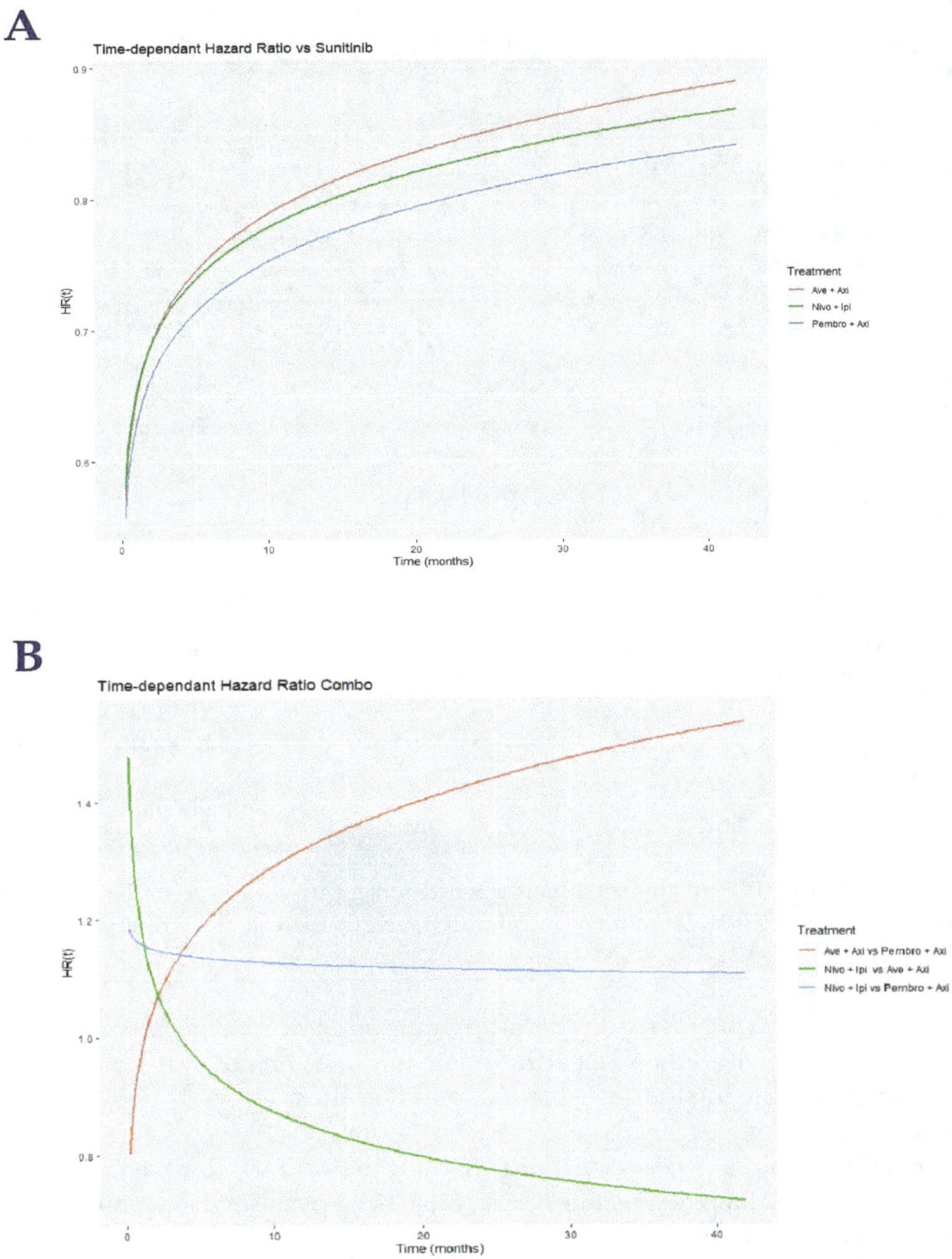

Figure 5. Time-dependent HRs for OS of combinations. (**A**) Time-dependent hazard ratio vs. sunitinib. Red: Ave-Axi vs. sunitinib, Green: Ipi-Nivo vs. sunitinib, Blue: Pembro-Axi vs. sunitinib. (**B**) Time-dependent hazard ratio between combinations. Red: Ave-Axi vs. Pembro-Axi, Green: Ipi-Nivo vs. Ave-Axi, Blue: Ipi-Nivo vs. Pembro-Axi.

The main observations resulting from the indirect pairwise comparison of the three combinations suggested a higher risk of death with Ipi-Nivo compared to Pembro-Axi throughout the study period (Figure 5B). The higher risk of death of Ipi-Nivo compared to Ave-Axi was only observed during the first 3 months, which decreased afterwards. Pembro-Axi appeared as a better option compared to Ave-Axi during the whole follow-up period (see parameter estimations, Table S5).

3.6. Exploratory Analysis of PFS in Sarcomatoid Patients

Upon indirect comparison, there was no significant difference between the trials, suggesting that these patients may respond well to all combinations (Figure 6), with all HRs close to 1.

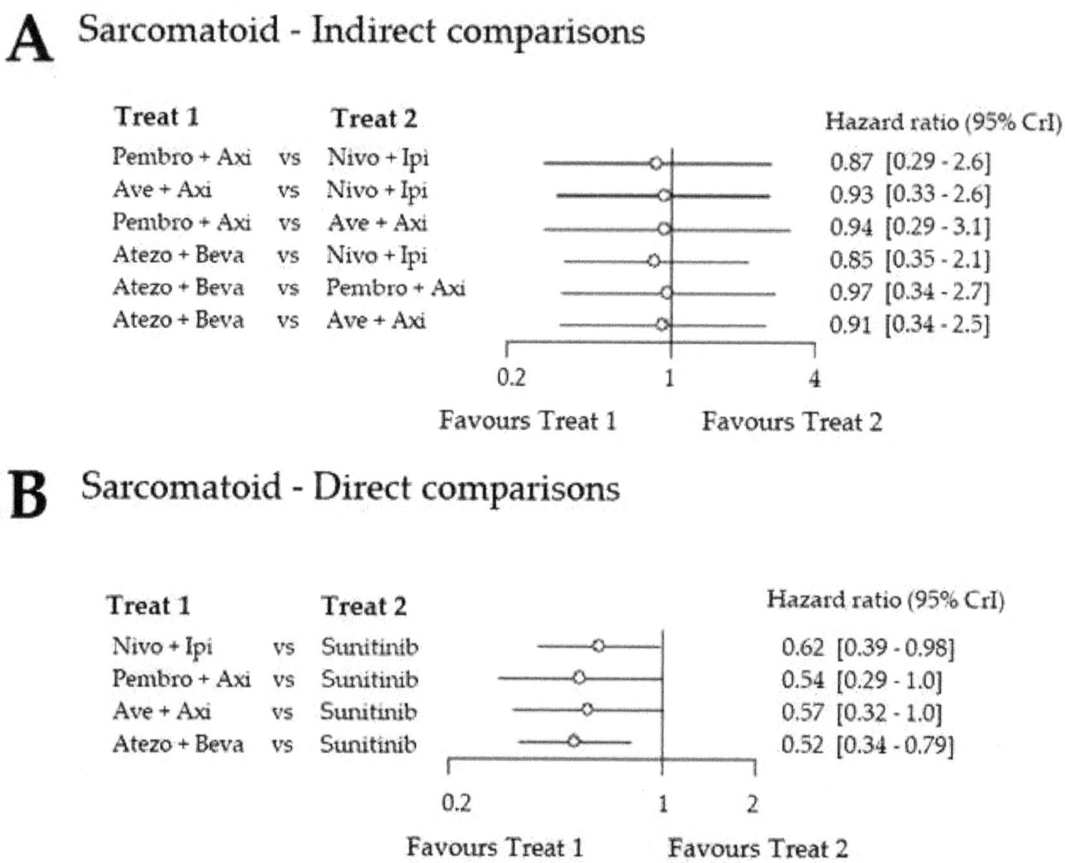

Figure 6. Forest plot of PFS in the sarcomatoid carcinoma population. (**A**) Direct comparisons. (**B**) Indirect comparisons. HRs of treatment in column A versus treatment in column B.

4. Discussion

The three combinations considered in this study may soon become new standards of care in the first-line setting for mRCC, without any clear rationale to prefer one over the other. We aimed to fill this knowledge gap by conducting indirect comparisons, and thus hopefully providing clinicians with critical aid in decision-making.

Network meta-analysis is a powerful and flexible method of comparing multiple different therapeutic strategies. To our knowledge, few NMAs have been published in an mRCC first-line setting. Andrew W. Hahn et al. concluded that cabozantinib, Pembro-Axi, and Ave-Axi were preferable for PFS, and Pembro-Axi appeared superior for OS in first-line mRCC [22]. However, their network included twelve different treatments and highly heterogeneous populations. A recent study by Wang et al. included all available first-line options representing no less than twenty-five heterogeneous studies, and concluded that Pembro-Axi was the preferred option with regards to OS, whereas cabozantinib was better with regards to PFS [23]. However, in the last study included, HRs were compared assuming sunitinib had the same effect across all the different trials, which did not reflect actual/observed data/results.

However, our approach significantly differed from these studies: we specifically focused our comparison on the efficacies of the three combinations with immune checkpoint inhibitors that have demonstrated a benefit in phase 3 trials (i.e., the drug combinations more likely to obtain a high-grade recommendation from academic societies and an approval from health authorities). We used the most recent data (up to August 2019) and employed both fixed- and random-effect models. Moreover, we used two different approaches to assess these different therapeutic options: a contrast-based and an arm-based approach. In our arm-based approach, we relaxed the assumption of a common effect of sunitinib to best model the actual trial differences. We also investigated models that may have taken into account various confounding factors, such as the between-study unbalanced prognostic risk groups, in order to allow for sufficient flexibility in the modelling of these new combinations complexities (e.g., by adding a covariance term to model the presence of axitinib in both CPI-TKI combinations, and/or to combine PFS and OS in a single model).

In our study, we compared three large multicenter phase 3 randomized controlled trials which included 2843 patients in total. In the contrast-based approach, Pembro-Axi was found to be the best option for the OS rate in the ITT population, whereas Pembro-Axi and Ave-Axi showed comparable efficacy for PFS, and Ave-Axi showed the best ORR efficacy. On the other hand, in the IMDC favorable risk group, Ave-Axi showed the most favorable results for PFS. Contrast-based approaches for both PFS and OS led to results close to what was reported in each independent updated study, due to the fact that only one study was available for each comparison and that we decided upon non-informative priors for treatment effects (i.e., no influencing data). In the arm-based approach (in the ITT population), Pembro-Axi seemed to be the preferable option only for the OS. We also observed that during the first 5 months of therapy, IO-TKI (immunotherapy and TKI) combinations exhibited a lower risk of progression compared with IO-IO combinations; however, Ipi-Nivo exhibited longer PFS in patients who did not progress during the first 5 months. This may be partially related to pseudo progression induced by the double IO combination, while having a high rate of complete response for the remaining patients in the CheckMate 214 trial.

Our study has both strengths and limitations. First, we focused on the new promising regimens, with results from published phase 3 randomized clinical trials, in order not to inflate population and design heterogeneity. Second, we used two different but complementary approaches for more consistent results: the contrast-based approach, which uses HRs as relative treatment effects and maintains the randomization structure within each study but requires strong assumptions. An arm-based approach is more likely to relax these assumptions, but the disadvantage is that it does not preserve the randomization structure. Moreover, in the contrast-based approach, HRs derived from the Cox model rely on the assumption of proportional hazards, which is commonly violated in many trials, leading to biased estimates. Arm-based methods do not rely on HR but need the parametric fit of Kaplan–Meier (KM) curves. Third, combinations may have more complex mechanisms of action than monotherapies, and to this end arm-based methods provide time-dependent HR, interpretations of which may help to decipher such mechanisms better than constant HR and decide which combination may be the best and when. One main limitation is the overall lack of data, which may reflect a potential uncontrolled bias; more studies comparing these regimens and/or individual patient data would be needed in order to improve the precision and heterogeneity of estimations. These additional data would also allow us to test for inconsistency (confirm concordance between direct and indirect comparisons), which was not possible in our current star-shaped network. IMDC subgroups and geographic regions may represent other confounding factors across comparisons; more studies are needed to adjust the NMA model and confirm our findings. We tried more complex multivariate NMAs to account for HRs per IMDC subgroup in one single model, but a lack of data for OS in each risk group prevented us from refining the final model. It could also have been relevant to consider PD-L1 expression, which may have differently influenced the PFS of the combinations, but given the different assays and thresholds used in each study, we could not proceed. Regarding toxicity, NMA using only counts of grade ≥ 3 events was too broad to efficiently compare toxicity between trials. Lastly, OS and possibly ORR data in the Javelin Renal 101 trial were still immature at the time of analysis; thus, the Ave-Axi combination ranking may change with a longer follow-up. Despite a comparable median follow-up, Pembro-Axi exhibited superiority in terms of OS, whereas Ave-Axi surprisingly did not. Our indirect comparison was indeed in favor of Pembro-Axi, but more updates and trials would be needed to further investigate this difference. Therefore, the results of our study should be interpreted cautiously given the underlying hypothesis and potential bias of the estimated effects.

Clinicians have concerns about sequencing and identifying predictive biomarkers. More follow-up and reported data from patients in second-line after IO-TKI and IO-IO combination treatments may be of great help to guide decisions about the line of treatment. Our NMA model can grow with each new trial to help decision-making. Other trial results are awaited, comparing pembrolizumab plus lenvatinib vs. everolimus plus lenvatinib vs. sunitinib (CLEAR, NCT02811861); triplet cabozantinib plus nivolumab plus ipilimumab vs. nivolumab plus ipilimumab (COSMIC-313, NCT03937219); and nivolumab plus cabozantinib vs. cabozantinib plus nivolumab plus ipilimumab vs. sunitinib (CheckMate 9ER, NCT03141177). Personalized-therapy-driven trials based on molecular profiling such as the BIONIKK trial (NCT02960906) may also provide new insights for clinical decision.

5. Conclusions

Our results support the importance of the IMDC risk score for the comparative efficacy assessment of new combinations in the first-line setting of metastatic clear-cell renal cell carcinoma. This is important given the lack of predictive validated biomarkers. Our results suggest a PFS, ORR, and OS superiority of IO-TKI, compared with IO-IO combinations, regardless of the IMDC risk group. In favorable risk-group patients, PFS and OS were superior with IO-TKI, but these differences vanished in the intermediate/poor risk group. Overall, based on the current evidence, pembrolizumab-axitinib may have a slight advantage over the two other combinations.

Author Contributions: Conceptualization, R.E. and Y.V.; Data curation, L.P.; Formal analysis, R.E. and L.P.; Investigation, Y.V.; Methodology, R.E. and L.P.; Supervision, R.E.; Validation, D.B., P.B., A.R., S.O. and Y.V.; Visualization, L.P.; Writing–original draft, R.E. and L.P.; Writing–review & editing, D.B., P.B., A.R., S.O. and Y.V. All authors have read and agreed to the published version of the manuscript.

References

1. Choueiri, T.K.; Motzer, R.J. Systemic Therapy for Metastatic Renal-Cell Carcinoma. *N. Engl. J. Med.* **2017**, *376*, 354–366. [CrossRef]
2. Iacovelli, R.; Ciccarese, C.; Bria, E.; Bimbatti, D.; Fantinel, E.; Mosillo, C.; Bisogno, I.; Brunelli, M.; Tortora, G.; Porta, C. Immunotherapy versus standard of care in metastatic renal cell carcinoma. A systematic review and meta-analysis. *Cancer Treat. Rev.* **2018**, *70*, 112–117. [CrossRef]
3. Labriola, M.K.; Batich, K.A.; Zhu, J.; McNamara, M.A.; Harrison, M.R.; Armstrong, A.J.; George, D.J.; Zhang, T. Immunotherapy Is Changing First-Line Treatment of Metastatic Renal-Cell Carcinoma. *Clin. Genitourin. Cancer* **2019**, *17*, e513–e521. [CrossRef] [PubMed]
4. Santoni, M.; Massari, F.; Di Nunno, V.; Conti, A.; Cimadamore, A.; Scarpelli, M.; Montironi, R.; Cheng, L.; Battelli, N.; Lopez-Beltran, A. Immunotherapy in renal cell carcinoma: Latest evidence and clinical implications. *Drugs Context* **2018**, *7*, 212528. [CrossRef] [PubMed]
5. Hutson, T.E.; Lesovoy, V.; Al-Shukri, S.; Stus, V.P.; Lipatov, O.N.; Bair, A.H.; Rosbrook, B.; Chen, C.; Kim, S.; Vogelzang, N.J. Axitinib versus sorafenib as first-line therapy in patients with metastatic renal-cell carcinoma: A randomised open-label phase 3 trial. *Lancet Oncol.* **2013**, *14*, 1287–1294. [CrossRef]
6. Choueiri, T.K.; Halabi, S.; Sanford, B.L.; Hahn, O.; Michaelson, M.D.; Walsh, M.K.; Feldman, D.R.; Olencki, T.; Picus, J.; Dakhil, S.; et al. Cabozantinib Versus Sunitinib As Initial Targeted Therapy for Patients With Metastatic Renal Cell Carcinoma of Poor or Intermediate Risk: The Alliance A031203 CABOSUN Trial. *J. Clin. Oncol.* **2017**, *35*, 591–597. [CrossRef]

7. Flippot, R.; Escudier, B.; Albiges, L. Immune Checkpoint Inhibitors: Toward New Paradigms in Renal Cell Carcinoma. *Drugs* **2018**, *78*, 1443–1457. [CrossRef]
8. Motzer, R.J.; Tannir, N.M.; McDermott, D.F.; Frontera, O.A.; Melichar, B.; Choueiri, T.K.; Plimack, E.R.; Barthélémy, P.; Porta, C.; Powles, T.; et al. Nivolumab plus Ipilimumab versus Sunitinib in advanced renal-cell carcinoma. *N. Engl. J. Med.* **2018**, *378*, 1277–1290. [CrossRef]
9. Rini, B.I.; Plimack, E.R.; Stus, V.; Gafanov, R.; Hawkins, R.; Nosov, D.; Pouliot, F.; Alekseev, B.; Soulières, D.; Vynnychenko, I.; et al. Pembrolizumab plus axitinib versus sunitinib for advanced renal-cell carcinoma. *N. Engl. J. Med.* **2019**, *380*, 1116–1127. [CrossRef] [PubMed]
10. Motzer, R.J.; Penkov, K.; Haanen, J.; Rini, B.; Albiges, L.; Campbell, M.T.; Venugopal, B.; Kollmannsberger, C.; Negrier, S.; Lee, J.L.; et al. Avelumab plus axitinib versus sunitinib for advanced renal-cell carcinoma. *N. Engl. J. Med.* **2019**, *380*, 1103–1115. [CrossRef] [PubMed]
11. Rini, B.I.; Powles, T.; Atkins, M.B.; Escudier, B.; McDermott, D.F.; Suarez, C.; Bracarda, S.; Stadler, W.M.; Donskov, F.; Hawkins, R.; et al. Atezolizumab plus bevacizumab versus sunitinib in patients with previously untreated metastatic renal cell carcinoma (IMmotion151): A multicentre, open-label, phase 3, randomised controlled trial. *Lancet* **2019**, *393*, 2404–2415. [CrossRef]
12. Heng, D.Y.; Xie, W.; Regan, M.M.; Harshman, L.C.; Bjarnason, G.A.; Vaishampayan, U.N.; Mackenzie, M.; Wood, L.; Donskov, F.; Rha, S.Y.; et al. External validation and comparison with other models of the International Metastatic Renal-Cell Carcinoma Database Consortium prognostic model: A population-based study. *Lancet Oncol.* **2013**, *14*, 141–148. [CrossRef]
13. Yip, S.M.; Wells, C.; Moreira, R.; Wong, A.; Srinivas, S.; Beuselinck, B.; Porta, C.; Sim, H.-W.; Ernst, D.S.; Yuasa, T.; et al. Checkpoint inhibitors in patients with metastatic renal cell carcinoma: Results from the International Metastatic Renal Cell Carcinoma Database Consortium. *Cancer* **2018**, *124*, 3677–3683. [CrossRef] [PubMed]
14. Escudier, B. Combination Therapy as First-Line Treatment in Metastatic Renal-Cell Carcinoma. *N. Engl. J. Med.* **2019**, *380*, 1176–1178. [CrossRef] [PubMed]
15. Hutton, B.; Salanti, G.; Caldwell, D.M.; Chaimani, A.; Schmid, C.H.; Cameron, C.; Straus, S.; Thoriund, K.; Jansen, J.P.; Mulrow, C.; et al. The PRISMA Extension Statement for Reporting of Systematic Reviews Incorporating Network Meta-analyses of Health Care Interventions: Checklist and Explanations. *Ann. Intern. Med.* **2015**, *162*, 777–784. [CrossRef]
16. Higgins, J.P.; Altman, D.G.; Gøtzsche, P.C.; Jüni, P.; Moher, D.; Oxman, A.D.; Savović, J.; Schulz, K.F.; Weeks, L.; Sterne, J.A.; et al. The Cochrane Collaboration's tool for assessing risk of bias in randomised trials. *BMJ* **2011**, *343*, d5928. [CrossRef]
17. Salanti, G.; Ades, A.E.; Ioannidis, J.P. Graphical methods and numerical summaries for presenting results from multiple-treatment meta-analysis: An overview and tutorial. *J. Clin. Epidemiol.* **2011**, *64*, 163–171. [CrossRef]
18. Dias, S.; Sutton, A.J.; Ades, A.E.; Welton, N.J. Evidence Synthesis for Decision Making 2. A Generalized Linear Modeling Framework for Pairwise and Network Meta-analysis of Randomized Controlled Trials. *Med. Decis. Mak.* **2013**, *33*, 607–617. [CrossRef]
19. Ouwens, M.J.; Philips, Z.; Jansen, J.P. Network meta-analysis of parametric survival curves. *Res. Synth Methods* **2010**, *1*, 258–271. [CrossRef]
20. Jansen, J.P. Network meta-analysis of survival data with fractional polynomials. *BMC Med. Res. Methodol.* **2011**, *11*, 61. [CrossRef]
21. van Valkenhoef, G.; Kuiper, J. *gemtc: Network Meta-Analysis Using Bayesian Methods*, R Package Version 0.8-2; Available online: https://cran.r-project.org/web/packages/gemtc/gemtc.pdf (accessed on 21 June 2020).
22. Hahn, A.W.; Klaassen, Z.; Agarwal, N.; Haaland, B.; Esther, J.; Xiang, Y.Y.; Wang, X.; Pal, S.K.; Wallis, C.J. First-line Treatment of Metastatic Renal Cell Carcinoma: A Systematic Review and Network Meta-analysis. *Eur. Urol. Oncol.* **2019**, *2*, 708–715. [CrossRef] [PubMed]
23. Wang, J.; Li, X.; Wu, X.; Wang, Z.; Zhang, C.; Cao, G.; Yan, T. Role of immune checkpoint inhibitor-based therapies for metastatic renal cell carcinoma in the first-line setting: A systematic review and Bayesian network analysis. *EBioMedicine* **2019**, *47*, 78–88. [CrossRef] [PubMed]

7

Targeting the Deterministic Evolutionary Trajectories of Clear Cell Renal Cell Carcinoma

Adam Kowalewski [1,*], Marek Zdrenka [2], Dariusz Grzanka [1] and Łukasz Szylberg [1,2]

[1] Department of Clinical Pathomorphology, Collegium Medicum in Bydgoszcz, Nicolaus Copernicus University in Torun, 85-067 Bydgoszcz, Poland; d_grzanka@cm.umk.pl (D.G.); l.szylberg@cm.umk.pl (Ł.S.)

[2] Department of Tumor Pathology and Pathomorphology, Oncology Centre-Prof. Franciszek Łukaszczyk Memorial Hospital, 85-796 Bydgoszcz, Poland; marek.zdrenka@cm.umk.pl

* Correspondence: kowalewskiresearch@gmail.com or 264643@stud.umk.pl

Simple Summary: In contrast to organismal evolution, human cancers are subjected to similar initial conditions and follow a limited range of possible evolutionary trajectories. Therefore, the repetitive nature of cancer evolution may prove to be its greatest weakness. Evolutionary trajectories of clear cell renal cell carcinoma (ccRCC) have been recently described. In this review, we will discuss the relevance of estimating the trajectory of ccRCC evolution as a readout for a response to therapy. Next, we will propose strategies to take advantage of the evolving nature of these tumors for patients' benefit.

Abstract: The emergence of clinical resistance to currently available systemic therapies forces us to rethink our approach to clear cell renal cell carcinoma (ccRCC). The ability to influence ccRCC evolution by inhibiting processes that propel it or manipulating its course may be an adequate strategy. There are seven deterministic evolutionary trajectories of ccRCC, which correlate with clinical phenotypes. We suspect that each trajectory has its own unique weaknesses that could be exploited. In this review, we have summarized recent advances in the treatment of ccRCC and demonstrated how to improve systemic therapies from the evolutionary perspective. Since there are only a few evolutionary trajectories in ccRCC, it appears feasible to use them as potential biomarkers for guiding intervention and surveillance. We believe that the presented patient stratification could help predict future steps of malignant progression, thereby informing optimal and personalized clinical decisions.

Keywords: clear cell renal cell carcinoma; ccRCC; RCC; kidney cancer; evolution; evolutionary trajectory; biomarker

---

1. Introduction

Renal cell carcinoma (RCC) is the eighth most commonly diagnosed cancer in the United States, with an estimated incidence of 74,000 new cases in 2020 [1]. The classic triad of flank pain, flank mass, and hematuria occurs only in 10% of cases [2]. Due to the ability of the kidney for functional compensation when part of it is destroyed, early detection from loss of function is usually impossible. As a result, RCC remains clinically occult for most of its course, and around one-third of patients present with metastatic disease at the time of diagnosis. Those with localized tumors have up to 40% risk of recurrence following complete resection [3,4]. Remarkable advances over the last decade contributed to the development of targeted therapies and immunotherapies that today represent a standard for unresectable RCC. Despite relatively high response rates to these agents, the vast majority of patients eventually experience cancer progression. The emergence of clinical resistance to currently available systemic therapies represents a significant challenge and forces us to rethink our approach to RCC.

The best-studied histological subtype is clear cell renal cell carcinoma (ccRCC), which is derived from the proximal convoluted tubule and accounts for approximately 70% of all cases [5]. A series of next-generation sequencing studies led to a better understanding of the genetic background of ccRCC [6–10]. The results of these studies uncovered a near-universal inactivation of the von Hippel-Lindau disease (*VHL*) tumor suppressor gene. Other frequent alterations involve histone-modifying genes, SWI/SNF complex, and PI3K/AKT/mTOR pathway. Moreover, an integrated, genome-wide analysis of copy-number changes and gene expression profiles in ccRCC identified 7 chromosomal regions of recurrent arm level or focal amplifications (1q, 2q, 5q, 7q, 8q, 12p, and 20q) and 7 regions of losses (1p, 3p, 4q, 6q, 8p, 9p, and 14q) [8].

The evolutionary landscape in ccRCC is dominated by intratumor heterogeneity (ITH) at a genetic, transcriptomic, and functional level [9]. The exome sequencing performed on multiple, spatially separate ccRCC samples revealed that that two-thirds of the somatic mutations are not shared between all the primary tumor regions [10]. Hence, single-biopsy analysis is likely to miss the key genetic events or misclassify them as clonal. Apart from the direct impact on diagnostic procedures and biomarkers development, ITH has significantly hindered our understanding of ccRCC evolution.

In comparison to other malignancies, ccRCC is characterized by a high prevalence of somatic copy number alterations (SCNAs) and a low burden of somatic substitutions [6,8,11,12]. The integrative analysis of the genetic and clinical data led to the identification of certain alterations with prognostic value, such as mutually exclusive mutations of *BAP1* and *PBRM1* [13–15]. These studies, although conducted on large cohorts of patients, did not determine the prognostic values of genetic alterations according to whether they were clonal or subclonal. Huang et al. were among the first to demonstrate the possibility of genomic subtyping of ccRCC [13]. Recently, Turajlic and colleagues provided a comprehensive model of ccRCC evolution [14], which might lay the foundation for the development of precision clinical management.

Cancer cells continuously undergo adaptive changes, and insensitivity to drugs arises due to genetic and epigenetic alterations that offer a survival advantage. While there is a number of pathways and networks a cancer cell has at its disposal, targeting individual components is likely to prove inadequate [15]. Instead, the ability to influence cancer evolution itself by inhibiting processes that propel it or manipulating its course might potentially put an end to cancer as a major health concern.

In this review, we will discuss the relevance of estimating the trajectory of ccRCC evolution as a readout for a response to therapy. Next, we will propose strategies to take advantage of the evolving nature of these tumors for patients' benefit.

2. The Origin, Evolution, and Routes to Metastasis of Clear Cell Renal Cell Carcinoma

2.1. *The Origin of Clear Cell Renal Cell Carcinoma*

Loss of the short arm of chromosome 3 is a nearly universal driver of ccRCC [16]. It occurs in childhood or adolescence, predominantly through chromothripsis. The deleted region encompasses at least four tumor suppressor genes, including *VHL*, *PBRM1*, *BAP1*, and *SETD2*. This earliest event produces a pool of a few hundred cells, which after decades of modest clonal expansion, acquire the necessary additional genetic alterations [17]. Chromosomal copies of deleted suppressor genes are often affected afterward, with inactivation of the second allele of *VHL* being the most common (65–80% of patients) [7,8,10]. In some cases, there are different driver mutations on the trunk of the phylogenetic tree, which, in contrast to 3p loss and *VHL* inactivation, trigger a substantial expansion [11,18].

2.2. *The Evolutionary Trajectories of Clear Cell Renal Cell Carcinoma*

On the basis of mutational ordering, timing, and co-occurrence, ccRCCs are classified into seven distinct evolutionary subtypes, or four groups, which correlate with clinical phenotypes [17,19].

These groups are distinguished by four features—variations in chromosomal complexity, ITH, model of tumor evolution, and metastatic potential. The variations in chromosomal complexity are measured as the fraction of the genome affected by SCNAs and expressed as a weighted genome instability index (wGII). ITH is measured as the ratio of subclonal drivers to clonal drivers [20].

Group 1 consists of primary tumors with *VHL* alteration as the sole driver event. They evolve in a "linear" fashion and are characterized by low both wGII and ITH. This mode of evolution is associated with indolent growth and low metastatic potential. Group 2 includes tumors in which early *PBRM1* mutation and subsequent *SETD2* mutation or PI3K pathway mutation or acquisition of SCNAs result in a "branched" evolutionary pattern. These are heterogeneous neoplasms with oligometastatic potential and attenuated progression. Clonal acquisition of multiple driver mutations (*VHL* plus ≥2 *BAP1, PBRM1, SETD2,* or *PTEN*) or the parallel *BAP1* mutation results in "punctuated" evolution. These tumors are characterized by high wGII but low ITH and belong to group 3. Punctuated evolution, driven mostly by high wGII, leads to rapid dissemination and is also observed among *VHL* wild-type tumors, which constitute the fourth group [14].

2.3. *The Routes to Metastasis of Clear Cell Renal Cell Carcinoma*

Metastasis competence is afforded by chromosome-level alterations that simultaneously affect the expression of hundreds of genes. These alterations provide a permissive genomic background for the selection of hallmark drivers of ccRCC metastasis and the loss of 9p and 14q [20]. Linear and branched evolution modes are analogous to Darwin's phyletic gradualism. On the other hand, punctuated evolution, as in punctuated equilibrium, is associated with rapid speciation events and considerable evolutionary changes. Thus, the acquisition of metastatic competence is far more likely through punctuated evolution.

3. Current Systemic Therapies for Renal Cell Carcinoma

Immunotherapy and/or tyrosine kinase inhibitors (TKI) constitute the standard of care for relapse or stage IV RCC. Appropriate clinical management depends on disease activity, according to the National Comprehensive Cancer Network (NCCN) Guidelines for Kidney Cancer. In favorable-risk patients, first-line treatments include a combination of axitinib plus pembrolizumab or monotherapy with pazopanib or sunitinib. For patients with poor- and intermediate-risk disease, the preferred regimen is ipilimumab with nivolumab or axitinib with pembrolizumab. Moreover, cabozantinib may be considered in a first-line setting, especially in cases with osseous metastatic RCC. Because of the significant toxicity of systemic therapies, a subset of asymptomatic patients with metastatic RCC may benefit from active surveillance.

A major advantage of immunotherapy is its potential to produce complete and durable responses in a subset of patients with advanced cancer, even after discontinuation of the drug. Indeed, despite the non-curative nature of systemic therapy in RCC, up to 9% of poor- and intermediate-risk patients may achieve a complete response, according to the results of subgroup analysis of CheckMate 214 clinical trial [18]. This rate could be further increased by introducing novel treatment modalities as well as better patient selection algorithms.

4. Strategies to Overcome the Evolution of Renal Cell Carcinoma

In the face of selective pressures, subpopulations of tumor cells with adaptive phenotypes emerge at the expense of others. The ability to predict the alterations in ITH along the temporal axis seems invaluable for the development of personalized therapy. In this section, we will provide a summary of recent strategies against RCC which, when contextualized within an evolutionary framework, could be significantly more effective.

4.1. *Cytoreductive Nephrectomy*

In select patients with metastatic RCC, primary nephrectomy is performed with cytoreductive intent. Apart from the alleviation of symptoms associated with larger masses, such intervention eliminates the reservoir of phenotypic tumor-cell diversity, minimizing the risk of further metastatic seeding from an evolving primary tumor [19]. While cytoreductive nephrectomy (CN) is associated with a significant risk of perioperative mortality (0–13%) and major complications (3–36%) [21], there is a great need to avoid unnecessary surgery in nonresponders.

Heng et al. examined the role of CN in metastatic RCC patients receiving targeted therapies in a retrospective study of data from the International Metastatic Renal Cell Carcinoma Database Consortium (IMDC). They found that patients with estimated overall survival (OS) of <12 months and those exhibiting fewer than 4 IMDC prognostic factors are not likely to benefit from CN [22]. From that time, several other observational studies demonstrated analogous results [23]. This data, however, must be treated with caution given the significant risk of selection bias inherent to their study designs, which potentially leads to misclassification of patients [24].

The role of CN continues to change amid a rapidly increasing armamentarium of systemic therapies. In the modern immuno-oncology era, CN is still a viable option, but careful patient selection is of paramount importance. The ongoing clinical trials are evaluating the use of deferred CN in patients receiving nivolumab and ipilimumab alone or alongside radiotherapy (NCT03977571, NCT04090710). These studies may help determine the most appropriate indications for CN.

4.2. *Adaptive Therapy*

In the case of disseminated cancer with no significant probability of cure, patient survival can be maximized if adaptive therapy is introduced. This strategy originates from mathematical models and aims at maintaining a stable tumor burden [25]. When drugs are administered sparingly and in a temporally dynamic fashion, a significant population of treatment-sensitive cells survives. These, due to their competitive advantage, suppress the proliferation of treatment-resistant populations under normal tumor conditions.

Adaptive therapy may play a role in metastatic RCC. Findings from a prospective phase II trial demonstrate active surveillance to be a viable initial strategy in patients with few adverse prognostic features [26]. Results from the SURTIME study, a randomized clinical trial comparing immediate vs deferred CN, revealed that deferred CN is a valid option for patients with the intermediate-risk disease and with general clinical conditions at baseline amenable to undergo surgery [27]. "Treatment-for-stability" may also be represented by an alternative schedule of sunitinib. The standard dosing schedule of sunitinib is 50 mg daily for 4 weeks, followed by 2 weeks off drug (schedule 4/2). However, according to a recent meta-analysis, the administration of sunitinib for 2 weeks followed by 1 week off (schedule 2/1) exhibited lower toxicity and lower rates of treatment discontinuation while maintaining comparable responses [28].

The full potential of adaptive therapy is yet to be witnessed. Frequency-dependent game-theoretic models of tumor evolution have enabled the introduction of three concepts to consider in the pursuit of designing a multi-drug adaptive approach [29]. These ideas focus on entrapping tumor evolution in periodic loops, limiting the evolutionary "absorbing region" reachable by the tumor and determining the optimal timing of drug administration. Each may contribute to the generation of new treatment schedules and comparisons to standards.

4.3. *Targeting Trunk Mutations*

The ability to target alteration present in all tumor cells is expected to diminish the odds of the escape of clonal branches. As previously described, inactivation of *VHL* constitutes the trunk event in ccRCC development while most of the other driver aberrations are subclonal. Apart from large chromosomal aberrations as in the cytogenetic 3p abnormalities, *VHL* inactivation may be caused by small deletions affecting the locus, or promoter methylation and epigenetic silencing [30]. pVHL, a *VHL* gene product, is essential in the cell's normal response to ischemic stress. Decreased expression of *VHL* results in the accumulation of hypoxia-inducible factor alpha (HIFα). Among the three known HIFα subunits, HIF2α is thought to be the core ccRCC driver since it upregulates a series of hypoxia-responsive genes [31–33]. The net effect is the activation of various kinase-dependent signaling pathways, such as MAPK/ERK and PI3K/AKT/mTOR [34]. While the most significant targets of *VHL* loss are the production of VEGF and PDGF, HIF2α has been regarded as undruggable for years [35,36]. Eventually, a structure-based design approach led to the identification of PT2385, a first-in-class HIF2α antagonist [37]. In a phase I dose-escalation clinical trial, PT2385 was found to be well-tolerated and demonstrated clinical activity in extensively pretreated ccRCC patients [38]. Its efficacy and safety are currently being evaluated in a phase II trial (NCT03108066). The primary objective of this trial is to assess the overall response rate in patients with VHL disease-associated ccRCC.

According to the mathematical model presented by Bozic et al., in the case of metastatic disease, monotherapy with a targeted agent offers no hope for recovery. Instead, combinations of two or more agents given simultaneously offer a small chance of cure, especially in the absence of cross-resistance mutations [39].

It is worth noting that the aforementioned drugs are directed against downstream effectors of *VHL*, hence, from an evolutionary point of view, there is a potential to better define the molecular target. Nicholson et al. found that inhibiting the cyclin-dependent kinases CDK4 and CDK6 impaired tumor growth in *VHL*-deficient ccRCC regardless of HIF2α dependency [40]. Abemaciclib, a CDK4/6 and PIM1 kinase inhibitor is currently being tested in phase I trial in combination with sunitinib in metastatic RCC (NCT03905889). Another compound that could represent a paradigm shift in targeted treatment is STF-62247. It has been shown to induce potent cytotoxic effects in *VHL*-deficient ccRCC cells, compared to their *VHL* wild-type counterparts [41]. The STF-62247-stimulated synthetic lethality occurs in a HIF-independent manner through autophagy; however, the mechanistic links between *VHL* and autophagy are incompletely understood [42].

4.4. Targeting Cancer Immune Evasion

Tumor cells interact with the immune system in a process called immunoediting, which consists of three phases: elimination, equilibrium, and escape [43]. Most of the tumor cells are destroyed in the first phase. Cells that cannot be eliminated enter the equilibrium in which they are selected through immune cell exhaustion and resistance to immune detection [44]. It is the longest of the three phases and, in ccRCC, manifests as a modest clonal expansion right after the 3p loss. The evolutionary pressure of immune predation may eventually lead to the development of mechanisms to escape immune responses. From that moment, malignant growth proceeds unrestrained. The ultimate goal of immunotherapy is to permanently reverse immune evasion strategies.

Recent phase III clinical trials led to the use of three immunotherapy-based combinations, including pembrolizumab, ipilimumab, and nivolumab, as a front-line for ccRCC [45]. These agents are highly effective, with a few patients achieving a durable complete response. The ongoing phase III clinical trials are currently testing different combinations of a checkpoint inhibitor plus a tyrosine kinase inhibitor (NCT02811861, NCT03937219) or IL-2 derivate (NCT03729245). Earlier phase studies are evaluating the potential of combining PD-1/PD-L1 inhibitors and antibodies directed against LAG-3 (NCT02996110, NCT03849469), TIM-3 (NCT02608268), or ICOS (NCT03693612, NCT03829501). An alternative approach is represented by the use of different cytokines (NCT02799095, NCT03063762) or personalized cancer vaccines (NCT03633110, NCT02950766).

ITH plays an essential role in shaping antitumor immune responses [43,44]. The highly heterogeneous tumors presumably escape immune surveillance because the reactive neoantigens undergo 'dilution' within the tumor, thereby leading to weaker antitumor immunity.

How do specific genomic features of ccRCC influence the clinical benefit from immunotherapy is under investigation. While tumor mutational burden (TMB) potentially increases ITH [46], a small study on 25 metastatic ccRCCs failed to confirm the association between TMB and response to immunotherapeutics [47]. Miao and colleagues found that truncating mutations in *PBRM1* were associated with significantly extended progression-free survival (PFS) and OS of patients with metastatic ccRCC treated with immune checkpoint inhibitors [48]. The underlying mechanism is probably related to increased sensitivity to T-cell-mediated cytotoxicity of *PBRM1*-mutant tumor cells [49]. This association was confirmed in an independent ccRCC cohort by a post hoc analysis of the CheckMate 025 randomized phase III study [50]. On the other hand, the exploratory analyses from JAVELIN Renal 101 and CheckMate 214 do not support this hypothesis [51,52]. The discrepant results are presumably due to the different populations studied, such as treatment-naïve versus VEGF-refractory [53].

4.5. *Modulating Genomic Instability*

Genomic instability of cancer cells drives genetic diversity required for the natural selection of adaptive traits, but there is a threshold beyond which cells cannot replicate successfully [54]. Hence, it is tempting to alter (increase or decrease) the frequency of mutations within the cancer genome.

RCC is characterized by a moderate level of genomic instability and the absence of mutations in canonical DNA damage response (DDR) genes, such as *RAD9*, *BRCA1*, or *TP53* [6,49]. As a result, RCC patients are commonly unresponsive to DNA-damaging therapies, such as chemo- or radiotherapy. For that reason, reducing genetic instability could be a more suitable approach. It can be achieved, among others, by constitutive activation of the transforming growth factor β (TGF-β) axis. TGF-β has been shown to inhibit DNA double-strand breaks (DSB) repair mechanisms to heighten the genetic diversity and adaptability of cancer cells [55]. In ccRCC cell cultures, TGF-β enhances proliferative capacity and promotes metastatic growth [56]. Early phase Ib clinical trial (NCT00356460) investigated the use of a monoclonal antibody against TGF-β fresolimumab in RCC patients and showed preliminary evidence of antitumor activity [57].

On the contrary, particular ccRCC driver genes do influence DDR and there is preclinical evidence to support the poly(ADP)-ribose polymerase (PARP) inhibition in *VHL*- or *BAP1*-mutated ccRCC [54,58,59]. Moreover, cells harboring *SETD2* mutation undergo synthetic lethal interaction with WEE1 blockade due to the depletion of nucleotide pools [60]. AZD1775, an experimental inhibitor of WEE1, is currently being evaluated for patients with *SETD2*-deficient tumors, including RCC (NCT03284385).

4.6. *Evolutionary Herding*

The tumor is less likely to be resistant to multiple drugs simultaneously, hence the combination therapy allows for the extermination of resistant cells before the emergence of further adaptive mechanisms. However, the use of two or more drugs simultaneously is strictly limited by the toxicity to normal tissues.

While checkpoint inhibitor and the antiangiogenic combination is a standard of care for metastatic ccRCC, there is a significant overlap in the toxicity profile of these drugs, with diarrhea, hypertension, and hepatotoxicity being among the most commonly presented [55,61]. These and other adverse effects may all contribute to treatment discontinuation or dose reduction. Moreover, there is frequently a need for additional medications, such as loperamide secondary to axitinib or high-dose corticosteroids for autoimmune colitis and hepatitis in case of checkpoint inhibitors. Then, drug–drug interactions become even harder to predict. Despite the toxicity issue, in most cases, cancer cells eventually develop multidrug resistance.

Any biological adaptation often involves trade-offs. In cancers, the cost of one resistance mechanism is likely to induce a population to be sensitive to an alternative therapy [62]. Evolutionary herding exploits this weakness by administering a combination of drugs in a particular order which enables to control the tumor cell population. When a second drug is administered, the clonal structure of the population is different from the start, and this may lead to enhanced sensitivity, or even complete tumor regression [63].

Since evolutionary herding alters the cellular composition of the tumor microenvironment, collateral drug sensitivity is likely to be persistent. Furthermore, this strategy is hardly influenced by stochastic perturbations and cell plasticity [64]. Acar et al. recently designed an experimental approach, in which evolution can be tightly controlled, monitored, and altered using drugs. It allows estimating evolutionary trade-offs and evaluating the effectiveness of patient-specific evolutionary herding strategies [65]. The suitability of evolutionary herding in RCC has not been tested yet.

5. Therapeutic Implications

As previously described, seven evolutionary trajectories can be distributed into four groups depending on the tumor's genomic characteristics, evolution mode, and clinical course. We suspect that each group has its own unique weaknesses that could be exploited. In Figure 1, we demonstrate the predicted effectiveness of evolution-targeted strategies against particular evolutionary trajectories of ccRCC.

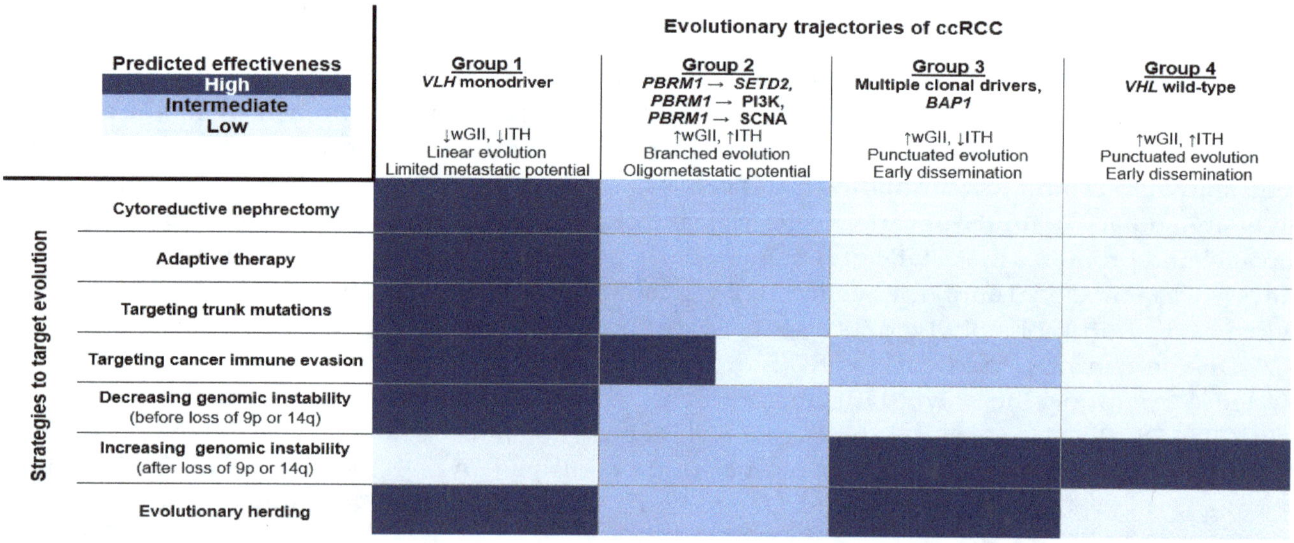

Figure 1. Predicted effectiveness of evolution-targeted strategies against particular evolutionary trajectories of clear cell renal cell carcinoma (ccRCC). Seven deterministic evolutionary trajectories are classified into four groups in terms of tumor's genomic characteristics, evolution mode, and clinical course. Loss of 9p or 14q represents the acquisition of metastatic competence. There are conflicting results regarding *PBRM1* mutation as a predictive biomarker of response to immunotherapy. The figure is based on assumptions about tumor biology and therapeutic options. ccRCC, clear cell renal cell carcinoma; wGII, weighted genome integrity index; ITH, intratumor heterogeneity.

While the benefit of upfront CN strictly depends on life expectancy, this procedure should be considered especially for Group 1 and, to a lesser extent, Group 2. Similarly, adaptive therapy that aims to enforce a stable tumor burden is expected to be highly effective against indolent cancers. Tumors from Group 1, in which *VHL* mutation is the sole driver event, are the best candidates for targeting trunk mutations. In Group 2, there is a limited number of trunk mutations, and this approach is still reasonable. As a general rule, ITH diminishes immune responses but tumors harboring *PBRM1* mutations (Group 2) could be highly vulnerable to immunotherapeutic agents. The predictive value of *PBRM1* mutation, however, is under debate and requires further investigation. Finally, decreased wGII is an indicator of a favorable response to immunotherapy, supporting its use in Group 1. In Figure 2, we illustrate how modulating genomic instability may affect ccRCC fitness. We suggest decreasing genomic instability before the loss of 9p or 14q, which represents the acquisition of metastatic competence. This approach is particularly attractive in Group 1, characterized by low wGII. In contrast, Groups 3 and 4, due to high wGII and a punctuated evolution pattern, are expected to respond to increasing genomic instability. Modulating genomic instability in Group 2 could be unsuitable because of high wGII and branched mode of evolution. Evolutionary herding aims to decrease ITH with each subsequent therapy. Hence, it should be considered in Groups 1 and 3. This strategy may also be adequate in Group 2 due to its indolent nature in comparison to Group 4.

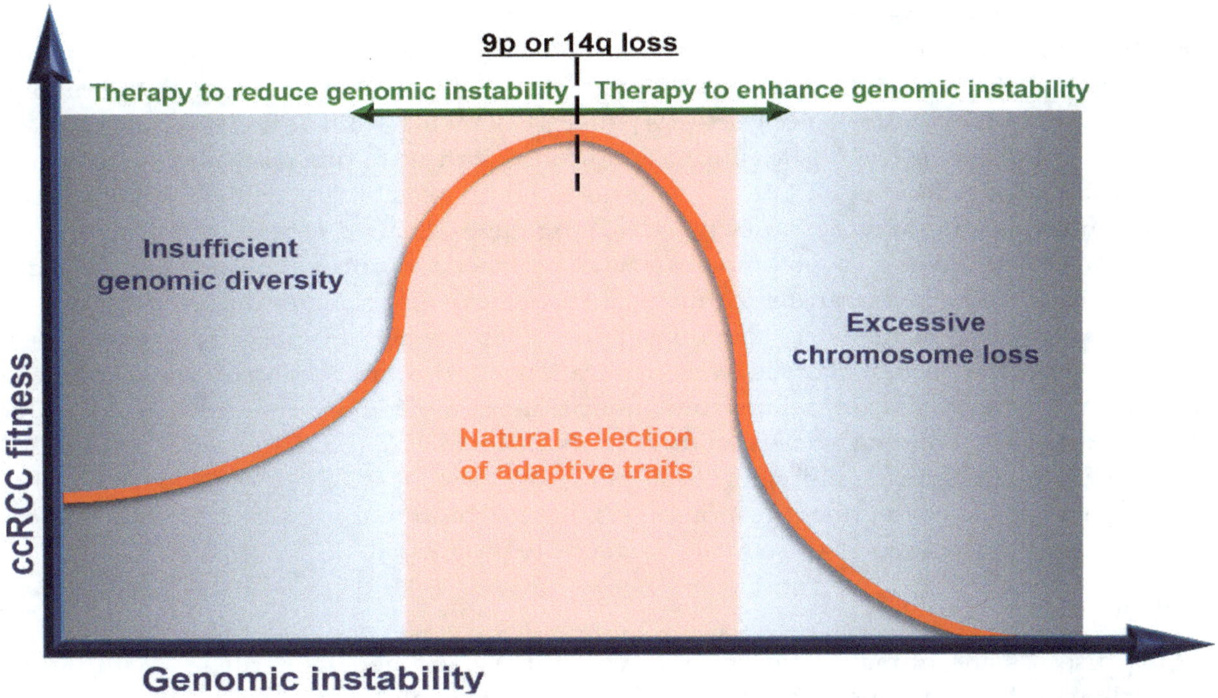

Figure 2. Modulating genomic instability to reduce ccRCC fitness. ccRCC fitness (vertical axis) is plotted against genomic instability (horizontal axis). There is an optimum range of genomic instability, in which ccRCC evolves. 9p or 14q loss represents the acquisition of metastatic competence and is a point of no return. Before this point is reached, decreasing genomic instability slows down cancer evolution. Once 9p or 14q is lost, increasing genome instability triggers extensive DNA damage and cell death.

6. Future Directions

Sequencing data obtained from spatial biopsies enable one to infer the phylogenetic tree structure and, in ccRCC, estimate the evolution trajectory. As a general rule, trunk alterations are found in all tumor cells and represent an ancestral event, while other modifications constitute the branches. The more regions sampled, the more branches will be found. In low-ITH cases, four biopsies would reflect the subclonal alteration with 75% accuracy. The gain in driver detection per additional sampling declines after eight, which is usually still not enough in cases with *PBRM1* mutation [14]. While molecular profiling of multiple specimens is not practical in the setting of clinical practice, the analysis of circulating tumor DNA (ctDNA) obtained from liquid biopsy represents a feasible alternative. Analysis of ctDNA enables identification of both clonal and subclonal tumor-specific mutations with high sensitivity and specificity, with detection rates comparable with those of traditional biopsies [61–66]. Furthermore, ctDNA has a relatively short half-life (approximately 2 h), allowing for the evaluation of tumor changes in real-time [67]. Finally, as minimally invasive, liquid biopsy eliminates the morbidity associated with the serial sampling of tumors. While qualitative and quantitative analyses of ctDNA have been extensively performed in RCC patients [68], liquid biopsy has not yet been used to capture RCC evolutionary trajectories.

The discovery of alternative evolutionary trajectories of RCC will provide a better insight into the underlying mechanisms of drug resistance. Some of these mechanisms may be closely related to geographic and environmental factors since patients from different regions have different genetic backgrounds and are exposed to different carcinogens. Huang et al. identified mutational signatures and SCNAs specific to Chinese or Japanese ccRCC patients [13]. In the first group, the alterations could be due to exposure to aristolochic acid, a common ingredient in many Chinese herbs [69]. The cause of unique genetic alterations in the Japanese cohort remains unexplained.

Novel techniques to perform an in-depth analysis of datasets, as well as larger-scale studies, will greatly expand our knowledge on the development of RCC. Recently, an original computational method, CONETT (CONserved Evolutionary Trajectories in Tumors), enabled the detection of three additional directions of evolution among ccRCCs [70]. Two of them terminate with a sequence alteration in gene *KDM5C* and one in *TSC1*. The clinical significance of these findings is yet to be determined.

Identification of hidden evolutionary patterns is made possible by artificial intelligence (AI). Caravagna and colleagues devised a machine-learning method called repeated evolution in cancer (REVOLVER), which allows to overcome the stochastic effects of cancer evolution and information noise [71]. This technique uses transfer learning (TL) to achieve reproducible disease prognosis based on next-generation sequencing (NGS) count data [70–73]. As a result, it is possible to classify patients on the basis of how their tumor evolved, with implications for the anticipation of disease progression.

According to the NCCN Guidelines for Kidney Cancer, molecular profiling does not influence decision-making. The ongoing phase 2 clinical trials, A-PREDICT (NCT01693822) and ADAPTeR (NCT02446860), incorporate a multiregional sampling of metastatic RCC prior to and during therapy to evaluate biomarkers of treatment response. Whether evolutionary trajectories could reflect the effectiveness of a particular anti-RCC strategy, remains to be elucidated.

7. Conclusions

Many diseases are intimately tied to our evolutionary and genetic heritage. With our better understanding of these conditions, we gradually acquire the evolutionary perspective, which turns out necessary for both prevention and treatment [74,75]. In contrast to organismal evolution, human cancers are subjected to similar initial conditions and follow a limited range of possible evolutionary trajectories. Therefore, the repetitive nature of cancer evolution may prove to be its greatest weakness.

Genomic characterization is currently paving the way for clinical decision-making in RCC. The problem of exceptional ITH could be minimized by multiregion biopsy or liquid biopsy. These tools not only provide insights into cancer genetic architecture but also allow the measurement of clonal evolution. Recent studies resolved the evolutionary features and subtypes underpinning the diverse clinical phenotypes of ccRCC. In this review, we have summarized recent advances in the treatment of ccRCC and demonstrated how each strategy could be improved from the evolutionary perspective. Since there are only a few deterministic evolutionary trajectories in ccRCC, it appears feasible to use them as potential biomarkers for guiding intervention and surveillance. We believe that the presented patient stratification could help predict future steps of malignant progression, thereby informing optimal and personalized clinical decisions.

Author Contributions: Conceptualization, writing—original draft preparation, writing—review and editing, A.K., M.Z., D.G., and Ł.S. All authors have read and agreed to the published version of the manuscript.

References

1. Ferlay, J.; Soerjomataram, I.; Dikshit, R.; Eser, S.; Mathers, C.; Rebelo, M.; Parkin, D.M.; Forman, D.; Bray, F. Cancer incidence and mortality worldwide: Sources, methods and major patterns in GLOBOCAN 2012. *Int. J. Cancer* **2015**, *136*, E359–E386. [CrossRef] [PubMed]
2. Cohen, H.T.; McGovern, F.J. Renal-cell carcinoma. *N. Engl. J. Med.* **2005**, *353*, 2477–2490. [CrossRef] [PubMed]
3. Lam, J.S.; Leppert, J.T.; Belldegrun, A.S.; Figlin, R.A. Novel approaches in the therapy of metastatic renal cell carcinoma. *World J. Urol.* **2005**, *23*, 202–212. [CrossRef] [PubMed]

4. Rajandram, R.; Bennett, N.C.; Morais, C.; Johnson, D.W.; Gobe, G.C. Renal cell carcinoma: Resistance to therapy, role of apoptosis, and the prognostic and therapeutic target potential of TRAF proteins. *Med. Hypotheses* **2012**, *78*, 330–336. [CrossRef] [PubMed]
5. Frew, I.J.; Moch, H. A Clearer View of the Molecular Complexity of Clear Cell Renal Cell Carcinoma. *Annu. Rev. Pathol. Mech. Dis.* **2015**, *10*, 263–289. [CrossRef] [PubMed]
6. Creighton, C.J.; Morgan, M.; Gunaratne, P.H.; Wheeler, D.A.; Gibbs, R.A.; Robertson, G.; Chu, A.; Beroukhim, R.; Cibulskis, K.; Signoretti, S.; et al. Comprehensive molecular characterization of clear cell renal cell carcinoma. *Nature* **2013**, *499*, 43–49. [CrossRef]
7. Varela, I.; Tarpey, P.; Raine, K.; Huang, D.; Ong, C.K.; Stephens, P.; Davies, H.; Jones, D.; Lin, M.-L.; Teague, J.; et al. Exome sequencing identifies frequent mutation of the SWI/SNF complex gene PBRM1 in renal carcinoma. *Nature* **2011**, *469*, 539–542. [CrossRef] [PubMed]
8. Beroukhim, R.; Brunet, J.P.; Di Napoli, A.; Mertz, K.D.; Seeley, A.; Pires, M.M.; Linhart, D.; Worrell, R.A.; Moch, H.; Rubin, M.A.; et al. Patterns of gene expression and copy-number alterations in von-Hippel Lindau disease-associated and sporadic clear cell carcinoma of the kidney. *Cancer Res.* **2009**, *69*, 4674–4681. [CrossRef]
9. Soultati, A.; Stares, M.; Swanton, C.; Larkin, J.; Turajlic, S. How should clinicians address intratumour heterogeneity in clear cell renal cell carcinoma? *Curr. Opin. Urol.* **2015**, *25*, 358–366. [CrossRef]
10. Gerlinger, M.; Rowan, A.J.; Horswell, S.; Math, M.; Larkin, J.; Endesfelder, D.; Gronroos, E.; Martinez, P.; Matthews, N.; Stewart, A.; et al. Intratumor heterogeneity and branched evolution revealed by multiregion sequencing. *N. Engl. J. Med.* **2012**, *366*, 883–892. [CrossRef]
11. Arai, E.; Sakamoto, H.; Ichikawa, H.; Totsuka, H.; Chiku, S.; Gotoh, M.; Mori, T.; Nakatani, T.; Ohnami, S.; Nakagawa, T.; et al. Multilayer-omics analysis of renal cell carcinoma, including the whole exome, methylome and transcriptome. *Int. J. Cancer* **2014**, *135*, 1330–1342. [CrossRef]
12. Gulati, S.; Martinez, P.; Joshi, T.; Birkbak, N.J.; Santos, C.R.; Rowan, A.J.; Pickering, L.; Gore, M.; Larkin, J.; Szallasi, Z.; et al. Systematic evaluation of the prognostic impact and intratumour heterogeneity of clear cell renal cell carcinoma biomarkers. *Eur. Urol.* **2014**, *66*, 936–948. [CrossRef]
13. Huang, Y.; Wang, J.; Jia, P.; Li, X.; Pei, G.; Wang, C.; Fang, X.; Zhao, Z.; Cai, Z.; Yi, X.; et al. Clonal architectures predict clinical outcome in clear cell renal cell carcinoma. *Nat. Commun.* **2019**, *10*, 1–10. [CrossRef]
14. Turajlic, S.; Xu, H.; Litchfield, K.; Rowan, A.; Horswell, S.; Chambers, T.; O'Brien, T.; Lopez, J.I.; Watkins, T.B.K.; Nicol, D.; et al. Deterministic Evolutionary Trajectories Influence Primary Tumor Growth: TRACERx Renal. *Cell* **2018**, *173*, 595.e11–610.e11. [CrossRef]
15. Hutchinson, L. Predicting cancer's next move. *Nat. Rev. Clin. Oncol.* **2014**, *11*, 61–62. [CrossRef]
16. Beroukhim, R.; Mermel, C.H.; Porter, D.; Wei, G.; Raychaudhuri, S.; Donovan, J.; Barretina, J.; Boehm, J.S.; Dobson, J.; Urashima, M.; et al. The landscape of somatic copy-number alteration across human cancers. *Nature* **2010**, *463*, 899–905. [CrossRef]
17. Mitchell, T.J.; Turajlic, S.; Rowan, A.; Nicol, D.; Farmery, J.H.R.; O'Brien, T.; Martincorena, I.; Tarpey, P.; Angelopoulos, N.; Yates, L.R.; et al. Timing the Landmark Events in the Evolution of Clear Cell Renal Cell Cancer: TRACERx Renal. *Cell* **2018**, *173*, 611.e17–623.e17. [CrossRef]
18. Motzer, R.J.; Tannir, N.M.; McDermott, D.F.; Arén Frontera, O.; Melichar, B.; Choueiri, T.K.; Plimack, E.R.; Barthélémy, P.; Porta, C.; George, S.; et al. Nivolumab plus Ipilimumab versus Sunitinib in Advanced Renal-Cell Carcinoma. *N. Engl. J. Med.* **2018**, *378*, 1277–1290. [CrossRef]
19. Flanigan, R.C.; Mickisch, G.; Sylvester, R.; Tangen, C.; van Poppel, H.; Crawford, E.D. Cytoreductive Nephrectomy in Patients With Metastatic Renal Cancer: A Combined Analysis. *J. Urol.* **2004**, *171*, 1071–1076. [CrossRef] [PubMed]
20. Turajlic, S.; Xu, H.; Litchfield, K.; Rowan, A.; Chambers, T.; Lopez, J.I.; Nicol, D.; O'Brien, T.; Larkin, J.; Horswell, S.; et al. Tracking Cancer Evolution Reveals Constrained Routes to Metastases: TRACERx Renal. *Cell* **2018**, *173*, 581–594.e12. [CrossRef]
21. Larcher, A.; Wallis, C.J.D.; Bex, A.; Blute, M.L.; Ficarra, V.; Mejean, A.; Karam, J.A.; Van Poppel, H.; Pal, S.K. Individualised Indications for Cytoreductive Nephrectomy: Which Criteria Define the Optimal Candidates? *Eur. Urol. Oncol.* **2019**, *2*, 365–378. [CrossRef]
22. Heng, D.Y.C.; Wells, J.C.; Rini, B.I.; Beuselinck, B.; Lee, J.L.; Knox, J.J.; Bjarnason, G.A.; Pal, S.K.; Kollmannsberger, C.K.; Yuasa, T.; et al. Cytoreductive nephrectomy in patients with synchronous metastases from renal cell carcinoma: Results from the International Metastatic Renal Cell Carcinoma Database Consortium. *Eur. Urol.* **2014**, *66*, 704–710. [CrossRef] [PubMed]

23. Graham, J.; Bhindi, B.; Heng, D.Y.C. The evolving role of cytoreductive nephrectomy in metastatic renal cell carcinoma. *Curr. Opin. Urol.* **2019**, *29*, 507–512. [CrossRef]
24. Laguna, M.P. Re: Cytoreductive nephrectomy in patients with synchronous metastases from renal cell carcinoma: Results from the international metastatic renal cell carcinoma database consortium: Editorial comment. *J. Urol.* **2015**, *193*, 1514–1515. [CrossRef]
25. Gatenby, R.A.; Silva, A.S.; Gillies, R.J.; Frieden, B.R. Adaptive therapy. *Cancer Res.* **2009**, *69*, 4894–4903. [CrossRef] [PubMed]
26. Rini, B.I.; Dorff, T.B.; Elson, P.; Rodriguez, C.S.; Shepard, D.; Wood, L.; Humbert, J.; Pyle, L.; Wong, Y.N.; Finke, J.H.; et al. Active surveillance in metastatic renal-cell carcinoma: A prospective, phase 2 trial. *Lancet Oncol.* **2016**, *17*, 1317–1324. [CrossRef]
27. Bex, A.; Mulders, P.; Jewett, M.; Wagstaff, J.; Van Thienen, J.V.; Blank, C.U.; Van Velthoven, R.; Del Pilar Laguna, M.; Wood, L.; Van Melick, H.H.E.; et al. Comparison of Immediate vs Deferred Cytoreductive Nephrectomy in Patients with Synchronous Metastatic Renal Cell Carcinoma Receiving Sunitinib: The SURTIME Randomized Clinical Trial. *JAMA Oncol.* **2019**, *5*, 164–170. [CrossRef]
28. Sun, Y.; Li, J.; Yang, X.; Zhang, G.; Fan, X. The Alternative 2/1 Schedule of Sunitinib is Superior to the Traditional 4/2 Schedule in Patients With Metastatic Renal Cell Carcinoma: A Meta-analysis. *Clin. Genitourin. Cancer* **2019**, *17*, e847–e859. [CrossRef]
29. West, J.; You, L.; Zhang, J.; Gatenby, R.A.; Brown, J.S.; Newton, P.K.; Anderson, A.R.A. Towards multidrug adaptive therapy. *Cancer Res.* **2020**, *80*, 1578–1589. [CrossRef]
30. Rathmell, W.K.; Chen, S. VHL inactivation in renal cell carcinoma: Implications for diagnosis, prognosis and treatment. *Expert Rev. Anticancer Ther.* **2008**, *8*, 63–73. [CrossRef]
31. Raval, R.R.; Lau, K.W.; Tran, M.G.B.; Sowter, H.M.; Mandriota, S.J.; Li, J.-L.; Pugh, C.W.; Maxwell, P.H.; Harris, A.L.; Ratcliffe, P.J. Contrasting Properties of Hypoxia-Inducible Factor 1 (HIF-1) and HIF-2 in von Hippel-Lindau-Associated Renal Cell Carcinoma. *Mol. Cell. Biol.* **2005**, *25*, 5675–5686. [CrossRef] [PubMed]
32. Gordan, J.D.; Bertout, J.A.; Hu, C.J.; Diehl, J.A.; Simon, M.C. HIF-2α Promotes Hypoxic Cell Proliferation by Enhancing c-Myc Transcriptional Activity. *Cancer Cell* **2007**, *11*, 335–347. [CrossRef]
33. Shen, C.; Kaelin, W.G. The VHL/HIF axis in clear cell renal carcinoma. *Semin. Cancer Biol.* **2013**, *23*, 18–25. [CrossRef]
34. Sakashita, N.; Takeya, M.; Kishida, T.; Stackhouse, T.M.; Zbar, B.; Takahashi, K. Expression of von Hippel-Lindau protein in normal and pathological human tissues. *Histochem. J.* **1999**, *31*, 133–144. [CrossRef]
35. Hofmann, F.; Marconi, L.S.O.; Stewart, F.; Lam, T.B.L.; Bex, A.; Canfield, S.E.; Ljungberg, B. Targeted therapy for metastatic renal cell carcinoma. *Cochrane Database Syst. Rev.* **2017**, *2017*. [CrossRef]
36. Koehler, A.N. A complex task? Direct modulation of transcription factors with small molecules. *Curr. Opin. Chem. Biol.* **2010**, *14*, 331–340. [CrossRef]
37. Wallace, E.M.; Rizzi, J.P.; Han, G.; Wehn, P.M.; Cao, Z.; Du, X.; Cheng, T.; Czerwinski, R.M.; Dixon, D.D.; Goggin, B.S.; et al. A small-molecule antagonist of HIF2α is efficacious in preclinical models of renal cell carcinoma. *Cancer Res.* **2016**, *76*, 5491–5500. [CrossRef]
38. Courtney, K.D.; Infante, J.R.; Lam, E.T.; Figlin, R.A.; Rini, B.I.; Brugarolas, J.; Zojwalla, N.J.; Lowe, A.M.; Wang, K.; Wallace, E.M.; et al. Phase I dose-escalation trial of PT2385, a first-in-class hypoxia-inducible factor-2a antagonist in patients with previously treated advanced clear cell renal cell carcinoma. *J. Clin. Oncol.* **2018**, *36*, 867–874. [CrossRef]
39. Bozic, I.; Reiter, J.G.; Allen, B.; Antal, T.; Chatterjee, K.; Shah, P.; Moon, Y.S.; Yaqubie, A.; Kelly, N.; Le, D.T.; et al. Evolutionary dynamics of cancer in response to targeted combination therapy. *Elife* **2013**, *2013*. [CrossRef]
40. Nicholson, H.E.; Tariq, Z.; Housden, B.E.; Jennings, R.B.; Stransky, L.A.; Perrimon, N.; Signoretti, S.; Kaelin, W.G. HIF-independent synthetic lethality between CDK4/6 inhibition and VHL loss across species. *Sci. Signal.* **2019**, *12*. [CrossRef] [PubMed]
41. Turcotte, S.; Chan, D.A.; Sutphin, P.D.; Hay, M.P.; Denny, W.A.; Giaccia, A.J. A Molecule Targeting VHL-Deficient Renal Cell Carcinoma that Induces Autophagy. *Cancer Cell* **2008**, *14*, 90–102. [CrossRef]
42. Jones, T.M.; Carew, J.S.; Nawrocki, S.T. Therapeutic targeting of autophagy for renal cell carcinoma therapy. *Cancers* **2020**, *12*, 1185. [CrossRef]
43. Dunn, G.P.; Old, L.J.; Schreiber, R.D. The Three Es of Cancer Immunoediting. *Annu. Rev. Immunol.* **2004**, *22*, 329–360. [CrossRef] [PubMed]
44. Kim, R.; Emi, M.; Tanabe, K. Cancer immunoediting from immune surveillance to immune escape. *Immunology* **2007**, *121*, 1–14. [CrossRef]

45. Rini, B.I.; Plimack, E.R.; Stus, V.; Gafanov, R.; Hawkins, R.; Nosov, D.; Pouliot, F.; Alekseev, B.; Soulières, D.; Melichar, B.; et al. Pembrolizumab plus Axitinib versus Sunitinib for Advanced Renal-Cell Carcinoma. *N. Engl. J. Med.* **2019**, *380*, 1116–1127. [CrossRef]
46. Wolf, Y.; Bartok, O.; Patkar, S.; Eli, G.B.; Cohen, S.; Litchfield, K.; Levy, R.; Jiménez-Sánchez, A.; Trabish, S.; Lee, J.S.; et al. UVB-Induced Tumor Heterogeneity Diminishes Immune Response in Melanoma. *Cell* **2019**, *179*, 219.e21–235.e21. [CrossRef]
47. Maia, M.C.; Almeida, L.; Bergerot, P.G.; Dizman, N.; Pal, S.K. Relationship of tumor mutational burden (TMB) to immunotherapy response in metastatic renal cell carcinoma (mRCC). *J. Clin. Oncol.* **2018**, *36*, 662. [CrossRef]
48. Miao, D.; Margolis, C.A.; Gao, W.; Voss, M.H.; Li, W.; Martini, D.J.; Norton, C.; Bossé, D.; Wankowicz, S.M.; Cullen, D.; et al. Genomic correlates of response to immune checkpoint therapies in clear cell renal cell carcinoma. *Science* **2018**, *359*, 801–806. [CrossRef]
49. Pan, D.; Kobayashi, A.; Jiang, P.; De Andrade, L.F.; Tay, R.E.; Luoma, A.M.; Tsoucas, D.; Qiu, X.; Lim, K.; Rao, P.; et al. A major chromatin regulator determines resistance of tumor cells to T cell-mediated killing. *Science* **2018**, *359*, 770–775. [CrossRef]
50. Braun, D.A.; Ishii, Y.; Walsh, A.M.; Van Allen, E.M.; Wu, C.J.; Shukla, S.A.; Choueiri, T.K. Clinical Validation of PBRM1 Alterations as a Marker of Immune Checkpoint Inhibitor Response in Renal Cell Carcinoma. *JAMA Oncol.* **2019**, *5*, 1631–1633. [CrossRef]
51. Motzer, R.J.; Robbins, P.B.; Powles, T.; Albiges, L.; Haanen, J.B.; Larkin, J.; Mu, X.J.; Ching, K.A.; Uemura, M.; Pal, S.K.; et al. Avelumab plus axitinib versus sunitinib in advanced renal cell carcinoma: Biomarker analysis of the phase 3 JAVELIN Renal 101 trial. *Nat. Med.* **2020**. [CrossRef]
52. Motzer, R.J.; Choueiri, T.K.; McDermott, D.F.; Powles, T.; Yao, J.; Ammar, R.; Papillon-Cavanagh, S.; Saggi, S.S.; McHenry, B.M.; Ross-Macdonald, P.; et al. Biomarker analyses from the phase III CheckMate 214 trial of nivolumab plus ipilimumab (N+I) or sunitinib (S) in advanced renal cell carcinoma (aRCC). *J. Clin. Oncol.* **2020**, *38*, 5009. [CrossRef]
53. Tucker, M.D.; Rini, B.I. Predicting response to immunotherapy in metastatic renal cell carcinoma. *Cancers* **2020**, *12*, 2662. [CrossRef]
54. Andor, N.; Maley, C.C.; Ji, H.P. Genomic instability in cancer: Teetering on the limit of tolerance. *Cancer Res.* **2017**, *77*, 2179–2185. [CrossRef]
55. Pal, D.; Pertot, A.; Shirole, N.H.; Yao, Z.; Anaparthy, N.; Garvin, T.; Cox, H.; Chang, K.; Rollins, F.; Kendall, J.; et al. TGF-β reduces DNA ds-Break repair mechanisms to heighten genetic diversity and adaptability of CD44+/CD24-cancer cells. *Elife* **2017**, *6*. [CrossRef]
56. Sitaram, R.T.; Mallikarjuna, P.; Landström, M.; Ljungberg, B. Transforming growth factor-β promotes aggressiveness and invasion of clear cell renal cell carcinoma. *Oncotarget* **2016**, *7*, 35917–35931. [CrossRef]
57. Morris, J.C.; Tan, A.R.; Olencki, T.E.; Shapiro, G.I.; Dezube, B.J.; Reiss, M.; Hsu, F.J.; Berzofsky, J.A.; Lawrence, D.P. Phase I study of GC1008 (Fresolimumab): A human anti-transforming growth factor-beta (TGFβ) monoclonal antibody in patients with advanced malignant melanoma or renal cell carcinoma. *PLoS ONE* **2014**, *9*. [CrossRef]
58. Okazaki, A.; Gameiro, P.A.; Christodoulou, D.; Laviollette, L.; Schneider, M.; Chaves, F.; Stemmer-Rachamimov, A.; Yazinski, S.A.; Lee, R.; Stephanopoulos, G.; et al. Glutaminase and poly(ADP-ribose) polymerase inhibitors suppress pyrimidine synthesis and VHL-deficient renal cancers. *J. Clin. Investig.* **2017**, *127*, 1631–1645. [CrossRef]
59. Yu, H.; Pak, H.; Hammond-Martel, I.; Ghram, M.; Rodrigue, A.; Daou, S.; Barbour, H.; Corbeil, L.; Hébert, J.; Drobetsky, E.; et al. Tumor suppressor and deubiquitinase BAP1 promotes DNA double-strand break repair. *Proc. Natl. Acad. Sci. USA* **2014**, *111*, 285–290. [CrossRef] [PubMed]
60. Pfister, S.X.; Markkanen, E.; Jiang, Y.; Sarkar, S.; Woodcock, M.; Orlando, G.; Mavrommati, I.; Pai, C.C.; Zalmas, L.P.; Drobnitzky, N.; et al. Inhibiting WEE1 Selectively Kills Histone H3K36me3-Deficient Cancers by dNTP Starvation. *Cancer Cell* **2015**, *28*, 557–568. [CrossRef]
61. Garje, R.; An, J.; Greco, A.; Vaddepally, R.K.; Zakharia, Y. The future of immunotherapy-based combination therapy in metastatic renal cell carcinoma. *Cancers* **2020**, *12*, 143. [CrossRef]
62. Hughes, D.; Andersson, D.I. Evolutionary consequences of drug resistance: Shared principles across diverse targets and organisms. *Nat. Rev. Genet.* **2015**, *16*, 459–471. [CrossRef] [PubMed]
63. Pluchino, K.M.; Hall, M.D.; Goldsborough, A.S.; Callaghan, R.; Gottesman, M.M. Collateral sensitivity as a strategy against cancer multidrug resistance. *Drug Resist. Updat.* **2012**, *15*, 98–105. [CrossRef]

64. Acar, A.; Nichol, D.; Fernandez-Mateos, J.; Cresswell, G.; Barozzi, I.; Hong, S.P.; Spiteri, I.; Stubbs, M.; Burke, R.; Stewart, A.; et al. Exploiting evolutionary herding to control drug resistance in cancer. *bioRxiv* **2019**, 566950. [CrossRef]
65. Acar, A.; Nichol, D.; Fernandez-Mateos, J.; Cresswell, G.D.; Barozzi, I.; Hong, S.P.; Trahearn, N.; Spiteri, I.; Stubbs, M.; Burke, R.; et al. Exploiting evolutionary steering to induce collateral drug sensitivity in cancer. *Nat. Commun.* **2020**, *11*. [CrossRef]
66. Lanman, R.B.; Mortimer, S.A.; Zill, O.A.; Sebisanovic, D.; Lopez, R.; Blau, S.; Collisson, E.A.; Divers, S.G.; Hoon, D.S.B.; Kopetz, E.S.; et al. Analytical and Clinical Validation of a Digital Sequencing Panel for Quantitative, Highly Accurate Evaluation of Cell-Free Circulating Tumor DNA. *PLoS ONE* **2015**, *10*, e0140712. [CrossRef] [PubMed]
67. Diehl, F.; Schmidt, K.; Choti, M.A.; Romans, K.; Goodman, S.; Li, M.; Thornton, K.; Agrawal, N.; Sokoll, L.; Szabo, S.A.; et al. Circulating mutant DNA to assess tumor dynamics. *Nat. Med.* **2008**, *14*, 985–990. [CrossRef]
68. Cimadamore, A.; Gasparrini, S.; Massari, F.; Santoni, M.; Cheng, L.; Lopez-Beltran, A.; Scarpelli, M.; Montironi, R. Emerging molecular technologies in renal cell carcinoma: Liquid biopsy. *Cancers* **2019**, *11*, 196. [CrossRef] [PubMed]
69. Rosenquist, T.A.; Grollman, A.P. Mutational signature of aristolochic acid: Clue to the recognition of a global disease. *DNA Repair (Amst.)* **2016**, *44*, 205–211. [CrossRef]
70. Hodzic, E.; Shrestha, R.; Malikic, S.; Collins, C.C.; Litchfield, K.; Turajlic, S.; Sahinalp, S.C. Identification of conserved evolutionary trajectories in tumors. *Bioinformatics* **2020**, *36*, i427–i435. [CrossRef]
71. Caravagna, G.; Giarratano, Y.; Ramazzotti, D.; Tomlinson, I.; Graham, T.A.; Sanguinetti, G.; Sottoriva, A. Detecting repeated cancer evolution from multi-region tumor sequencing data. *Nat. Methods* **2018**, *15*, 707–714. [CrossRef]
72. Pan, S.J.; Yang, Q. A survey on transfer learning. *IEEE Trans. Knowl. Data Eng.* **2010**, *22*, 1345–1359. [CrossRef]
73. Hajiramezanali, E.; Dadaneh, S.Z.; Karbalayghareh, A.; Zhou, M.; Qian, X. Bayesian multi-domain learning for cancer subtype discovery from next-generation sequencing count data. *Adv. Neural Inf. Process. Syst.* **2018**, *2018*, 9115–9124.
74. Greaves, M. Darwinian medicine: A case for cancer. *Nat. Rev. Cancer* **2007**, *7*, 213–221. [CrossRef]
75. Nesse, R.M. How is Darwinian medicine useful? *West. J. Med.* **2001**, *174*, 358–360. [CrossRef] [PubMed]

8

Cysteine Cathepsins Inhibition Affects their Expression and Human Renal Cancer Cell Phenotype

Magdalena Rudzińska [1,†], Alessandro Parodi [1,†], Valentina D. Maslova [2], Yuri M. Efremov [3], Neonila V. Gorokhovets [1], Vladimir A. Makarov [1], Vasily A. Popkov [4], Andrey V. Golovin [1,2,5], Evgeni Y. Zernii [1,4] and Andrey A. Zamyatnin Jr. [1,4,*]

1 Institute of Molecular Medicine, Sechenov First Moscow State Medical University, 119991 Moscow, Russia; magdda.rudzinska@gmail.com (M.R.); aparodi.sechenovuniversity@gmail.com (A.P.); gorokhovets@gmail.com (N.V.G.); known.sir@yandex.ru (V.A.M.); golovin.andrey@gmail.com (A.V.G.); zerni@belozersky.msu.ru (E.Y.Z.)
2 Faculty of Bioengineering and Bioinformatics, Moscow State University, 119992 Moscow, Russia; valmarfgecnf@gmail.com
3 Institute for Regenerative Medicine, Sechenov University, 119991 Moscow, Russia; yu.efremov@gmail.com
4 Belozersky Institute of Physico-Chemical Biology, Lomonosov Moscow State University, 119992 Moscow, Russia; popkov.vas@gmail.com
5 Shemyakin-Ovchinnikov Institute of Bioorganic Chemistry, Russian Academy of Sciences, 117997 Moscow, Russia
* Correspondence: zamyat@belozersky.msu.ru
† Authors contributed equally.

Abstract: Renal cancer would greatly benefit from new therapeutic strategies since, in advanced stages, it is refractory to classical chemotherapeutic approaches. In this context, lysosomal protease cysteine cathepsins may represent new pharmacological targets. In renal cancer, they are characterized by a higher expression, and they were shown to play a role in its aggressiveness and spreading. Traditional studies in the field were focused on understanding the therapeutic potentialities of cysteine cathepsin inhibition, while the direct impact of such therapeutics on the expression of these enzymes was often overlooked. In this work, we engineered two fluoromethyl ketone-based peptides with inhibitory activity against cathepsins to evaluate their potential anticancer activity and impact on the lysosomal compartment in human renal cancer. Molecular modeling and biochemical assays confirmed the inhibitory properties of the peptides against cysteine cathepsin B and L. Different cell biology experiments demonstrated that the peptides could affect renal cancer cell migration and organization in colonies and spheroids, while increasing their adhesion to biological substrates. Finally, these peptide inhibitors modulated the expression of LAMP1, enhanced the expression of E-cadherin, and altered cathepsin expression. In conclusion, the inhibition of cysteine cathepsins by the peptides was beneficial in terms of cancer aggressiveness; however, they could affect the overall expression of these proteases.

Keywords: cysteine cathepsins; cysteine cathepsin inhibitors; lysosome; renal cancer

1. Introduction

Cysteine cathepsins (Cts) are lysosomal proteases belonging to the C1 family of papain-like enzymes. They are responsible for the degradation and turnover of cellular [1] and extracellular [2] proteins, covering an essential role in maintaining cell and tissue homeostasis. Different enzymes with endo-, exo-, and endo/exopeptidase activity [3] compose the Cts family. Their proteolytic properties rely on a residue of cysteine in their active site, while other cathepsins are characterized by the presence of aspartic acid or serine amino acid [4]. Cathepsin expression is dysregulated in many pathological conditions, including cancer [5], and their overexpression is traditionally associated with the acquisition of a more aggressive tumor phenotype [6].

Cts, in particular, were shown to play a pivotal role in cancer invasiveness [7], tumor cell communication [8], apoptosis [9], and autophagy [10]. Considering that the Cts family includes 11 different members, only a few of them were tested extensively as tumor pharmacological targets, and, despite the overall scientific opinion, current data regarding the positive or negative contribution of Cts to cancer disease are contradictory [4,11–16]. For example, in the lysosomes, they can contribute to the proper function of autophagy, rescuing the cells from exogenous and endogenous stress [17]. In contrast, when they were found free in the cell cytoplasm, they could induce apoptosis through a caspase-independent mechanism of cellular death [9,18]. The role of Cts in cancer disease was shown to depend on their activation state [19] and cellular location [20].

Nevertheless, conclusive progress in the field is hampered by potential redundant and compensatory activities [21] both within the different members of the Cts family [21] and between other cathepsins/proteases [22]. Most of the research performed by far, unveiled the role of single Cts in cancer disease, with few further considerations on how the investigated inhibitors, the genetic silencers, or modifications affected the overall biology of the cells and the expression of the targeted enzymes. These considerations are pivotal to the correct designing of more effective pharmacological interventions and evaluate their long term effects.

To address these questions, we designed two small fluoromethyl ketone (FMK)-containing peptides to broadly inhibit the activity against these enzymes. The designing of these inhibitors was inspired by a well-known substrate of the papain-like cysteine protease Triticain-α, derived from *Triticum aestivum* (wheat) [23]. This peptide consists of four amino acids Acetyl-Pro-Leu-Val-Gln (Ac-PLVQ), while the inhibitor sequences are Acetyl-Pro-Leu-Val-Glu-FMK (Ac-PLVE-FMK) and Acetyl-Val-Leu-Pro-Glu-FMK (Ac-VLPE-FMK) (Figure 1a). The working mechanism of both inhibitors should be the same as other selective irreversible cysteine proteinase inhibitors like Z-VAD-FMK (Figure 1b) [24], as well as other FMK-containing drugs. In this class of inhibitors, the FMK group forms a covalent bond with the catalytic cysteine, with the fluorine ion leaving [25,26]. As a model of tumor disease, we chose human renal cancer since this pathology showed aberrant expression of some members of the Cts family [27]. Additionally, further progress in kidney tumor disease depends on the discovery of new targetable markers [28] since when the diagnosis is performed at an advanced stage, the survival rate is low [29], and traditional chemotherapy is ineffective [30]. Investigation on Cts inhibition in this cancer model is rare, and to our knowledge, no comprehensive study in relation to phenotypic and enzymatic alterations has ever been performed. In this work, we tested the biological impact of our inhibitory peptides on the biology of human renal cancer cells, with a focus on the overall lysosomal compartment. We demonstrated that the general inhibition of Cts over longer time periods does not affect the cell proliferation rate. Still, it can affect the overall biology of human renal cancer cells, as well as impacting on the overall Cts expression.

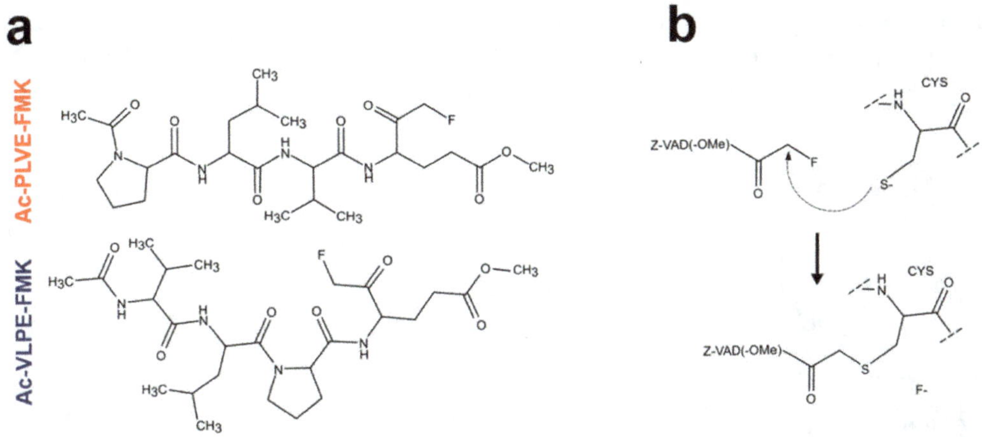

Figure 1. The structure and working mechanism of Ac-PLVE- fluoromethyl ketone (FMK) and Ac-VLPE-FMK inhibitors: (**a**) Inhibitory peptides structure and (**b**) their working mechanism based on Z-VAD-FMK inhibitor.

2. Results

2.1. Computational Modeling of the Peptide Inhibitory Properties on Cts Activity

A docking simulation to predict the interactions of the inhibitors with the binding site of the Cts was performed with the protein-ligand docking software PLANTS [31]. Both Ac-PLVE-FMK and Ac-VLPE-FMK were docked into CtsB, L, and W active sites at pH 4.5, 6.5, and 7.2 since pH can influence the protein interactions through the protonation of the ionizable residues [32]. CtsB and L were chosen as enzymatic models because they have endo and endo/exopeptidase activity, respectively, addressing all the Cts proteolytic mechanisms. They were also shown to play a pivotal role in renal cancer malignancy, and their overexpression was associated with a more aggressive cancer phenotype [33–35]. On the other hand, CtsW represents a poorly investigated protease in renal cancer. In contrast, in other investigations, it was shown to preferentially locate in the endothelial reticulum [36], and it is evolutionarily distinguished from CtsB and L [37], representing, therefore, optimal negative control for our research.

Fifty poses per binding site for each ligand were obtained. The analysis revealed that our inhibitors did not bind with the proteases in the pre-reaction state with the fluorine atom of the FMK group in a 3.5 Å radius from the HD2 hydrogen atom of the catalytic histidine and with the carbon atom of the fluoromethyl group in a 3.5 Å radius from the SG atom of the catalytic cysteine. The non-covalent binding energy of the peptides to the proteases is substantially lower than the energy of one covalent bond. Thus, the conformation suitable for covalent bonding may be far from the optimal peptide position in the non-covalent mode. To find non-covalent interactions potentially leading to covalent bond formation, we analyzed the crystal structure of Z-VAD-FMK, covalently bonded to the cysteine protease *Marasmius oreades agglutinin* (PDB id 5D61). In this case, the oxygen atom of the FMK group interacts via hydrogen bonds with the oxyanion hole of the enzyme, formed by the catalytic cysteine backbone N and NE1 atom of Trp-208. For further docking simulations, we added a distance constraint between the oxygen atom of the FMK group of our inhibitors and two hydrogen atoms from the oxyanion holes in the Cts structures. This adjustment allowed for obtaining poses close to the pre-reaction state for both inhibitors. The resulting poses demonstrated that Ac-PLVE-FMK tends to occupy S2 binding sites with either Val or Leu residues, depending on the backbone conformation. The C-terminal Glu residue fitted in the groove around site S1′. However, the N-terminal residue did not bind in S3 or S4 sites and laid closer to the protein surface. Ac-VLPE-FMK instead, tended to bind in S1′-S2′ sites of Cts with its N-terminal residues' sidechains. Thus, both inhibitors should occupy mostly hydrophobic substrate-binding pockets by Val and Leu side chains. Representative docking of the peptides with the CtsB, L, and W at pH 4.5 is shown in Figure 2a–c. According to the docking score, both inhibitors are less likely to bind in the pre-reaction state, capable of covalent bond formation with CtsW confirming its potential role as a negative control (Figure 2d). Ac-VLPE-FMK also has a weaker binding with all Cts than Ac-PLVE-FMK, possibly due to the lack of conformation variability around Pro residue.

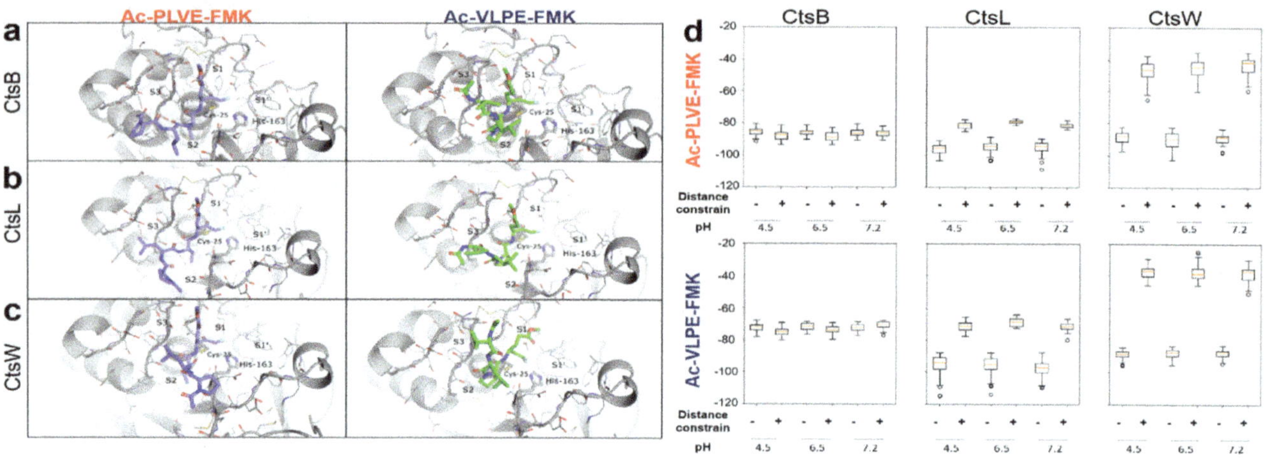

Figure 2. Binding poses of designed inhibitors to cysteine cathepsins (Cts). Docking of the peptides in (**a**) CtsB,(**b**) CtsL, (**c**) CtsW (pH 4.5). Hydrogen atoms are omitted for better depiction. Catalytic Cysteine and Histidine are shown in thick sticks. Inhibitors are shown in purple or green. S1-S3 and S1′ binding pockets are labeled. (**d**) Binding scores (PLANTS Chemplp energy units) for Ac-PLVE-FMK and Ac-VLPE-FMK docking results at different pH levels with and without distance constraints.

2.2. *Assessment of Peptide Inhibitory Properties on Cts Activity via Biochemical Assays*

Ac-PLVE-FMK and Ac-VLPE-FMK inhibitory properties were evaluated against human recombinant CtsL and B. These recombinant enzymes were expressed in *E. coli* via plasmid transformation and further purification, using nickel-nitrilotriacetic acid (Ni-NTA) sepharose. Gel zymography assay was used to provide a preliminary evaluation of the ability of these recombinant proteins to degrade the gelatin substrate previously embedded in the gel (Supplementary Figure S1). Following Coomassie staining, the Cts were detectable as single bands. As expected, a translucent area was evident, due to the substrate digestion in the proximity of the proteins. Then, the recombinant proteins were tested for their ability to digest the Triticain-α substrate Ac-PLVQ via fluorescent protease activity assay, previously optimized by our group [23]. This probe was conjugated with the fluorogenic chromophore 7-amino-4-methylcoumarin (Ac-PLVQ-AMC). After proteolytic cleavage, it emits a detectable fluorescent signal.

Both human recombinant CtsB and L (20 nM each) were able to cleave the probe Ac-PLVQ-AMC (50 μM) and increase the fluorescent signal detection (red line). In the same experimental conditions, performed in the presence of Ac-PLVE-FMK or Ac-VLPE-FMK (2 μM), the intensity of the fluorescent signal was significantly affected (Supplementary Figure S2—blue and green line, respectively).

To evaluate the inhibitory properties of the peptides directly on the human renal cancer cells, we firstly assessed the impact of Ac-PLVE-FMK and Ac-VLPE-FMK on the cell viability of 769-P and A498 cells to determine the working concentrations for further experiments. The peptides were easily dispersed in water and administered at increasing doses to both cell lines for 72 h (Figure 3a,b). The inhibitors showed cytostatic properties on both cell lines only within 48 h of treatment when all the concentrations used negatively impacted on cell proliferation, in particular in the case of 769-P cells. However, after 72 h of incubation, cell viability increased, reaching values not significantly different from the control cells. Further experiments were performed using a concentration of 20 μM. To understand if the peptides could affect the activity of caspase proteases, we tested their effect on cell viability in combination with the chemotherapeutic paclitaxel (PXT) in both the cell lines. The cell line A498 did not result in high mortality even when the cells were treated with PXT alone (data not shown), confirming previously published data [38]. However, in the case of 769-P cells, the ability of the PXT to kill cancer cells was evident after 72 h of treatment at a concentration of 100 nM. When the treatment with PXT was performed in combination with the peptides (20 μM), no significant differences were observed (Supplementary Figure S3). Next, we evaluated the effect of the peptides on renal cancer cell proteolytic activity against the fluorogenic probe Ac-PLVQ-AMC. In this case, 769-p and A498 cells were treated for 30 min with Ac-PLVE-FMK or Ac-VLPE-FMK and were then exposed for 10 min to the substrate Ac-PLVQ-AMC prior fluorescence microscopy analysis (Figure 3c,d). As depicted by the pictures, both the peptides were effective in inhibiting the generation of the fluorescence derived from the cleavage of the substrate in both the cell lines and fluorimetric analysis confirmed that they significantly inhibited the probe degradation. Overall, these data demonstrate that the peptides do not considerably interfere with cell viability and that their inhibitory properties do not affect the proteolytic activity of the proteases that are involved in cell apoptosis; however, they can effectively interfere with the cellular Cts.

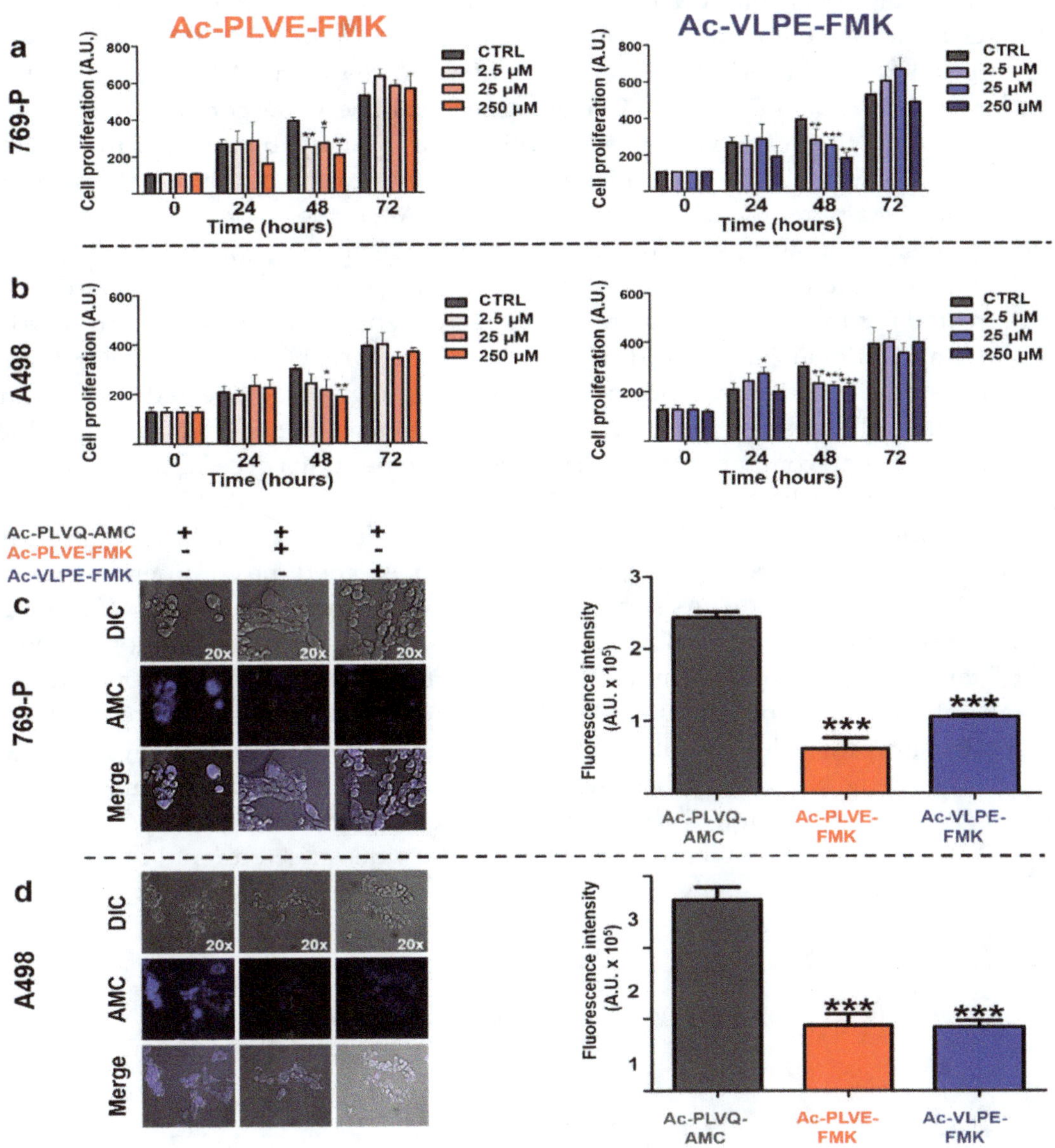

Figure 3. The effect of the peptide inhibitors on human 769-P and A498 renal cancer cell proliferation and proteolytic activity. (**a**) 769-P and (**b**) A498 cells were treated with increasing doses of Ac-PLVE-FMK (red bars) and Ac-VLPE-FMK (blue bars) (2.5–250 μM). Cell proliferation was measured after 24, 48,

and 72 h via MTT (3-(4,5-dimethylthiazol-2-yl)-2,5-diphenyltetrazolium bromide) assay. Data represent the mean (±S.D.) of at least three independent experiments, each performed in triplicate. (**c**) Fluorescence microscopy evaluation and quantification of the cell proteolytic activity in 769-P and (**d**) A498 cells towards the fluorogenic substrate Ac-PLVQ-AMC in the absence or presence of Ac-PLVE-FMK and Ac-VLPE-FMK. The cells were seeded in a 96- well plate and after exposure to the peptides for 30 min prior incubation with the fluorescent substrate Ac-PLVQ-AMC for 10 min. Data are expressed as mean (±S.D.), and significance was calculated through one-way ANOVA followed by Dunnet's test. * = $p < 0.05$, ** = $p < 0.01$, *** = $p < 0.001$.

2.3. Effect of the Inhibitory Peptides on Human Tumor Cell Biology

The effective inhibition of specific members of the Cts family was associated with changes in cancer cell properties, such as a decrease in cell invasiveness and migration properties in different tumors, including renal cancer cell lines [39–41]. For this reason, various tests were used to evaluate potential changes in cancer cell biology following treatment with the inhibitory peptides. Firstly, we assessed the ability of renal cancer cells to generate colonies. 769-P and A498 cells were treated with the inhibitors for a total of 2 days (20 μM) before being seeded at very low confluency in 10 cm diameter dishes. After cell seeding, the treatment with the peptides was prolonged for an additional 10 days until colony formation was detectable, and identification and quantification of the colonies were performed through Crystal Violet staining. Even though in the case of A498, the colonies were smaller than with 769P cells, both the inhibitors were effective in significantly decreasing colony numbers, as shown in Figure 4a,b. Next, we evaluated the ability of the inhibitory peptides to affect spheroids formation. The cells were treated for 48 h with the Cts inhibitors (20 μM) before being seeded in Matrigel-coated 96-well plates for an additional 7 days. Additionally, in this case, A498 spheroid size and number were smaller than 769-P cells, and the presence of the inhibitors negatively affected the total number of spheroids in both the cell lines (Figure 4c,d), reaching highly significant decreasing values in 769P cells. It is worth noting that, compared to untreated cells, the peptides decreased spheroid size, while increasing their circularity in both the cell lines (Supplementary Figure 4a,b). Finally, we evaluated the ability of the inhibitors to contrast the motility of the cells in a classical scratch healing assay. Human renal cancer cells were seeded and grown until they reached the confluency when a gap was artificially created with a 200 μM tip. As shown in Figure 4e,f, the inhibitors were efficient in a similar fashion in decreasing the gap closure velocity, both at 8 and 24 h after the formation of the scratch. In light of the registered changes in cell phenotype, we hypothesized that the inhibition of Cts could have impacted on cell adhesion to biological substrates. Human renal cancer cells were treated for 48 h before assessing their adhesion properties on collagen IV and Matrigel. Both the peptides induced an increase in cell adhesion on both the biological substrates (Figure 5a,b), and these properties were accompanied by changes in cell stiffness, evaluated through atomic force microscopy analysis (Supplementary Figure S5a,b). Overall, these data demonstrated that the peptides affected renal cancer cell biology.

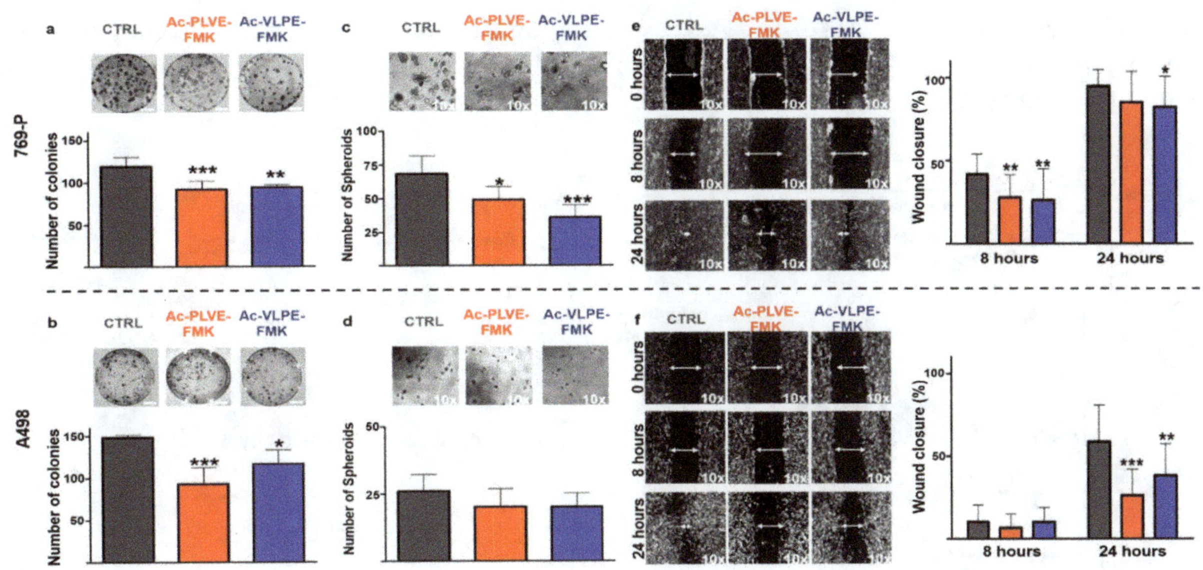

Figure 4. Effect of the peptides on renal cancer cell biology: colony formation assay of (**a**) 769-P and (**b**) A498 under treatment with Ac-PLVE-FMK and Ac-VLPE-FMKI. The cells were treated for 48 h with 20 μM inhibitors and seeded into 10 culture dishes (10 cm diameter) at low confluency where they grew with or without the peptides for an additional 10 days. Representative images of the colony formation assay and quantitative data analysis are shown in the graph. (**c**) 769P and (**d**) A498 spheroid formation evaluated after 7 days of culture on Matrigel coated dishes. The graph is showing the number of spheroids. (**e**) 769-p and (**f**) A498 scratch assay. The graph shows the cell migration rate. All pictures were taken under 10× magnification. Data are expressed as mean (±S.D.), and significance was calculated through one-way ANOVA followed by Dunnet's test. * = $p < 0.05$, ** = $p < 0.01$, *** = $p < 0.001$.

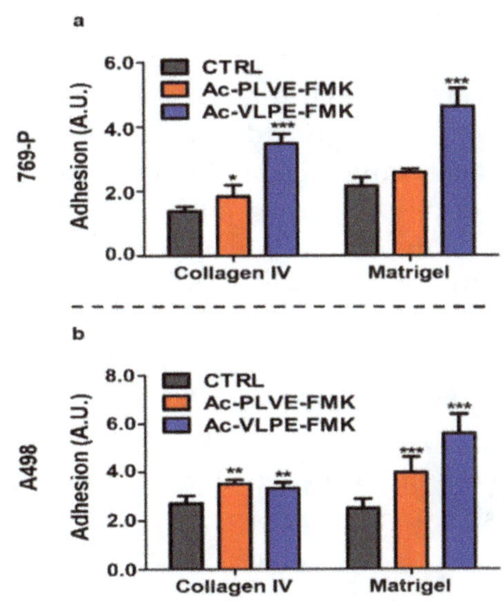

Figure 5. Effect of Cts inhibitors on renal cancer cell adhesion on biological coatings: (**a**) adhesion 769-P and (**b**) A498 cells to collagen IV and Matrigel after treatment with the inhibitors. Data are expressed as mean (±S.D.), and significance was calculated through one-way ANOVA followed by Dunnet's test. * = $p < 0.05$, ** = $p < 0.01$, *** = $p < 0.001$.

2.4. Effect of the Inhibitory Peptides on E-Cadherin and SNAIL1

The collected data indicated that Ac-PLVE-FMK and Ac-VLPE-FMK could affect the overall renal cancer cell phenotype. These properties could be the result of the modulation of the effectors controlling EMT, as previously shown in other tumor models [40,42–44]. To test this hypothesis, the cells were treated with the inhibitors for 24, 48, and 72 h by changing the media every day, and they were tested for E-cadherin and SNAIL1 expression (Figure 6; detail information of western blots can be seen in Supplementary Figure S7).

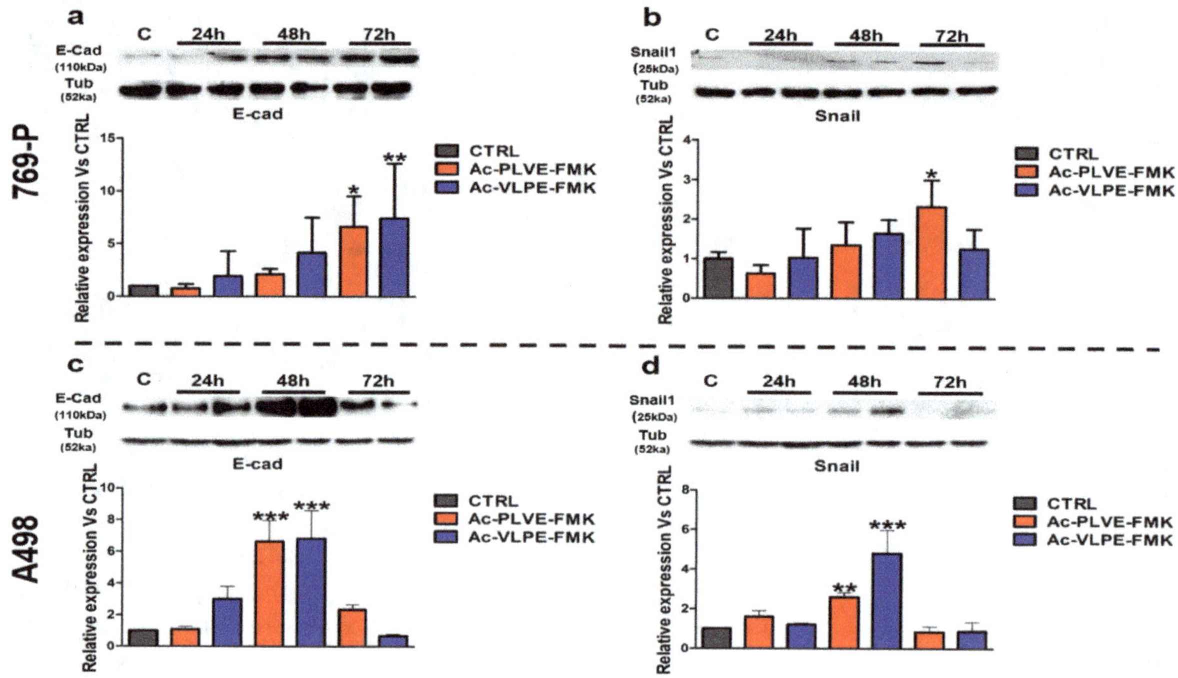

Figure 6. Effects of the peptides on E-cadherin and SNAIL1 protein expression: (**a**,**b**) protein expression of E-cadherin and SNAIL1 in 769-P and (**c**,**d**) A498 cells after 24, 48, and 72 h of treatment with the peptides. Data are represented as mean ± SD of at least three replicates. Significance was calculated through one-way ANOVA, followed by Dunnet's test.

These markers are critical players in the control of EMT, and they are associated with opposite effects on the cancer cell phenotype. While E-cadherin is considered a marker of differentiation, working against EMT (favoring mesenchymal-epithelial transition, as known as MET), SNAIL1 is associated with the acquisition of an undifferentiated phenotype. Both the peptides increased the protein expression of E-cadherin in the first 48 h in both the cell lines (Figure 6). At 72 h, the values of E-cadherin further increased in 769P cells, while decreased in A498 cells. On the other hand, SNAIL1 increased significantly at 72 h only in the case of 769P cells treated with AC-PLVE-FMK, while dropped to values more similar to the control upon treatment with Ac-VLPE-FMK and in A498 cells with both the peptides. More importantly, in both the cell lines, E-cadherin and SNAIL1 followed a similar trend in response to the treatments. Taken together, these data demonstrated that the inhibitory peptides could affect the cell phenotype, involving the genes that control EMT. These phenomena could be at the base of the observed cell adhesion and motility properties, considering that E-cadherin showed the highest increase after treatment, compared to untreated CTRL.

2.5. Impact of the Peptides on Lysosomal Biology

To evaluate the potential changes to the lysosomal compartment, we measured the expression of Lysosome Associated Membrane Protein 1 (LAMP-1) over 72 h of treatment. This protein is usually associated with the lysosomal membrane, and it is universally recognized as a marker of these organelles. Western blotting analysis demonstrated a very different effect of the peptides on the modulation of this marker in the two cell lines. In 769-P cells, both the inhibitors significantly increased the expression of this lysosomal biomarker at all the considered time points, reaching significant peaks at 48 h of treatment and generally increasing this marker in all the considered time points. Additionally, Ac-VLPE-FMK demonstrated to be more efficient than Ac-PLVE-FMK in increasing the expression of LAMP-1 (Figure 7a). These data were corroborated by confocal microscopy analysis, confirming that at 48 h, both the peptides increased LAMP-1 expression (Figure 7b), while at 72 h, the content of LAMP-1 decreased towards control levels. On the other hand, LAMP-1 protein expression in A498 cells was significantly affected during the first 48 h, and it was characterized by a substantial recovery at 72 h, reaching values slightly higher than CTRL levels (Figure 7c,d). A similar trend in both the cell lines was observed by analyzing the endolysosomal compartment integrity through Neutral red assay (Supplementary Figure S6) and LysoTracker red fluorescence measurement where we registered slightly increasing and decreasing values only at 48 h of treatment for 769-P and A498 cells, respectively.

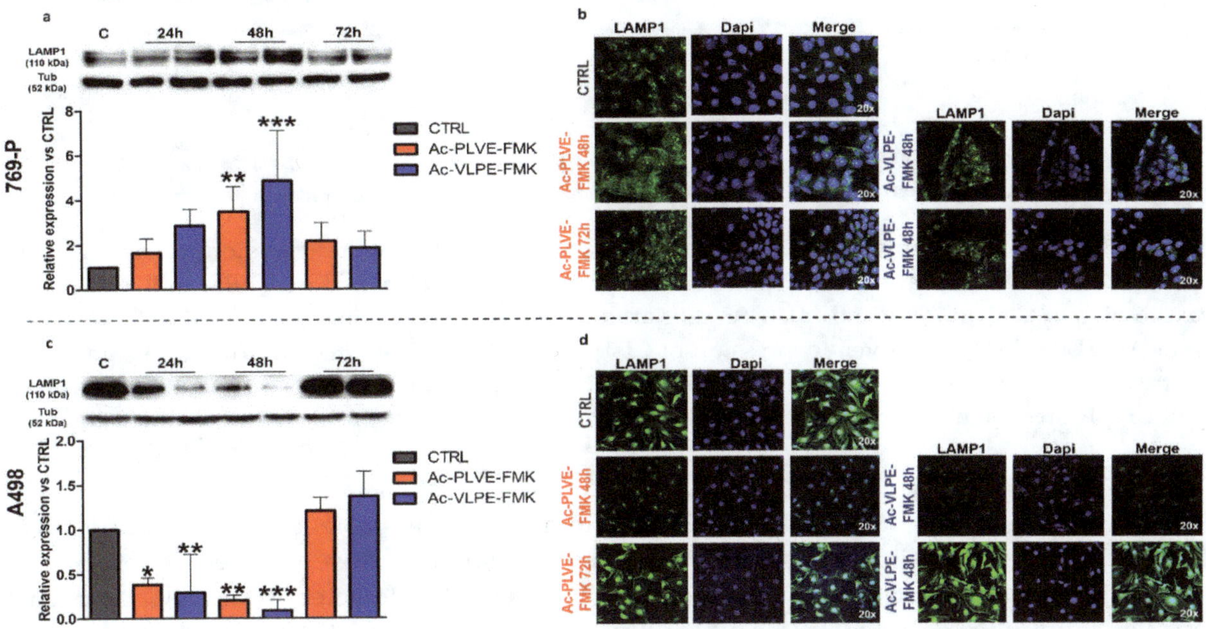

Figure 7. Effect of the peptides on LAMP-1 protein expression: (**a**) Western blotting analysis of LAMP-1 after treatment with PLVE and VLPE (20 μM) for 24, 48, and 72 h in 769-P cells. (**b**) Confocal microscopy evaluation of LAMP-1 expression after 48 and 72 h of treatment with PLVE and VLPE (20 μM) in 769-P cells. (**c**) Western blotting analysis of LAMP-1 after treatment with PLVE and VLPE (20 μM) for 24, 48, and 72 h in A498 cells. (**d**) Confocal microscopy evaluation of LAMP-1 expression after 48 and 72 h of treatment with PLVE and VLPE (20 μM) in A498 cells. Data are represented as mean ± SD of at least three replicates. Significance was calculated through one-way ANOVA followed by Dunnet's test. * = $p < 0.05$, ** = $p < 0.01$, *** = $p < 0.001$.

Next, we evaluated the protein expression of CtsB, L, and W (Figure 8). In both the cell lines, the Cts protein expression was similar. In particular, CtsB and L increased significantly at the later time points of treatment with both the peptides (Figure 8a–d). In contrast, in the case of CtsW, the peptides negatively affected the protein expression in 769-P cells, while no particular differences were detected in A498 cells (Figure 8e,f). Other tested Cts were modulated in their protein expression similarly to CtsB and L. Overall, these experiments indicated that the peptides could affect the biology of the lysosomal compartment and the expression of Cts. The only exception to this rule was represented by CtsW, which did not show a high affinity for the peptides, and its expression was negatively affected by the peptides only in 769-P cells, while no substantial differences were registered in A498 cells.

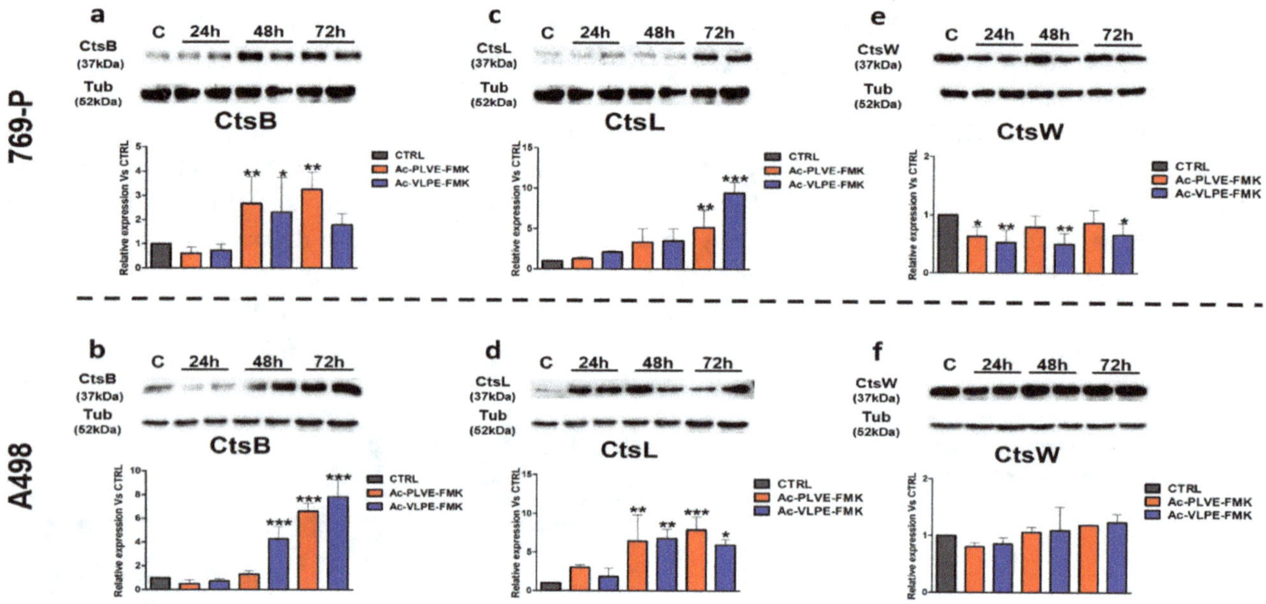

Figure 8. Effect of the peptides on CtsB, L, and W expression: (**a**) protein expression of CtsB in 769-P and (**b**) A498 cells after 24, 48, and 72 h of treatment with Ac-PLVE-FMK and Ac-VLPE-FMK. (**c**) protein expression of CtsL in 769-P and (**d**) A498 cells after 24, 48, and 72 h of treatment with Ac-PLVE-FMK and Ac-VLPE-FMK. (**e**) Protein expression of CtsB in 769-P and (**f**) A498 cells after 24, 48, and 72 h of treatment with Ac-PLVE-FMK and Ac-VLPE-FMK. Data are represented as mean ± S.D. of at least three replicates. Significance was calculated through one-way ANOVA followed by Dunnet's test.

3. Discussion

Cts are universally considered as key players in maintaining proteostasis regulation, and their proteolytic activity is traditionally associated with the lysosomes. However, their sphere of action is not limited just to the lumen of these organelles. They were also detected in the cell cytoplasm [45], nucleus [46], and when secreted, in the extracellular space [46], regulating important processes like autophagy [47], apoptosis [48], gene expression [49], cell signaling [50], and angiogenesis [51]. In this scenario, a potential contribution of Cts in tumor disease is practically obvious, and the first pieces of evidence regarding their role in cancer were published in the late 80s [52]. In the case of renal cancer, the upregulation of CtsB was shown to decrease three- and five-year patient survival rates [33], and CtsK was shown to be overexpressed in renal cell carcinoma patients with Xp11 translocation [53]. Despite detailed data regarding the role of specific Cts in tumor disease, this family of proteases counts 11 members with redundant and compensatory activities, as shown in autoimmune diseases [54] and or thyroglobulin processing [55], respectively. For this reason, strategies aimed at specifically inhibiting the activity of a single Cts member could result in a low impact on cancer cell biology, as well as a limited understanding of the role of these proteases in tumor disease. More importantly, current literature generally did not focus on understanding the impact of the Cts inhibitors on the overall expression of these proteases. In this context, the investigation performed in renal cancer represents an additional novelty since specific studies in the field are very rare in this disease model.

In this work, we designed peptide-based inhibitors that could universally inhibit the action of Cts. Ac-PLVE-FMK and Ac-VLPE-FMK derive from the well-known substrate of the Triticain-α cysteine protease Ac-PLVQ, which was extensively used by our group in previous work to define the activity of this enzyme through fluorimetric assay [23]. The proposed inhibition mechanism is based on FMK-containing drugs, which are known as selective and efficient cysteine protease inhibitors [56]. Molecular docking is a powerful computational approach commonly employed to predict the binding poses and affinities of various ligands to macromolecules. Ligand conformations, obtained in the docking procedure, allow for estimating the interactions required for successful binding and provide insights for further improvements in ligand design. However, this method has limitations, since it does not allow for predicting the occurrence of covalent bonds between macromolecules and ligands [57]. In our case, both Ac-PLVE-FMK and Ac-VLPE-FMK were designed to bind the catalytic cysteine in the Cts covalently; however, the docking model can only estimate the interactions between the peptides and the Cts in the pre-reaction binding.

In the simulation, Ac-PLVE-FMK and Ac-VLPE-FMK tend to occupy the S2 binding site of Cts with aliphatic side chains and form hydrogen bonds by the peptide backbone atoms of the respective residues. However, the N-terminal amino acids of the peptides tend to form fewer contacts with the Cts proteins. Thus, the designed inhibitor molecules can be further improved by the rational design of their N-terminus. According to the docking results, Ac-VLPE-FMK appears to be a weaker binder to all the Cts we considered (see Figure 2d), since the Pro residue hinders the movement of this peptide, thereby reducing the possibility of its proper pre-reaction binding. Thus, Ac-PLVE-FMK theoretically represents a more promising target for further improvement.

Both peptides showed a similar efficiency in inhibiting the activity of recombinant human CtsB and L. More importantly, they demonstrated pronounced inhibitory properties in vitro directly on the cells, implying their ability to penetrate the cell membrane with moderate cytostatic effects only registered during the first 48 h of treatment. Previous work performed with the multi-Cts inhibitor E64 on pancreatic cells showed only a moderated cytotoxic effect, which reached a plateau phase after 48 and 72 h [58]. In general, Cts inhibitors cannot be considered very potent cytostatic molecules. However, as demonstrated in other works, they could increase chemotherapy efficacy [59], even though when used in combination with PXT our peptides did not increase cell toxicity in a significant way. We exclude, however, that the peptides lost their potency over time because the treatments were administered afresh every day. Therefore, we conclude that our peptides do not have a significant impact on renal cancer cell viability.

On the other hand, Cts activity was shown as a modulator of invasive properties, including cellular adhesion [8], anchorage-independent growth [60], colony formation [61], and motility [44] of cells. Our data support this evidence in both the human renal cancer cell lines tested with the peptides, decreasing their ability to migrate in a scratch assay, while increasing their adhesion to biological substrates. It is important to note that differences in cell spreading, associated with more potent cellular adhesive force, can be accompanied by decreased cell migration [62,63]. Additionally, the peptides inhibited colony and spheroid formation, phenomena that can be favored by Cts activity [44,64]. These effects could be a result of an increased E-cadherin expression, a protein involved in cell adhesion, and considered as a marker of differentiation during MET, which increased upon treatment with both the peptides, reaching significant levels at the later time points. A previous work [65] demonstrated that in renal cancer spheroid formation, a down-regulation of E-cadherin occurs, highlighting its potential contribution to the detected anti-spheroid and colony formation properties shown by our peptides.

Interestingly, the inhibitory proteolytic properties of our peptides impacted on Cts homeostasis. We observed different variations in the expression of LAMP-1. At 48 h of treatment with both the peptides, LAMP-1 increased in 769-P cells, while it decreased in A498 cells. However, at 72 h, both the cell lines were characterized by an increase in LAMP-1 expression, even though it did not reach significant levels. These data were corroborated by further fluorescent microscopy analysis as well as by the evaluation of the endosomal compartment integrity performed through neutral red assay and LysoTracker Red. An increase in LAMP-1 expression after CtsB and L knock out was similarly registered in mouse embryonic fibroblast cells [66] and bone marrow-derived macrophages [67].

More importantly, the peptides affected Cts turnover by inducing two different trends in their expression. The CtsB and L expression increased over time after treatment with the peptides in both the cell lines. On the other hand, CtsW protein expression was very stable, and in the case of 769-P cells, it decreased. We can speculate that in the case of CtsB and L, the proteolytic inhibition, induced by the peptides, was counterbalanced by an over-expression of these proteins. This rule was not to apply to CtsW that probably follows other mechanisms of expression regulation [37]. In addition, our data demonstrated a weaker interaction of the inhibitors in the case of the CtsW active site. Compared to other Cts, CtsW was shown to be significantly localized in the endoplasmic reticulum of immune cells [36], and this evidence could form the basis of its differential regulation.

From the pharmacological standpoint, the development of these inhibitors could provide new avenues of research to develop targeted therapies aimed at inhibiting cancer cell proteostasis while impacting their overall phenotype since they showed to affect cell migration and increasing adhesion and expression of E-Cadherin.

Future work is required to take into consideration the potential side effects of this treatment strategy and its impact on cancer biology in vivo, evaluating the peptides' synergistic effects with current chemotherapeutics, as well as revealing their effects on renal cancer spreading. In addition, more insights are necessary to evaluate their overall effect on the endolysosomal compartment stability, integrity, function (i.e., autophagy) as well on the cell metabolism. On the other hand, the generation of new Cts inhibitors could provide fundamental insights into understanding lysosomal biology and lysosomal-related conditions. In particular, more evidence is necessary to unveil the role of the inhibitors in regulating Cts expression as well as lysosomal turnover, as previously demonstrated by other works [58].

4. Materials and Methods

4.1. Docking Studies

Crystal structures of CtsB (6AY2) and L (2XU4) were obtained from the PDB databank. The CtsW structure was predicted using Modeller [68,69]. CtsB was used as a template structure. All protein structures were protonated with PROPKA at PDB2PQR server at pH 4.5, 6.5, and 7.2 [69]. Ligand structures were built and optimized in the GAFF force field using Avogadro [70,71].

Docking was performed using PLANTS [72]. The Chemplp scoring function was used in combination with search speed 1. The binding center was set at the SG atom of catalytic cysteine of all considered Cts. Both catalytic cysteine and histidine were set as flexible. When docking with constraints, simple distance constraints between the oxygen atom in the FMK group and atoms H in the catalytic cysteine or amine hydrogens of Gln-23/19/20 in CtsB/L/W were used. The constraint was applied for the distance between 1 and 3 Å. For each ligand, five poses per run were obtained. Ten runs per pH per protein per ligand were made.

4.2. Protein Expression and Purification

Total RNA extract from retinoblastoma J79 cells was used to obtain cDNA. A pair of oligonucleotides (TATACATATGCGGAGCAGGCCCTCTTTC and CTCGAGTTAGATCTTTTCCCAGTACTG) was used for the amplification of DNA fragment containing CtsB, the product of which was ligated into pET15b (Merck Millipore, Billerica, MA, USA) using NdeI and XhoI. DNA fragment containing CtsL was amplified using a pair of oligonucleotides (TATAGCTAGCACTCTAACATTTGATCACAGTTT and ATTAAGCTTTCACACAGTGGGGTAGCTG) and ligated into pET28a (+) (Merck Millipore, Billerica, MA, USA) using NheI and HindIII. After the transformation of obtained vectors into Rosetta gammy B(DE3) cells (Merck Millipore, Billerica, MA, USA), these *E. coli* strains were used for the expression of 6His-tagged CathB or CathL using a procedure described by Gorokhovets et al. (2017) for the expression of 6His-tagged papain-like cysteine protease triticain-α [23]. CtsB or CtsL from the insoluble fraction were purified using Ni-NTA sepharose and then refolded using the methods described in detail for protease triticain-α in Gorokhovets et al. (2017).

4.3. Gelatin Zymography

A 5× non-reducing loading buffer (0.05% bromophenol blue, 10% SDS, 1.5 M Tris, 50% glycerol) was added to all recombinant proteins: CtsL and B and prior to loading. Then, the proteins were resolved by 12% SDS-polyacrylamide gels containing 0.2% gelatin at 4 °C. Gels were removed, and enzymes were refolded for four washes in 2.5% Triton-X100, 15 min each. Next, the gels were washed twice and incubated in activating buffer (NaAc, pH 4.8, 1 mM EDTA, and 20 mM L-cysteine hydrochloride monohydrate) for 24 h at 37 °C. In the morning, the gels were fixed for 1 h in 50% methanol with 10% acetic acid and then stained for 1 h in Coomassie (10% acetic acid, 25% isopropanol, 4.5% Coomassie Blue). The gels were destained in 10% isopropanol and 10% acetic acid and scanned using the Bio-Rad ChemiDoc MP Imaging System.

4.4. Cathepsin Inhibitors

Specific inhibitors for cysteine Cts were developed with the help of computer-graphic modeling, based on the structure of the proteins. The two peptides, Ac-PLVE-FMK and Ac-VLPE-FMK were selected as the specific inhibitors, that provide a binding affinity to Cts and can block their activity. The inhibitors were synthesized by Pepmic (Pepmic Suzhou Jiangsu, China).

4.5. Enzymatic Kinetic Studies

The activity of recombinant CtsL and B was detected by the hydrolysis of the fluorogenic substrate Ac-Pro-Leu-Val-Gln- 7-amino-4-methylcoumarin (AMC) (Pepmic Suzhou Jiangsu, China). A total of 20 nM of each protein was mixed in a 96-well plate with 0.1 M sodium acetic buffer (100 mM NaCl, 0.5% DMSO, 0.6 mM EDTA pH 4.6) in the presence or absence of cysteine Cts inhibitor at a final concentration of 2 μM. The substrate was added to a final concentration of 50 μM, and its hydrolysis was continuously measured for 12 min using a CLARIOstar® Plus plate reader (BMG Labtech Ortenberg Baden-Württemberg, Germany) at excitation and emission wavelengths of 353 and 442 nm, respectively.

4.6. Cell Culture

The human renal cancer cell line lines 786-P, A498 were obtained from Dr. Vadim Pokrovsky (purchased from American Type Culture Collection). The cells were cultured in RPMI 1640, supplemented with 10% fetal bovine serum and 1% mixture of antibiotics penicillin-streptomycin (all from Gibco, Waltham, MA, USA) at 5% CO_2 and 37 °C in a humidified chamber. Cells were grown to confluence and harvested by trypsinization, using a 0.25 mg/mL trypsin/EDTA solution (ThermoFisher, Carlsbad, CA, USA) and resuspended in the fresh culture medium. Viable cells were enumerated on the Countess II FL Automated Cell Counter (ThermoFisher, Waltham, MA, USA), following Trypan Blue staining. The cell lines were tested for mycoplasma contamination regularly, using the Molecular Probes™ MycoFluor Mycoplasma Detection Kit (ThermoFisher, Waltham, MA, USA).

4.7. MTT

The cell number was evaluated by counting viable cells using the MTT (3-(4,5-dimethylthiazol-2-yl)-2,5-diphenyltetrazolium bromide) colorimetric assay. A total of 2×10^4 cells/well were seeded on independent 96-well plates for each time point (0, 24, 48, and 72 h), with five replicates and treated with two inhibitors (2.5–250 μM). Then, 10 μL of the MTT reagent was added to each well, and cells were incubated for another 5 h. Next, the absorbance value was measured using a CLARIOstar® Plus plate reader (BMG Labtech, Ortenberg, Germany) at 490 nm. Triplicate wells were assayed, and S.D.s were determined.

4.8. RNA Extraction and cDNA Synthesis

Total RNA was extracted from cells using the Total RNA isolation kit (Evrogen, Moscow, Russia). Complementary DNA (cDNA) was transcribed from mRNA using a cDNA synthesis kit (Evrogen, Moscow, Russia), according to the manufacturer's protocols. For RT reaction 1 μg of total RNA was used with optical density OD260/OD280 1.7-2.0 measured with NanoDrop One (ThermoFisher, Waltham, MA, USA).

4.9. *Western Blot Analysis*

Cells were seeded in RPMI containing 10% FBS and cultured for 24 h. Next, 30 μM of inhibitors were added to the culture medium and incubated for 24, 48, and 72 h. Control cells were treated with 0.01% DMSO. At all time points the samples were lysed in 50 mM Tri-HCl (pH 8.0), 100 mM NaCl, 0.5% NP-40, 1% Triton X-100, 1× protease inhibitor cocktail (ThermoFisher, Waltham, MA, USA). The 50 μg of protein lysates were separated by electrophoresis on a 12% SDS-PAGE gel and transferred to the PFDF membranes. The expression of cysteine Cts, LAMP-1, E-cadherin, and SNAIL1 were identified by a reaction with specific primary antibodies (CtsB-Ab190077, Abcam, UK; CtsL-Ab95154, Abcam, UK; CtsW Ab191083; LAMP-1- Ab24170, Abcam, UK; SNAIL1 Ab216347, Abcam, UK and e-cadherin-612131, BD Sciences Franklin Lakes, NJ, USA) which were resuspended in 5% non-fat milk in PBST (all Cts 1:3000, LAMP-1, SNAIL1 and E-cadherin 1:1000) and incubated O/N. The next day, the membranes were washed three times with PBST and incubated for 1 h with secondary antibodies (P-GAR Iss (Goat pAb to rabbit IgG (HRP), Abcam, UK or Rabbit Ab to mouse, Abcam, UK; both 1:5000) in 5% non-fat milk in PBST. After an additional wash (three times with PBS), reactive bands were detected by chemiluminescence (Bio-Rad, Irvine, CA, USA). As a loading control, the membranes were incubated with a polyclonal anti-tubulin antibody (1:5000; Ab52866, Abcam, UK) identically.

4.10. *Immunofluorescence Staining*

The cells were treated for 48 and 72 h, then were fixed in 4% PFA/PBS for 15 min and permeabilized in 0.25% Triton®X-100 for 10 min. After blocking the non-specific sites in 2% BSA/PBS-T, the immunofluorescence was performed overnight with primary antibody anti-LAMP-1 (1:100, Abcam, Eugene, OR, USA) incubation, followed by incubation with the appropriate fluorophore-labeled secondary antibody Donkey anti-Rabbit IgG (H+L) ReadyProbes™, Alexa Fluor 488 (1:500; ThermoFisher, USA). The cells were then counterstained with nuclear dye DAPI and visualized under a fluorescent and/or confocal microscope (Olympus BX51, Shinjuku, Tokyo, Japan, and AxioObserver Z1, Zeiss, Oberkochen, Germany) using oil-immersion lenses.

4.11. *AFM Measurements*

Before the AFM experiments, the 50,000 cells were seeded per dish and treated for 48 and 72 h with inhibitors. The AFM measurements were performed at 37 °C, using a commercial atomic force microscope Bioscope Resolve AFM (Bruker, Billerica, MA, USA) combined with an inverted optical microscope (Carl Zeiss, Ulm, Germany). The PeakForce QNM-Live Cell cantilevers (PFQNM-LC-A-CAL, Bruker AFM Probes, USA) with a pre-calibrated spring constant (in a range of 0.06–0.08 N/m) and a 70 nm tip radius was used. The deflection sensitivity (nm/V) was calibrated from the thermal using the pre-calibrated value of the spring constant. The nanomechanical maps were acquired in the force volume mode with a typical map size of 80 × 80 microns and 40 × 40 measurement points [73]. For the force curves, a vertical ramp distance was 3 μm, a vertical piezo speed was 183 μm/s, and the trigger force was 0.5–1 nN. The Young's modulus (E) was calculated by fitting the force curves with the Hertz model with a bottom-effect correction [73,74].

4.12. *Scratch Assay*

The cells were treated for 48 h with Cts inhibitors in a six-well plate. At experimental time zero, a scratch of culture monolayer was made in each well using a pipette tip. The monolayers were washed with PBS to remove detached cells and cell debris and next refilled with growth medium, including Cts inhibitors. The wells were imaged at time zero and again 6 and 24 h later. Using ImageJ, a measurement was taken for how much the denuded area had filled after 6 and 24 h.

4.13. Colony-Forming Assay

769-P and A498 cells were treated 48 h with 30 μM Ac-PLVE-FMK or Ac-VLPE-FMK, next calculated, and 300 cells were placed on 10 cm plates. Cells were maintained in the completed medium with inhibitors for the 10 days, then fixed with 4% paraformaldehyde and stained with 0.4% Crystal Violet solution, finally photographed.

4.14. Spheroids Formation Assay

The 769-P cells were treated for 48 h with Cts inhibitors and next suspended in 2% Matrigel in the total medium containing 30 μM Ac-PLVE-FMK or Ac-VLPE-FMK. The 100 prepared cells were seeded in 96-well microplates on top of 50 μL Matrigel (Corning, NY, USA) and incubated for 6 days. The formed spheroids were imaged under an Olympus IX71 microscope, and their number, size, and circularity were measured using ImageJ software. Each experiment had two replicates and was repeated three times.

4.15. Adhesion

The 96-well plates were coated with either 15 μg/mL collagen IV (Imtek, Moscow, Russia) or Matrigel 0.5% in RPMI-1640 (Corning, NY, USA) and stored at 4 °C O/N. On the day of the assay, plates were washed twice with PBS and 40,000 cells/well were seeded and incubated for 50 min at 37 °C. Adherent cells were fixed and stained with 0.2% crystal violet/10% ethanol and read at 485 nm on a microplate reader. All the experiments were performed in triplicate.

4.16. LysoTracker Red Fluorescence Measurement

First, 1.5×10^4 769-P or A498 cells were seeded in 96-well plates in full medium. The day after the cells were treated with the peptides for 3 consecutive days to establish 24, 48, and 72 h groups of treatment. LysoTracker Red fluorescence intensity was measured via microplate reader following the protocols described in [75] and applying Ex/Em = 570/600. The cells were incubated with 75 nM of LysoTracker red for 1 h.

4.17. Statistical Analysis

All experiments were repeated at least three times. Data are reported as mean ± SD. Data were analyzed using one-way ANOVA, followed by Dunnet's test (GraphPad, Prism 6.00 for Windows, Graf Pad software, San Diego, CA, USA). The p-value of <0.05 was considered statistically significant. with *, similarly $p < 0.01$ with ** and $p < 0.001$ with ***.

5. Conclusions

Recently, it has been recognized that the pathogenic function of Cts in cancerogenesis is far more complicated than initially conceived [76]. Experimental studies have shown that many Cts are overexpressed in different tumor types, frustrating every attempt to precisely correlate the role of single Cts with the disease development [77]. In this work, we generated two novel peptides with wide-ranging inhibitory properties towards Cts that could provide new resources to develop new treatments. In particular, they could improve current treatments for conditions such as renal cancer that is resistant to standard chemotherapeutic approaches and could benefit from novel targeted therapies [30,78]. Despite their low cytostatic power, these small inhibitors demonstrated broad inhibiting properties, high membrane permeability, minimal toxicity, and above all, a significant impact on cancer cell phenotype.

Our data demonstrated that the peptides could inhibit Cts activity in two different human renal cancer cell lines impacting their motility, anchorage-independent growth, colony formation, and their adhesion. More importantly, this strategy affected Cts expression, and this evidence should be taken into consideration when similar treatment strategies are designed for cancer and other diseases.

Supplementary Materials:
Figure S1: Detection of recombinant human CtsL and B activity through gelatin zymography assay. Recombinant purified human CtsL and B were loaded on the gelatin-gel zymogram. The Cts were activated through incubation of gel in an activating buffer (pH 4.8). Further staining with Coomassie brilliant blue G-250 showed the induction of proteolytic activity as bright white bands on dark background in correspondence with the bands of the enzymes, Figure S2. Determination of the peptide inhibitory properties against human purified CtsB and L. The activities of human recombinant CtsB and L, were measured via fluorimetric analysis by exploiting the fluorogenic properties of the Triticain-α substrate Ac-PLVQ-AMC. In the assay, the 20 nM of recombinant human CtsL and CtsB were incubated with 50 μM substrate without Cts inhibitors (red line) and with Ac-PLVE-FMK and Ac-VLPE-FMK (blue and green line, respectively) at a concentration of 2 μM. Fluorescence was measured as relative as relative fluorescence unit (RFU), Figure S3. Combined effect of PXT and the inhibitors on 769-P proliferation: 769-P cells were treated with 100 nM of PXT alone or in combination with 20 μM of Ac-PLVE and Ac-VLPE and cell proliferation was measured after 24, 48, and 72 h via MTT assay. Data represent the mean (± S.D.) of three independent experiments, each performed in triplicate, Figure S4. Spheroids size and circularity: (**a**,**b**) size and circularity of 769-P and (**c**,**d**) A498 cells upon treatment with Ac-PLVE-FMK and Ac-VLPE-FMK. Data represent the mean (±S.D.) of three independent experiments, each performed in triplicate, Figure S5. Effect of Cts inhibitory peptides on cell stiffness: representative optical phase contrast image of cells (first row) and stiffness maps determined by indentation (Young's modulus) of 769-P cells (second row) with and without treatment with PLVE and VLPE. Calibration bars represent 25 μm. The graph shows the values of Young's modulus of all analyzed samples, data are expressed as mean (± S.D.) and significance was calculated through one-way ANOVA followed by Dunnet's test. * = $p < 0.05$, ** = $p < 0.01$, Figure S6. The effect of the peptide inhibitors on human 769-P and A498 renal cancer cell on lysosomes integrity. (**a**) 769-P and (**b**) A498 cells were treated with increasing doses of Ac-PLVE-FMK (red bars) and Ac-VLPE-FMK (blue bars) (2.5–250 μM). NR uptake was measured after 24, 48, and 72 h via MTT assay. (**c**) LysoTracker red evaluation in 769-P and (**d**) A498 cells after 24, 48, and 72 h with the inhibitors (20 μM). Data represent the mean (± S.D.) of at least three independent experiments, each performed in triplicate, Figure S7. Uncropped western blots.

Author Contributions: Conceptualization, A.A.Z., M.R. and A.P.; methodology, M.R., A.P., Y.M.E., N.V.G., V.A.M., E.Y.Z.; software, V.D.M., A.V.G.; validation A.A.Z., A.P., M.R.; formal analysis, A.P., M.R.; investigation, M.R., A.P., V.D.M., A.V.G., A.A.Z.; resources, A.A.Z.; data curation, M.R., A.P.; writing—original draft preparation, A.P., M.R.; writing—review and editing, A.P., M.R., A.A.Z., V.D.M., A.V.G., Y.M.E., E.Y.Z.; visualization, V.A.P., M.R.; supervision, A.A.Z.; project administration, A.A.Z.; funding acquisition, A.A.Z. All authors have read and agreed to the published version of the manuscript.

Acknowledgments: We thank Peter S. Timashev for fruitful discussions in relation to this paper.

References

1. Nägler, D.K.; Ménard, R. Family C1 cysteine proteases: Biological diversity or redundancy? *Biol. Chem.* **2003**, *384*, 837–843. [CrossRef] [PubMed]
2. Fonović, M.; Turk, B. Cysteine cathepsins and extracellular matrix degradation. *Biochim. Biophys. Acta (BBA)-Gen. Subj.* **2014**, *1840*, 2560–2570. [CrossRef] [PubMed]
3. Verma, S.; Dixit, R.; Pandey, K.C. Cysteine proteases: Modes of activation and future prospects as pharmacological targets. *Front. Pharmacol.* **2016**, *7*, 107. [CrossRef] [PubMed]
4. Rudzińska, M.; Parodi, A.; Soond, S.M.; Vinarov, A.Z.; Korolev, D.O.; Morozov, A.O.; Daglioglu, C.; Tutar, Y.; Zamyatnin, A.A. The role of cysteine cathepsins in cancer progression and drug resistance. *Int. J. Mol. Sci.* **2019**, *20*, 3602. [CrossRef]
5. Gocheva, V.; Joyce, J.A. Cysteine cathepsins and the cutting edge of cancer invasion. *Cell Cycle* **2007**, *6*, 60–64. [CrossRef]
6. Chen, S.; Dong, H.; Yang, S.; Guo, H. Cathepsins in digestive cancers. *Oncotarget* **2017**, *8*, 41690. [CrossRef]
7. Jennifer, E.K.; Mamoun, A.; Bonnie, F.S. Unraveling the role of proteases in cancer. *Clin. Chim. Acta* **2000**, *291*, 113–135.
8. Kos, J.; Jevnikar, Z.; Obermajer, N. The role of cathepsin X in cell signaling. *Cell Adhes. Migr.* **2009**, *3*, 164–166. [CrossRef]
9. Chwieralski, C.; Welte, T.; Bühling, F. Cathepsin-regulated apoptosis. *Apoptosis* **2006**, *11*, 143–149. [CrossRef]
10. Lamparska-Przybysz, M.; Gajkowska, B.; Motyl, T. Cathepsins and B.I.D. are involved in the molecular switch between apoptosis and autophagy in breast cancer MCF-7 cells exposed to camptothecin. *J. Physiol. Pharmacol.* **2005**, *56*, 159.
11. Bengsch, F.; Buck, A.; Günther, S.; Seiz, J.; Tacke, M.; Pfeifer, D.; Von Elverfeldt, D.; Sevenich, L.; Hillebrand, L.; Kern, U. Cell type-dependent pathogenic functions of overexpressed human cathepsin B in murine breast cancer progression. *Oncogene* **2014**, *33*, 4474–4484. [CrossRef] [PubMed]

12. Ruffell, B.; Affara, N.I.; Cottone, L.; Junankar, S.; Johansson, M.; DeNardo, D.G.; Korets, L.; Reinheckel, T.; Sloane, B.F.; Bogyo, M. Cathepsin C is a tissue-specific regulator of squamous carcinogenesis. *Genes Dev.* **2013**, *27*, 2086–2098. [CrossRef] [PubMed]
13. Sudhan, D.R.; Siemann, D.W. Cathepsin L targeting in cancer treatment. *Pharmacol. Ther.* **2015**, *155*, 105–116. [CrossRef] [PubMed]
14. Zhang, L.; Wang, H.; Xu, J. Cathepsin S as a cancer target. *Neoplasma* **2015**, *62*, 16–26. [CrossRef] [PubMed]
15. Vasiljeva, O.; Turk, B. Dual contrasting roles of cysteine cathepsins in cancer progression: Apoptosis versus tumour invasion. *Biochimie* **2008**, *90*, 380–386. [CrossRef]
16. Petushkova, A.; Savvateeva, L.; Korolev, D.; Zamyatnin, A. Cysteine cathepsins: Potential applications in diagnostics and therapy of malignant tumors. *Biochemistry* **2019**, *84*, 746–761. [CrossRef]
17. Zhang, J.; Zhou, W.; Lin, J.; Wei, P.; Zhang, Y.; Jin, P.; Chen, M.; Man, N.; Wen, L. Autophagic lysosomal reformation depends on mTOR reactivation in H2O2-induced autophagy. *Int. J. Biochem. Cell Biol.* **2016**, *70*, 76–81. [CrossRef]
18. Mediavilla-Varela, M.; Pacheco, F.J.; Almaguel, F.; Perez, J.; Sahakian, E.; Daniels, T.R.; Leoh, L.S.; Padilla, A.; Wall, N.R.; Lilly, M.B. Docetaxel-induced prostate cancer cell death involves concomitant activation of caspase and lysosomal pathways and is attenuated by LEDGF/p75. *Mol. Cancer* **2009**, *8*, 68. [CrossRef]
19. Giusti, I.; D'Ascenzo, S.; Millimaggi, D.; Taraboletti, G.; Carta, G.; Franceschini, N.; Pavan, A.; Dolo, V. Cathepsin B mediates the pH-dependent proinvasive activity of tumor-shed microvesicles. *Neoplasia* **2008**, *10*, 481. [CrossRef]
20. Sullivan, S.; Tosetto, M.; Kevans, D.; Coss, A.; Wang, L.; O'Donoghue, D.; Hyland, J.; Sheahan, K.; Mulcahy, H.; O'Sullivan, J. Localization of nuclear cathepsin L and its association with disease progression and poor outcome in colorectal cancer. *Int. J. Cancer* **2009**, *125*, 54–61. [CrossRef]
21. Akkari, L.; Gocheva, V.; Quick, M.L.; Kester, J.C.; Spencer, A.K.; Garfall, A.L.; Bowman, R.L.; Joyce, J.A. Combined deletion of cathepsin protease family members reveals compensatory mechanisms in cancer. *Genes Dev.* **2016**, *30*, 220–232. [CrossRef] [PubMed]
22. Schurigt, U.; Hummel, K.M.; Petrow, P.K.; Gajda, M.; Stöckigt, R.; Middel, P.; Zwerina, J.; Janik, T.; Bernhardt, R.; Schüler, S. Cathepsin K deficiency partially inhibits, but does not prevent, bone destruction in human tumor necrosis factor–transgenic mice. *Arthritis Rheum. Off. J. Am. Coll. Rheumatol.* **2008**, *58*, 422–434. [CrossRef] [PubMed]
23. Gorokhovets, N.V.; Makarov, V.A.; Petushkova, A.I.; Prokopets, O.S.; Rubtsov, M.A.; Savvateeva, L.V.; Zernii, E.Y.; Zamyatnin, A.A., Jr. Rational design of recombinant papain-like cysteine protease: Optimal domain structure and expression conditions for wheat-derived enzyme triticain-α. *Int. J. Mol. Sci.* **2017**, *18*, 1395. [CrossRef] [PubMed]
24. Fransolet, M.; Henry, L.; Labied, S.; Noël, A.; Nisolle, M.; Munaut, C. In vitro evaluation of the anti-apoptotic drug Z-VAD-FMK on human ovarian granulosa cell lines for further use in ovarian tissue transplantation. *J. Assist. Reprod. Genet.* **2015**, *32*, 1551–1559. [CrossRef]
25. Rasnick, D. Synthesis of peptide fluoromethyl ketones and the inhibition of human cathepsin B. *Anal. Biochem.* **1985**, *149*, 461–465. [CrossRef]
26. Arafet, K.; Ferrer, S.; Moliner, V. First quantum mechanics/molecular mechanics studies of the inhibition mechanism of cruzain by peptidyl halomethyl ketones. *Biochemistry* **2015**, *54*, 3381–3391. [CrossRef]
27. Cocchiaro, P.; De Pasquale, V.; Della Morte, R.; Tafuri, S.; Avallone, L.; Pizard, A.; Moles, A.; Pavone, L.M. The multifaceted role of the lysosomal protease cathepsins in kidney disease. *Front. Cell Dev. Biol.* **2017**, *5*, 114. [CrossRef]
28. Golovastova, M.O.; Korolev, D.O.; Tsoy, L.V.; Varshavsky, V.A.; Xu, W.-H.; Vinarov, A.Z.; Zernii, E.Y.; Philippov, P.P.; Zamyatnin, A.A. Biomarkers of renal tumors: The current state and clinical perspectives. *Curr. Urol. Rep.* **2017**, *18*, 3. [CrossRef]
29. Blecher, G.; McDermott, K.; Challacombe, B. Renal cancer. *Surgery* **2019**, *37*, 508–512.
30. Makhov, P.; Joshi, S.; Ghatalia, P.; Kutikov, A.; Uzzo, R.G.; Kolenko, V.M. Resistance to systemic therapies in clear cell renal cell carcinoma: Mechanisms and management strategies. *Mol. Cancer Ther.* **2018**, *17*, 1355–1364. [CrossRef]
31. Korb, O.; Stutzle, T.; Exner, T.E. Empirical scoring functions for advanced protein—Ligand docking with PLANTS. *J. Chem. Inf. Modeling* **2009**, *49*, 84–96. [CrossRef] [PubMed]

32. Kilambi, K.P.; Reddy, K.; Gray, J.J. Protein-protein docking with dynamic residue protonation states. *PLoS Comput. Biol.* **2014**, *10*. [CrossRef] [PubMed]
33. Chen, C.-H.; Bhasin, S.; Khanna, P.; Joshi, M.; Joslin, P.M.; Saxena, R.; Amin, S.; Liu, S.; Sindhu, S.; Walker, S.R. Study of Cathepsin B inhibition in VEGFR TKI treated human renal cell carcinoma xenografts. *Oncogenesis* **2019**, *8*, 1–18. [CrossRef] [PubMed]
34. Giuliano, S.; Cormerais, Y.; Dufies, M.; Grépin, R.; Colosetti, P.; Belaid, A.; Parola, J.; Martin, A.; Lacas-Gervais, S.; Mazure, N.M. Resistance to sunitinib in renal clear cell carcinoma results from sequestration in lysosomes and inhibition of the autophagic flux. *Autophagy* **2015**, *11*, 1891–1904. [CrossRef] [PubMed]
35. Uhlen, M.; Zhang, C.; Lee, S.; Sjöstedt, E.; Fagerberg, L.; Bidkhori, G.; Benfeitas, R.; Arif, M.; Liu, Z.; Edfors, F. A pathology atlas of the human cancer transcriptome. *Science* **2017**, *357*, eaan2507. [CrossRef]
36. Wex, T.; Bühling, F.; Wex, H.; Günther, D.; Malfertheiner, P.; Weber, E.; Brömme, D. Human cathepsin W, a cysteine protease predominantly expressed in N.K. cells, is mainly localized in the endoplasmic reticulum. *J. Immunol.* **2001**, *167*, 2172–2178. [CrossRef]
37. Wex, T.; Levy, B.; Brömme, D. Human cathepsins W and F form a new subgroup of cathepsins that is evolutionary separated from the cathepsin B-and L-like cysteine proteases. In *Cellular Peptidases in Immune Functions and Diseases 2*; Springer: Berlin, Germany, 2002; Volume 477, pp. 271–280.
38. Jung, Y.-S.; Chun, H.-Y.; Yoon, M.-H.; Park, B.-J. Elevated estrogen receptor-α in VHL-deficient condition induces microtubule organizing center amplification via disruption of BRCA1/Rad51 interaction. *Neoplasia* **2014**, *16*, 1070–1081. [CrossRef]
39. Elie, B.T.; Pechenyy, Y.; Uddin, F.; Contel, M. A heterometallic ruthenium–gold complex displays antiproliferative, antimigratory, and antiangiogenic properties and inhibits metastasis and angiogenesis-associated proteases in renal cancer. *JBIC J. Biol. Inorg. Chem.* **2018**, *23*, 399–411. [CrossRef]
40. Sevenich, L.; Schurigt, U.; Sachse, K.; Gajda, M.; Werner, F.; Müller, S.; Vasiljeva, O.; Schwinde, A.; Klemm, N.; Deussing, J. Synergistic antitumor effects of combined cathepsin B and cathepsin Z deficiencies on breast cancer progression and metastasis in mice. *Proc. Natl. Acad. Sci. USA* **2010**, *107*, 2497–2502. [CrossRef]
41. Kuester, D.; Lippert, H.; Roessner, A.; Krueger, S. The cathepsin family and their role in colorectal cancer. *Pathol.-Res. Pract.* **2008**, *204*, 491–500. [CrossRef]
42. Gondi, C.S.; Rao, J.S. Cathepsin B as a cancer target. *Expert Opin. Ther. Targets* **2013**, *17*, 281–291. [CrossRef] [PubMed]
43. Lechner, A.M.; Assfalg-Machleidt, I.; Zahler, S.; Stoeckelhuber, M.; Machleidt, W.; Jochum, M.; Nägler, D.K. RGD-dependent binding of procathepsin X to integrin αvβ3 mediates cell-adhesive properties. *J. Biol. Chem.* **2006**, *281*, 39588–39597. [CrossRef] [PubMed]
44. Wang, J.; Chen, L.; Li, Y.; Guan, X.-Y. Overexpression of cathepsin Z contributes to tumor metastasis by inducing epithelial-mesenchymal transition in hepatocellular carcinoma. *PLoS ONE* **2011**, *6*. [CrossRef] [PubMed]
45. Vidak, E.; Javoršek, U.; Vizovišek, M.; Turk, B. Cysteine cathepsins and their extracellular roles: Shaping the microenvironment. *Cells* **2019**, *8*, 264. [CrossRef]
46. Tamhane, T.; Lu, S.; Maelandsmo, G.M.; Haugen, M.H.; Brix, K. Nuclear cathepsin L activity is required for cell cycle progression of colorectal carcinoma cells. *Biochimie* **2016**, *122*, 208–218. [CrossRef]
47. Araujo, T.F.; Cordeiro, A.V.; Vasconcelos, D.A.; Vitzel, K.F.; Silva, V.R. The role of cathepsin B in autophagy during obesity: A systematic review. *Life Sci.* **2018**, *209*, 274–281. [CrossRef]
48. De Castro, M.; Bunt, G.; Wouters, F. Cathepsin B launches an apoptotic exit effort upon cell death-associated disruption of lysosomes. *Cell Death Discov.* **2016**, *2*, 1–8. [CrossRef]
49. De Mingo, Á.; De Gregorio, E.; Moles, A.; Tarrats, N.; Tutusaus, A.; Colell, A.; Fernandez-Checa, J.C.; Morales, A.; Marí, M. Cysteine cathepsins control hepatic NF-κ B-dependent inflammation via sirtuin-1 regulation. *Cell Death Dis.* **2016**, *7*, e2464. [CrossRef]
50. Huang, C.-C.; Lee, C.-C.; Lin, H.-H.; Chang, J.-Y. Cathepsin S attenuates endosomal EGFR signalling: A mechanical rationale for the combination of cathepsin S and EGFR tyrosine kinase inhibitors. *Sci. Rep.* **2016**, *6*, 1–12. [CrossRef]
51. Sudhan, D.R.; Rabaglino, M.B.; Wood, C.E.; Siemann, D.W. Cathepsin L in tumor angiogenesis and its therapeutic intervention by the small molecule inhibitor KGP94. *Clin. Exp. Metastasis* **2016**, *33*, 461–473. [CrossRef]

52. Sheahan, K.; Shuja, S.; Murnane, M.J. Cysteine protease activities and tumor development in human colorectal carcinoma. *Cancer Res.* **1989**, *49*, 3809–3814. [PubMed]
53. Ross, H.; Argani, P. Xp11 translocation renal cell carcinoma. *Pathology* **2010**, *42*, 369–373. [CrossRef]
54. Allan, E.R.O.; Yates, R.M. Redundancy between cysteine cathepsins in murine experimental autoimmune encephalomyelitis. *PLoS ONE* **2015**, *10*. [CrossRef] [PubMed]
55. Friedrichs, B.; Tepel, C.; Reinheckel, T.; Deussing, J.; von Figura, K.; Herzog, V.; Peters, C.; Saftig, P.; Brix, K. Thyroid functions of mouse cathepsins B, K, and L. *J. Clin. Investig.* **2003**, *111*, 1733–1745. [CrossRef] [PubMed]
56. Shaw, E.; Angliker, H.; Rauber, P.; Walker, B.; Wikstrom, P. Peptidyl fluoromethyl ketones as thiol protease inhibitors. *Biomed. Biochim. Acta* **1986**, *45*, 1397–1403.
57. Saikia, S.; Bordoloi, M. Molecular docking: Challenges, advances and its use in drug discovery perspective. *Curr. Drug Targets* **2019**, *20*, 501–521. [CrossRef]
58. Jung, M.; Lee, J.; Seo, H.-Y.; Lim, J.S.; Kim, E.-K. Cathepsin inhibition-induced lysosomal dysfunction enhances pancreatic beta-cell apoptosis in high glucose. *PLoS ONE* **2015**, *10*. [CrossRef]
59. Bell-McGuinn, K.M.; Garfall, A.L.; Bogyo, M.; Hanahan, D.; Joyce, J.A. Inhibition of cysteine cathepsin protease activity enhances chemotherapy regimens by decreasing tumor growth and invasiveness in a mouse model of multistage cancer. *Cancer Res.* **2007**, *67*, 7378–7385. [CrossRef]
60. Bian, B.; Mongrain, S.; Cagnol, S.; Langlois, M.J.; Boulanger, J.; Bernatchez, G.; Carrier, J.C.; Boudreau, F.; Rivard, N. Cathepsin B promotes colorectal tumorigenesis, cell invasion, and metastasis. *Mol. Carcinog.* **2016**, *55*, 671–687. [CrossRef]
61. Zhang, L.; Wei, L.; Shen, G.; He, B.; Gong, W.; Min, N.; Zhang, L.; Duan, Y.; Xie, J.; Luo, H. Cathepsin L is involved in proliferation and invasion of ovarian cancer cells. *Mol. Med. Rep.* **2015**, *11*, 468–474. [CrossRef]
62. Mirza, A.A.; Kahle, M.P.; Ameka, M.; Campbell, E.M.; Cuevas, B.D. MEKK2 regulates focal adhesion stability and motility in invasive breast cancer cells. *Biochim. Biophys. Acta (BBA)-Mol. Cell Res.* **2014**, *1843*, 945–954. [CrossRef] [PubMed]
63. Webb, K.; Hlady, V.; Tresco, P.A. Relationships among cell attachment, spreading, cytoskeletal organization, and migration rate for anchorage-dependent cells on model surfaces. *J. Biomed. Mater. Res. An Off. J. Soc. Biomater. Jpn. Soc. Biomater.* **2000**, *49*, 362–368. [CrossRef]
64. Pišlar, A.; Nanut, M.P.; Kos, J. Lysosomal cysteine peptidases–molecules signaling tumor cell death and survival. *Semin. Cancer Biol.* **2015**, *35*, 168–179. [CrossRef] [PubMed]
65. Zhang, Y.; Sun, B.; Zhao, X.; Sun, H.; Cui, W.; Liu, Z.; Yao, X.; Dong, X. Spheres derived from the human SN12C renal cell carcinoma cell line are enriched in tumor initiating cells. *J. Exp. Clin. Cancer Res.* **2016**, *35*, 163. [CrossRef] [PubMed]
66. Cermak, S.; Kosicek, M.; Mladenovic-Djordjevic, A.; Smiljanic, K.; Kanazir, S.; Hecimovic, S. Loss of Cathepsin B and l leads to lysosomal dysfunction, NPC-like cholesterol sequestration and accumulation of the key Alzheimer's proteins. *PLoS ONE* **2016**, *11*. [CrossRef] [PubMed]
67. Yang, G.; Sun, X.; Liu, J.; Feng, L.; Liu, Z. Light-responsive, singlet-oxygen-triggered on-demand drug release from photosensitizer-doped mesoporous silica nanorods for cancer combination therapy. *Adv. Funct. Mater.* **2016**, *26*, 4722–4732. [CrossRef]
68. Eswar, N.; Webb, B.; Marti-Renom, M.A.; Madhusudhan, M.; Eramian, D.; Shen, M.Y.; Pieper, U.; Sali, A. Comparative protein structure modeling using Modeller. *Curr. Protoc. Bioinform.* **2006**, *15*, 831–860. [CrossRef]
69. Dolinsky, T.J.; Nielsen, J.E.; McCammon, J.A.; Baker, N.A. PDB2PQR: An automated pipeline for the setup of Poisson–Boltzmann electrostatics calculations. *Nucleic Acids Res.* **2004**, *32*, W665–W667. [CrossRef]
70. Hanwell, M.D.; Curtis, D.E.; Lonie, D.C.; Vandermeersch, T.; Zurek, E.; Hutchison, G.R. Avogadro: An advanced semantic chemical editor, visualization, and analysis platform. *J. Cheminformatics* **2012**, *4*, 17. [CrossRef]
71. Wang, J.; Wolf, R.M.; Caldwell, J.W.; Kollman, P.A.; Case, D.A. Development and testing of a general amber force field. *J. Comput. Chem.* **2004**, *25*, 1157–1174. [CrossRef]
72. Korb, O.; Stützle, T.; Exner, T.E. PLANTS: Application of ant colony optimization to structure-based drug design. In Proceedings of the International Workshop on Ant Colony Optimization and Swarm Intelligence, Brussels, Belgium, 4–7 September 2006; pp. 247–258.

73. Efremov, Y.M.; Shpichka, A.; Kotova, S.; Timashev, P. Viscoelastic mapping of cells based on fast force volume and PeakForce Tapping. *Soft Matter* **2019**, *15*, 5455–5463. [CrossRef] [PubMed]
74. Garcia, P.D.; Garcia, R. Determination of the elastic moduli of a single cell cultured on a rigid support by force microscopy. *Biophys. J.* **2018**, *114*, 2923–2932. [CrossRef] [PubMed]
75. Xu, M.; Liu, K.; Swaroop, M.; Sun, W.; Dehdashti, S.J.; McKew, J.C.; Zheng, W. A phenotypic compound screening assay for lysosomal storage diseases. *J. Biomol. Screen.* **2014**, *19*, 168–175. [CrossRef] [PubMed]
76. Sobotič, B.; Vizovišek, M.; Vidmar, R.; Van Damme, P.; Gocheva, V.; Joyce, J.A.; Gevaert, K.; Turk, V.; Turk, B.; Fonović, M. Proteomic identification of cysteine cathepsin substrates shed from the surface of cancer cells. *Mol. Cell. Proteom.* **2015**, *14*, 2213–2228. [CrossRef]
77. Tan, G.-J.; Peng, Z.-K.; Lu, J.-P.; Tang, F.-Q. Cathepsins mediate tumor metastasis. *World J. Biol. Chem.* **2013**, *4*, 91. [CrossRef]
78. Rini, B.I.; Campbell, S.C.; Escudier, B. Renal cell carcinoma. *Lancet* **2009**, *373*, 1119–1132. [CrossRef]

9

Clinical and Pathological Characteristics of Metastatic Renal Cell Carcinoma Patients Needing a Second-Line Therapy

Nicola Longo [1], Marco Capece [1], Giuseppe Celentano [1,*], Roberto La Rocca [1], Gianluigi Califano [1], Claudia Collà Ruvolo [1], Carlo Buonerba [2], Fabio Esposito [1], Luigi Napolitano [1], Francesco Mangiapia [1], Ferdinando Fusco [3], Vincenzo Mirone [1] and Massimiliano Creta [1]

[1] Department of Neurosciences, Science of Reproduction and Odontostomatology, University of Naples Federico II, 80131 Naples, Italy; nicola.longo@unina.it (N.L.); marco.capece@unina.it (M.C.); roberto.larocca@unina.it (R.L.R.); gianl.califano2@gmail.com (G.C.); claudia.collaruvolo@unina.it (C.C.R.); fabio.esposito2@unina.it (F.E.); luigi.napolitano12@studenti.unina.it (L.N.); francesco.mangiapia@unina.it (F.M.); mirone@unina.it (V.M.); massimiliano.creta@unina.it (M.C.)

[2] Department of Clinical Medicine and Surgery, University of Naples Federico II, 80131 Naples, Italy; carlo.buonerba@unina.it

[3] Department of Woman, Child and General and Specialized Surgery, Urology Unit, University of Campania 'Luigi Vanvitelli', 80131 Naples, Italy; ferdinando.fusco@unicampania.it

* Correspondence: giuseppe.celentano2@unina.it

Simple Summary: The management of metastatic renal cell carcinoma (mRCC) represents a clinical challenge. Progression or toxicity may occur during first-line treatments and many patients require a second-line option. Given the expanding options for second-line therapies clinicians are faced with the challenge to individualize treatment. We performed a systematic review in order to summarize available evidences about the clinicopathological profile of mRCC patients who receive a second-line therapy. We identified twenty-nine studies enrolling 7650 patients. Discontinuation of first-line therapy was due to progression in the majority of patients with 77.8% patients harboring ≥2 metastatic sites. Most patients had a good performance status, their age ranged from 55 to 70 years and their prognostic profile revealed a good or intermediate disease in most cases. Tailoring of second-line treatment strategies based on these features is strongly advocated.

Abstract: A high percentage of patients with metastatic renal cell carcinoma (mRCC) require a second-line option. We aimed to summarize available evidences about the clinicopathological profile of mRCC patients who receive a second-line therapy. A systematic review was performed in August 2020. We included papers that met the following criteria: original research; English language; human studies; enrolling mRCC patients entering a second-line therapy. Twenty-nine studies enrolling 7650 patients (73.5% male, mean age: 55 to 70 years) were included. Clear cell histology was reported in 74.4% to 100% of cases. Tyrosine kinase inhibitors, immunotherapy, bevacizumab, mTOR inhibitors, and chemotherapy were adopted as first line option in 68.5%, 29.2%, 2.9%, 0.6%, and 0.2% of patients, respectively. Discontinuation of first-line therapy was due to progression and toxicity in 18.4% to 100% and in 17% to 48.8% of patients, respectively. Eastern Cooperative Oncology Group performance status score was 0 or 1 in most cases. Most prevalent prognostic categories according to the International Metastatic RCC Database Consortium and Memorial Sloan–Kettering Cancer Centre score were intermediate and good. About 77.8% of patients harboured ≥2 metastatic sites. In conclusion, patients who enter a second-line therapy are heterogeneous in terms of a clinical-pathological profile. Tailoring of second-line treatment strategies is strongly advocated.

Keywords: metastatic; renal cell carcinoma; second line therapy

1. Introduction

Renal cell carcinoma (RCC) accounts for about 3% of all cancers, with the highest incidence occurring in Western countries [1–3]. Approximately 25% of patients with RCC present with metastatic disease at diagnosis and up to 20% of those treated for early-stage disease will experience recurrence [1–3]. The overall incidence of metastatic RCC (mRCC) continues to rise by 2% per year. The landscape of therapy for patients with mRCC, has evolved dramatically over the past decade [2]. Prior to 2005, immunotherapy with interleukin-2 (IL-2) and interferon-α (IFN-α) represented the mainstay of therapy and median overall survival was about 1 year [2]. In 2005, the Food and Drug Administration approved sorafenib, the first vascular endothelial growth factor receptor (VEGFR)-targeted tyrosine kinase inhibitor (TKI) for RCC. The approval was closely followed by the introduction of several additional agents for advanced mRCC including other VEGFR-TKIs as well as mammalian target of rapamycin (mTOR) inhibitor therapies. These agents improved median survival estimates to approximately 2.5–3 years [2]. However, the management of mRCC still represents a clinical challenge [3]. Indeed, progression during first-line treatments may occur due to biological resistance mechanisms, and up to 60% of patients with mRCC require a second-line option with different mechanisms of action [3,4]. Moreover, treatment might be interrupted in some patients due to toxicity. In the second-line setting, treatment strategies have initially focused on vascular endothelial growth (VEGF) inhibition or switching toward inhibition of mechanistic target of mTOR [3]. Traditional second-line approaches include the mTOR inhibitor everolimus and axitinib, a selective VEGFR TKI [3]. Since 2015, three new second-line treatments have become available: cabozantinib, a TKI, nivolumab, an immuniocheckpoint inhibitor (ICI), and lenvatinib, a TKI used in combination with everolimus [3]. Given the expanding options for second-line therapies clinicians are facing with the challenge to individualize treatment [3]. Indeed, no conclusive data exist with respect to potential sequencing. The knowledge of demographic and clinical profile of patients with mRCC who enter a second-line therapy is considered of benefit for researchers involved in the identification of novel pharmacological strategies and for clinicians who are asked to personalize treatment strategies [5]. Currently, despite several evidences about molecular mechanisms involved in drug resistance to first-line therapy and clinical efficacy of second-line options in patients with mRCC, there are few evidences describing their demographic and clinical profile of mRCC patients who need a second-line regimen. The present systematic review aims to summarize available evidences about the clinicopathological profile of mRCC patients undergoing a second-line therapy.

2. Evidence Acquisition

This analysis was conducted and reported according to the general guidelines recommended by the Primary Reporting Items for Systematic Reviews and Meta-analyses (PRISMA) statement [6]. On August 2020 we performed a literature review to search for published studies demographic and clinical-pathological profile of mRCC patients who receive a second-line regimen. The search was performed in the Medline (US National Library of Medicine, Bethesda, MD, USA), Scopus (Elsevier, Amsterdam, The Netherlands) databases, and Web of Science Core Collection (Thomson Reuters, Toronto, ON, Canada). The following terms were combined to capture relevant publications: renal cell carcinoma (RCC), metastatic, resistant, toxicity, second line. We included full papers published in the last 15 years that met the following criteria: reporting original research; English language; human studies; enrolling mRCC patients who enter a second-line therapy. Reference lists in relevant articles and reviews were also screened for additional studies. Abstracts (with no subsequent full-text publications) and unpublished studies were not considered. Two authors (GC, CCR) reviewed the records separately and individually to select relevant publications, with any discrepancies resolved by a third author

(NL). The following data were extracted from the studies included: first author, year of publication, enrollment period, sample size, ethnic origin, age, gender, tumor histology, tumor stage and grade, prior nephrectomy, first-line regimen, first-line progression free survival, first-line objective response rate, reasons for discontinuation, Eastern Cooperative Oncology Group performance status (ECOG PS) score, Memorial Sloan-Kettering Cancer Centre (MSKCC) score, International Metastatic Renal Cell Carcinoma Database Consortium (IMDC) score, number and site of metastatic sites, second line regimen. The quality of included studies was assessed using the Methodological Index for Non-Randomized Studies (MINORS) and the Jadad scores for non-randomized and randomized studies, respectively [7,8]. Ethical approval and patients' consent were not required for the present study.

3. Evidence Synthesis

The search strategy revealed a total of 745 results. The screening of the titles and the abstracts defined 75 papers eligible for inclusion. Further assessment of eligibility, based on the study of the full-text papers, led to the exclusion of 46 papers. Twenty-nine studies were then included in the final analysis [9–37] (Figure 1).

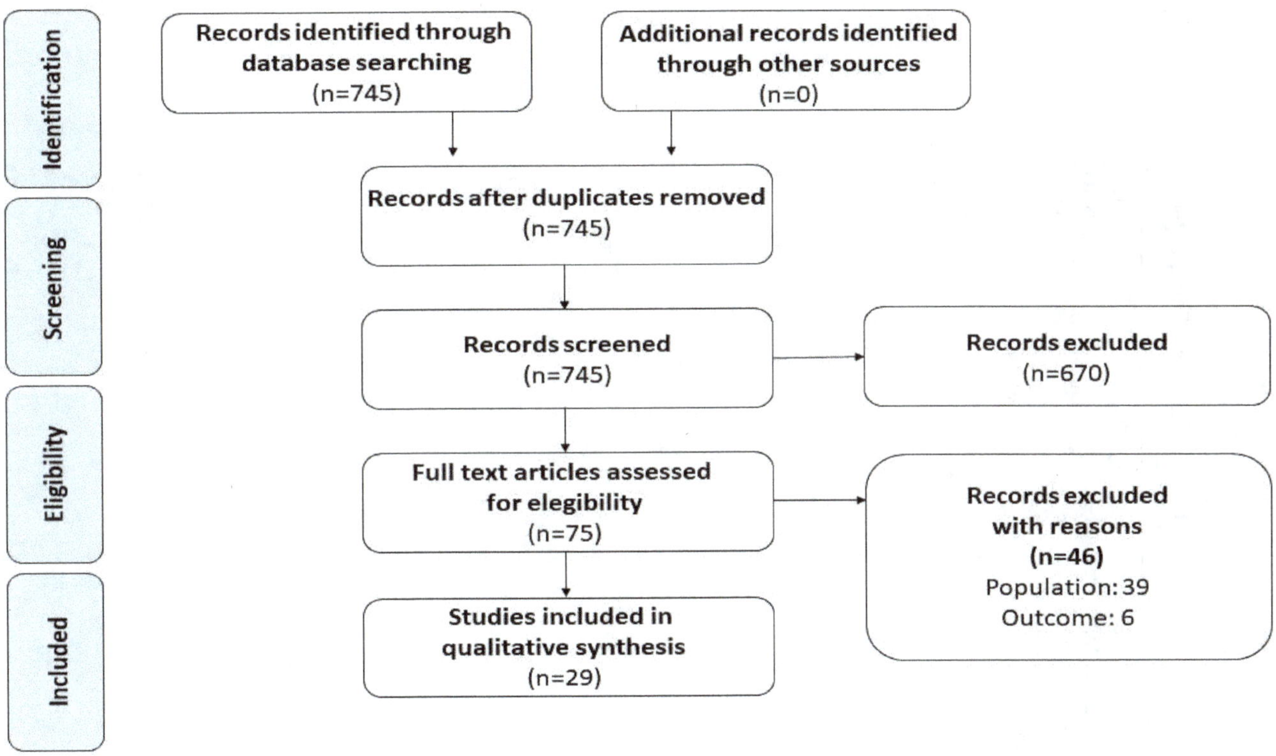

Figure 1. Flow diagram of the systematic review.

Specifically, seven studies were randomized control trials (RCT) with Jadad score ranging from 1 to 5, six were prospective and 16 were retrospective, with methodological index for non-randomized studies (MINORS) score ranging from 8 to 18 (Table 1).

Table 1. Patients' demographics and tumor characteristics.

Author (Year)	Study Design	Study Period	Jadad Score	MINOR Score	Sample Size (*n*)	Ethnic Origin (*n*)	Age at Progression Mean (Range)	Male:Female	Histology of Primary Tumour (%)	T-Stage (%)	Fuhrman or WHO/ISUP Grade (%)	Nephrectomy *n* (%)
Suzuki (2020) (a) [10]	R	2016–2019	-	14	41	n/a	70 (46–88)	33:8	Clear Cell (82.9) Other (17.1)	n/a	n/a	34 (82.9)
Suzuki (2020) (b) [10]					39		67 (39–87)	29:10	Clear Cell (74.4) Other (25.6)			34 (87.2)
Tomita (2020) [11]	P	2017–2020	-	-	35	n/a	63 (42–84)	24:11	Clear Cell (100)	n/a	n/a	34 (97.1)
Hamieh (2020) [12]	P	n/a–2019	-	-	7	Caucasian (7)	57 (39–63)	7:0	Clear Cell (100)	n/a	n/a	6 (86.0)
Yoshida (2019) [13]	R	n/a–2018	-	8	6	n/a	65.2 (49–83)	5:1	Clear Cell (83.3) Acquried cystic disease associated RCC (16.7)	T1b (16.6) T2 (16.6) T3a (66.6)	n/a	6 (100)
Shah (2019) [14]	R	2015–2018		11	70	n/a	59 (44–75)	50:20	Clear Cell (100)	n/a	n/a	60 (86.0)
Bersanelli (2019) [15]	R	2005–2011	-	12	150	n/a	n/a	115:35	Clear Cell (77.0) Papillary (13.5) Pure sarcomatoid (5.4) Sarcomatoid component (13.0) Others (4.0)	T1 (6.0) T2 (14.0) T3 (58.0) T4 (8.7)	n/a	129 (86.0)
Hasanov (2019) [16]	P	2013–2019	-	-	9	White or Caucasian (8) Hispanic or Latino (1)	59 (53–73)	5:4	Clear Cell (100)	n/a	n/a	8 (89.0)

Table 1. *Cont.*

Author (Year)	Study Design	Study Period	Jadad Score	MINOR Score	Sample Size (*n*)	Ethnic Origin (*n*)	Age at Progression Mean (Range)	Male:Female	Histology of Primary Tumour (%)	T-Stage (%)	Fuhrman or WHO/ISUP Grade (%)	Nephrectomy *n* (%)
Semrad (2018) (a) [17]	RCT	2012–2018	3	-	17	White (9) American Indian/Alaska native (2) Black (2) Hispanic (4)	64 (49–76)	13:4	Clear Cell (100)	n/a	n/a	n/a
Semrad (2018) (b) [17]					18	White (12) Asian/Pacific Islander (1) Black (1) Hispanic (4)	59 (46–74)	14:4				
Auvray (2018) [18]	R	2015–2018		12	33	n/a	61 (40–77)	23:10	Clear Cell (100)	n/a	n	25 (76.0)
Ishihara (2017) [19]	R	2007–2016	-	9	60	n/a	n/a	42:18	Clear Cell (76.7) Other (23.3)	n/a	n/a	n/a
Lakomy (2017) [20]	R	2014–2016	-	13	1029	n/a	59 (33–81)	740:248	Clear Cell (94.1) Papillary (4.85) Other (1.05)	n/a	n/a	849 (85.9)
Eggers (2017) [9]	R	2005–2012	-	10	105	n/a	n/a	74:31	Clear Cell (83.2) Papillary (4.3) Other (4.4)	T1 (15.2) T2 (21.0) T3 (40.0) T4 (3.8)	G1 (8.6) G2/3: (80.9)	n/a
Davis (2016) [21]	R	2003–2015		10	1516	n/a	n/a	1110:406	Clear Cell (89.0) Other (11.0) Sarcomatoid component (11.0)	n/a	n/a	1256 (83.0)

Table 1. *Cont.*

Author (Year)	Study Design	Study Period	Jadad Score	MINOR Score	Sample Size (*n*)	Ethnic Origin (*n*)	Age at Progression Mean (Range)	Male:Female	Histology of Primary Tumour (%)	T-Stage (%)	Fuhrman or WHO/ISUP Grade (%)	Nephrectomy *n* (%)
D'Aniello (2016) [22]	R	2014–2016	-	8	62	n/a	62 (36–86) *	55:7	Clear Cell (94.2) Other (4.8)	n/a	n/a	54 (87.1)
Motzer (2015) (a) [23]	RCT	2012–2013	4	-	51	n/a	61 (44–79)	35:16	Clear Cell (100)	n/a	n/a	44 (86.0)
Motzer (2015) (b) [23]					52		64 (41–79)	39:13				43 (83.0)
Motzer (2015) (c) [23]					50		59 (37–77)	38:12				48 (96.0)
Choueiri (2015) (a) [24]	RCT	2013–2014	3	-	330	White (269) Asian (21) Black (6) Other (19) Not reported (15) Missing (0)	63 (32–86)	253:77	n/a	n/a	n/a	284 (86.0)
Choueiri (2015) (b) [24]					328	White (263) Asian (26) Black (3) Other (13) Not reported (22) Missing (1)	62 (31–84)	241:86				280 (85.0)
Bergmann (2015) [25]	P	2009–2013	-	-	334	n/a	68 (22–89)	250:84	Clear Cell (88.0) Non-Clear Cell (7.0) Missing (5.0)	n/a	n/a	300 (90.0)

Table 1. *Cont.*

Author (Year)	Study Design	Study Period	Jadad Score	MINOR Score	Sample Size (*n*)	Ethnic Origin (*n*)	Age at Progression Mean (Range)	Male:Female	Histology of Primary Tumour (%)	T-Stage (%)	Fuhrman or WHO/ISUP Grade (%)	Nephrectomy *n* (%)
Hutson (2014) (a) [26]	RCT	2007–2011	4	-	259	White (178) Asian (38) Other (43)	60 (19–82)	193:66	Clear Cell (83.0) Non-Clear Cell (17.0)	n/a	n/a	223 (86.0)
Hutson (2014) (b) [26]					253	White (163) Asian (50) Other (40)	61 (21–80)	192:61	Clear Cell (82.0) Non-Clear Cell (18.0)			219 (87.0)
Signorovitch (2014) [27]	R	2019–2012	-	12	281	n/a	n/a	182:99	Clear Cell (84.0) Non-Clear Cell (16.0)	n/a	n/a	130 (46.3)
Wong (2014) [28]	R	2011	-	13	534	White (421) Others (113)	64 (34–88)	376:158	Clear Cell (89.0) Non-Clear Cell (11.0)	n/a	n/a	89 (16.7)
Park (2012) [29]	R	2005–2011		14	83	n/a	55 (26–84)	61:22	Clear Cell (78.0) Non-Clear Cell (22.0)	n/a	n/a	67 (81.0)
Busch (2013) [30]	R	2005–2011	-	18	103	n/a	n/a	67:36	Clear Cell (86.0) Non-Clear Cell (10.0) Unknown (7.0)	n/a	n/a	100 (97.0)
Trask (2011) [31]	RCT	2006	1	-	62	White (60) Asian (1) Other (1)	n/a	42:20	Clear Cell (82.2) Other (17.8)	T4 (95.1) Other (4.9)	n/a	62 (100)
Rini (2011) (a) [32]	RCT	2008–2010	4	-	361	White (278) Black (1) Asian (77) Other (5)	61 (20–82)	265:96	Clear Cell (100)	n/a	n/a	n/a
Rini (2011) (b) [32]					362	White (278) Black (1) Asian (77) Other (5)	61 (22–80)	258:104				
Zimmerman (2009) [33]	R	2005–2006	-	12	22	n/a	61 (39–78)	16:6	Clear Cell (100)	n/a	n/a	12 (54.5)

Table 1. *Cont.*

Author (Year)	Study Design	Study Period	Jadad Score	MINOR Score	Sample Size (*n*)	Ethnic Origin (*n*)	Age at Progression Mean (Range)	Male:Female	Histology of Primary Tumour (%)	T-Stage (%)	Fuhrman or WHO/ISUP Grade (%)	Nephrectomy *n* (%)
Di Lorenzo (2009) [34]	P	2006–2008	-	-	52	n/a	60 (40–78)	35:17	Clear Cell (86.5) Papillary (9.6) Sarcomatoid (3.8)	n/a	n/a	49 (94.2)
Tamaskar (2008) [35]	R	n/a	-	12	30	n/a	62 (42–77)	24:6	Clear Cell (93.3) Papillary + Clear Cell (6.6)	n/a	n/a	30 (100)
Motzer (2006) [36]	P	2003	-	-	63	n/a	60 (24–87)	43:20	Clear Cell (87.0) Papillary (6.0) Sarcomatoid variant (2.0) Unknown (5.0)	n/a	n/a	58 (92.0)
Escudier (2004) (a) [37]	RCT	2003–2005	5	-	451	n/a	58 (19–86)	315:58	Clear Cell (100)	n/a	n/a	422 (94.0)
Escudier (2004) (b) [37]					452		59 (29–84)	340:59	Clear Cell (100)			421 (93.0)

MINORS: Methodological Index for Non-Randomized Studies; P: prospective; R: retrospective, RCT: randomized controlled trial; RCC: renal cell carcinoma; n/a: not available; *: median (IQR).

3.1. *Patients' Demographics and Tumor Characteristics*

A total of 7650 patients who received second line therapy from 2003 to 2019 were included in the final analysis. Davis et al. [21] recorded the largest sample size (n = 1516), while Yoshida et al. [13] the smallest (n = 6). The patients' demographics and characteristics of the tumour was not fully reported for all 7650 patients included and are summarized in Table 1. Mean age ranged from 55 to 70 years (range 19–89). Most of the patients included were white (n = 1671 out of 2143 reported (77.9%)), male (n = 5604, 73.5%) and with clear cell histology (ranged from 74.4% to 100%). Fuhrman or WHO/ISUP grade was only reported by one author [9]. Most patients (40.0% to 95.1%) had a ≥T3 stage disease. A total of 5371 (79.0% of 6793 reported) underwent nephrectomy. The percentage of patients who underwent prior nephrectomy ranged from 16.7% to 100%. Included studies failed to provide data about the type (radical vs. cytoreductive) and timing (upfront vs. delayed) of nephrectomy.

3.2. *Treatment History*

Details about first-line treatment history are described in Table 2.

3.2.1. First Line Therapy

All the studies, except one [9], reported the first-line therapy drugs and the relative number of patients (n = 9027). Of those, 6187 patients (68.5%) received TKI (Sunitinib: 4528 (73.1%), Sorafenib: 880 (14.2%), Pazopanib: 637 (10.3%), Axitinib: 134 (2.1%), Tivozanib: 7 (0.1%), Cabozanitinib: 1 (0.01%)). Immunotherapy was administrated in 2637 (29.2%) patients (Interleukin and/or Interferon (1462, 55.4%), non-specified cytokine (1026, 38.9%), ICIs (149, 5.6%)). Moreover, 262 (2.9%) patients received Bevacizumab. In 59 patients (0.6%) mTOR inhibitors (Temsirolimus: 53 (89.8%), Everolimus: 6 (10.2%)) were administrated. Finally, 17 (0.2%) patients received chemotherapy (Thalidomide: 6 (35.3%), Lenalidomide: 5 (29.4%), Capecitabine: 3 (17.6%), Gemcitabine: 3 (17.6%)).

3.2.2. Progression Free Survival (PFS) and Objective Response Rates

Median PFS under first-line therapy was reported in 10 studies and ranged from 1.5 to 13.3 months. First-line response rate was reported in 5 studies (419 patients). In details, complete response (CR), partial response (PR), stable disease (SD) and progression disease (PD) was reported in 3 (0.7%), 94 (22.4%), 199 (47.5%) and 123 (29.3%) patients, respectively.

3.2.3. Reason for Discontinuation

Reasons for discontinuation of first-line therapy were reported in 6 studies (262 patients). Specifically, 51 (19.4%) and 211 (80.6%) discontinued first line therapy because of toxicity and disease progression, respectively.

3.3. *Disease Characteristics at Initiation of Second Line Therapy*

Details about disease characteristics before starting second line therapy are described in Table 2.

Table 2. Treatment history and disease characteristics at initiation of second line therapy.

Author (Year)	First Line Regimen (n)	Reason for Discontinuation n (%)		First-line PFS (Months) Mean (Range)	First-Line Response Rate (%)	ECOG PS Score (n)	Prognostic Category n (%)			Metastatic Sites (n)	Involved Metastatic Sites (n)	Second Line Regimen (%)
		Toxicity	Progression				Favorable /Good	Intermediate	Poor			
Suzuki (2020) (a) [10]	Sunitinib (18) Pazopanib (19) Sorafenib (2) Temsirolimus (2)	20 (48.8)	21 (51.2)	12.7(6.2–45.1)	n/a	n/a	3 (7.3) #	24 (58.5) #	14 (34.2) #	1 (23) ≥2 (18)	n/a	Axitinib 41 (100)
Suzuki (2020) (b) [10]	Sunitinib (20) Pazopanib (18) Sorafenib (1)	11 (28.2)	28 (71.8)	13.3 (7.1 -16.9)	n/a		2 (25.1) #	23 (59.0) #	14 (35.9) #	1 (21) ≥2 (18)		Nivolumab 39 (100)
Tomita (2020) [11]	Sunitinib (24) Axitinib (18) Pazopanib (7) Nivolumab (11) Avelumab (3) Pembrolizumab (1)	n/a	n/a	n/a	n/a	n/a	11 (31.4) °	19 (62.9) °	5 (14.3)	1 (6) 2 (11) ≥3 (3)	Bone (8) Lung (21) Liver (9) Lung or liver, and bone (25) Lymph node (11) Other (15)	Cabozantinib 35 (100)
Hamieh (2020) [12]	Sunitinib (2) Pazopanib (1) Ipilimumab + Nivolumab (3) Cabozantinib (1)	n/a	n/a	1.5 (0.8 -3.0)	n/a	n/a	0 (0) #	4 (57.1) #	3 (42.8) #	n/a	Lung (6) Bone (3) Brain (4) Liver (1)	Lenvatinib + Everolisimus 7 (100)
Yoshida (2019) [13]	Sorafenib (2) Sunitinib (3) IL2 (1) + Nivolumab	n/a	n/a	n/a	n/a	n/a	0 (0) #	6 (100) #	0 (0) #	1 (2) 2 (3) 3 (1)	Lung (n/a) Lymph node (n/a) Right adrenal gland (n/a)	Axitinib 6 (100)
Shah (2019) [14]	Anti-PD-(L)1 single agent (12) PD-1 + CTLA-4 blockade (33) PD-(L)1 + anti-VEGF therapy (25)	12 (17.0)	58 (83.0)	n/a	n/a	n/a	8 (11.0) #	48 (69.0) #	14 (20.0) #	n/a	Lung (61) Bone (35) Liver (12) Lymph node (48) Adrenal gland (22)	Pazopanib 19 (27) Sunitinib 6 (9) Axitinib 25 (36) Cabozantinib 20 (28)

Table 2. *Cont.*

Author (Year)	First Line Regimen (*n*)	Reason for Discontinuation *n* (%)		First-line PFS (Months) Mean (Range)	First-Line Response Rate (%)	ECOG PS Score (*n*)	Prognostic Category *n* (%)			Metastatic Sites (*n*)	Involved Metastatic Sites (*n*)	Second Line Regimen (%)
		Toxicity	Progression				Favorable /Good	Intermediate	Poor			
Bersanelli (2019) [15]	Sunitinib (150)	n/a (26.3)	n/a (61.7)	n/a	n/a	n/a	16 (10.7) °	95 (63.7) °	28 (18.9) °	1 (19) 2 (33) ≥3 (48)	Lung (70) Lymph node (59) Bone (31) Liver (25) Brain (11) Renal bed (9)	VEGF -TKI (n/a) mTORI (n/a)
Hasanov (2019) [16]	Sunitinib (7) Everolimus (6) Pazopanib (6) Temsirolimus (4) Capecitabine (3) Gemcitabine (3) Axitinib (2) Bevacizumab (1) Sorafenib (1) Tivozanib (1)	n/a	n/a	1.8 (0.8–3.6)	n/a	0 (6) 1 (2) 2 (1)	1 (11.0) °	6 (67) °	2 (22) °	1 (1) 2 (3) 3 (1) 4 (2) 6 (1) 10 (1)	Lung (8) Mediastinum (4) Liver (3) Lymph node (2) Chest wall (1)	Carfilzomib 9 (100)
Semrad (2018) (a) [17]	Bevacizumab (5) Pazopanib (6) Sorafenib (2) Sunitinib (4)	n/a	n/a	n/a	n/a	0 (12) 1 (5)	n/a			n/a	n/a	Trebabanib 17 (48.5)
Semrad (2018) (b) [17]	Bevacizumab (10) Pazopanib (5) Sorafenib (2) Sunitinib (1)					0 11) 1 (7)						Trebabanib + anti VEGF 18 (51.5)
Auvray (2018) [18]	Nivolumab -ipilimumab (33)	8 (24.2)	25 (75.8)	8.0 (5.0–13.0)	n/a	n/a	4 (12.1) #	23 (69.7) #	6 (18.2) #	n/a	n/a	Sunitinib 17 (51.5) Axitinib 8 (24.2) Pazopanib 6 (18.2) Cabozantinib 2 (6.1)
Ishihara (2017) [19]	Sunitinib (37) Sorafenib (21) Pazopanib (2)	0 (0)	60 (100)	n/a	n/a	n/a	9 (15.0) °	44 (73.3) °	7 (11.7) °	1 (18) ≥2 (42)	Lung (50) Liver (10) Bone (12) Lymph node (19)	Sunitinib13 (21.6) Sorafenib 2 (3.69) Axitinib 30 (50) Pazopanib 3 (5) Temsirolimus 4 (6.7) Everolimus 8 (13.3)

Table 2. *Cont.*

Author (Year)	First Line Regimen (*n*)	Reason for Discontinuation *n* (%)		First-line PFS (Months) Mean (Range)	First-Line Response Rate (%)	ECOG PS Score (*n*)	Prognostic Category *n* (%)			Metastatic Sites (*n*)	Involved Metastatic Sites (*n*)	Second Line Regimen (%)
		Toxicity	Progression				Favorable /Good	Intermediate	Poor			
Lakomy (2017) [20]	Bevacizumab + interferon-alpha (35) Sorafenib (232) Sunitinib (655) Temsirolimus (23) Pazopanib (84)	n/a	n/a	10 (n/a)	n/a	0 (182) 1 (487) 2 (46) 3 (1) Unknown (272)	361 (36.5) °	573 (58.0) °	54 (5.46) °	n/a	n/a	Everolimus 520 (50.5) Sorafenib 240 (23.3) Sunitinib 228 (22.1) Axitinib 29 (2.8) Pazopanib 10 (0.97) Temsirolimus 1 (0.09) Bevacizumab + interferon-alpha 1 (0.09)
Eggers (2017) [9]	Sunitinib (n/a) Sorafenib (n/a) Axitinib (n/a) Pazopanib (n/a) Cytokine (n/a)	n/a	n/a	n/a	n/a	0 (75) ≥1 (8) n/a (22)	8 (7.6) °	30 (28.6) °	2 (1.9) °	1 (44) >1 (41) n/a (20)	n/a	n/a
Davis (2016) [21]	Sunitinib (1068) Sorafenib (279) Axitinib (4) Bevacizumab (55) Pazopanib (110)	n/a	n/a	8.1 (3.9-16.0)	n/a	n/a	329 (22) °	902 (60) °	285 (19) °	n/a	n/a	Sunitinib 278 (18.0) Sorafenib 325 (21.0) Axitinib 107 (7.1) Pazopanib 120 (7.9) Cabozantinib 16 (1.1) Bevacizumab 28 (1.8) Temsirolimus 133 (8.8) Everolimus 403 (27.0) INF/IL-2 13 (0.9) Clinical trial drugs 93 (6.1)
D'Aniello (2016) [22]	Sunitinib (62)	n/a	n/a	7.18 (4.04-13.4)	n/a	0 (42) 1 (18) 2 (2)	15 (24.2) °	43 (69.4) °	4 (6.5) °	n/a	Lung: (29) Bone: (8) Liver: (4) Lymph-node: (9) Other: (12)	Axitinib 62 (100)

Table 2. *Cont.*

Author (Year)	First Line Regimen (*n*)	Reason for Discontinuation *n* (%)		First-line PFS (Months) Mean (Range)	First-Line Response Rate (%)	ECOG PS Score (*n*)	Prognostic Category *n* (%)			Metastatic Sites (*n*)	Involved Metastatic Sites (*n*)	Second Line Regimen (%)
		Toxicity	Progression				Favorable /Good	Intermediate	Poor			
Motzer (2015) (a) [23]	Axitinib (1) Bevacizumab (0) Pazopanib (9) Sorafenib (1) Sunitinib (36) Tivozanib (3) Other (1)				CR 1 (2) PR 14 (28) SD 20 (39) PD 7 (14) n/a 9 (18)	0 (27) 1 (24)	12 (24.0) °	19 (37.0) °	20 (39.0) °	1 (18) 2 (15) ≥3 (18)	Bone (12) Liver (10) Lung (27) Lymph nodes (25)	Lenvatinib + Everolimus 51 (100)
Motzer (2015) (b) [23]	Axitinib (2) Bevacizumab (1) Pazopanib (13) Sorafenib (0) Sunitinib (35) Tivozanib (1) Other (0)	n/a	n/a	n/a	PR 10 (19) SD 28 (54) PD 10 (19) n/a 4 (8)	0 (29) 1 (23)	11 (21.0) °	18 (35.0) °	23 (44.0) °	1 (9) 2 (15) ≥3 (28)	Bone (13) Liver (14) Lung (35) Lymph nodes (31)	Single agent Lenvatinib 52 (100)
Motzer (2015) (c) [23]	Axitinib (0) Bevacizumab (4) Pazopanib (13) Sorafenib (2) Sunitinib (28) Tivozanib (2) Other (1)				PR 10 (20) SD 21 (42) PD 15 (30) n/a 9 (8)	0 (28) 1 (22)	12 (24.0) °	19 (38.0) °	19 (38.0) °	1 (5) 2 (15) ≥3 (30)	Bone (16) Liver (13) Lung (35) Lymph nodes (33)	Single agent Everolimus 50 (100)
Choueiri (2015) (a) [24]	Sunitinib (210) Pazopanib (144) Axitinib (52) Sorafenib (21) Bevacizumab (5) IL-2 (20) Interferon alfa (19) Nivolumab (17)	n/a	n/a	n/a	n/a	0 (226) 1 (104)	150 (45.0) °	137 (42.0) °	43 (13.0) °	n/a	n/a	Cabozantinib 330 (50.1)

Table 2. *Cont.*

Author (Year)	First Line Regimen (*n*)	Reason for Discontinuation *n* (%)		First-line PFS (Months) Mean (Range)	First-Line Response Rate (%)	ECOG PS Score (*n*)	Prognostic Category *n* (%)			Metastatic Sites (*n*)	Involved Metastatic Sites (*n*)	Second Line Regimen (%)
		Toxicity	Progression				Favorable /Good	Intermediate	Poor			
Choueiri (2015) (b) [24]	Sunitinib (205) Pazopanib (136) Axitinib (55) Sorafenib (31) Bevacizumab (11) IL-2 (29) Interferon alfa (24) Nivolumab (14)					0 (217) 1 (111)	150 (46.0) °	135 (41.0) °	43 (13.0) °			Everolimus 328 (49.9)
Bergmann (2015) [25]	Sunitinib (260) Sorafenib (68) Pazopanib (12) Bevacizumab (41) Cytokines (33)	n/a	n/a	n/a	n/a	n/a	84 (35.0) °	134 (56.0) °	20 (8.0) °	n/a	Lung (226) Lymph node (145) Bone (125) Liver (87) Adrenal gland (47)	Everolimus 334 (100)
Hutson (2014) (a) [26]	Sunitinib (259)	n/a	n/a	n/a	n/a	0 (103) 1 (150) Other (6)	50 (19.0) °	178 (69.0) °	31 (12.0) °	n/a	n/a	Temsirolsimus 259 (100)
Hutson (2014) (b) [26]	Sunitinib (253)					0 (113) 1 (139) Other (1)	44 (17.0) °	177 (70.0) °	32 (13.0) °			Sorafenib 253 (100)
Signorovitch (2014) [27]	Sunitinib (206) Sorafenib (49) Pazopanib (26)	n/a	n/a	n/a	n/a	0 (40) ≥1 (234)	67 (23.8) °	138 (49.1) °	30 (10.7) °	n/a	Lung (232) Lymph nodes (152) Bone (148) Liver (76) Adrenal gland (35) Soft tissue (49) Central nervous system (13) Other (6)	Everolimus 138 (49.1) Temsirolimus 64 (22.8) Sorafenib 20 (7.1) Sunitinib 16 (5.7) Pazopanib 35 (12.5) Axitinib 8 (2.8)

Table 2. *Cont.*

Author (Year)	First Line Regimen (*n*)	Reason for Discontinuation *n* (%)		First-line PFS (Months) Mean (Range)	First-Line Response Rate (%)	ECOG PS Score (*n*)	Prognostic Category *n* (%)			Metastatic Sites (*n*)	Involved Metastatic Sites (*n*)	Second Line Regimen (%)
		Toxicity	Progression				Favorable /Good	Intermediate	Poor			
Wong (2014) [28]	Sunitinib (459) Sorafenib (50) Pazopanib (25)	n/a	n/a	n/a	n/a	n/a		n/a		n/a	Lung (379) Lymph nodes (146) Bone (262) Liver (164) Adrenal gland (77) Soft tissue (49) Central nervous system (16)	Everolimus 233 (43.6) Temsirolsimus 178 (33.3) Sorafenib 123 (23.0)
Park (2012) [29]	Sunitinib (60) Sorafenib (16) Pazotinib (7)	n/a	0	n/a	≥ SD 66 (79.0) PD 14 (17.0) n/a 4 (5.0)	n/a		n/a		≤2 (44) ≥3 (39)	n/a	VEGF TKI 41 (49.4) mTORI: 42 (50.6)
Busch (2013) [30]	Sunitinib (20) Sorafenib (12) Bevacizumab (3) Pazopanib (1)	n/a	19 (18.4)	9.1 (6.8–11.5)	CR 1 (1.9) PR 22 (21.4) SD 42 (40.8) PD 47 (40.8)	0 (69) 1 (10) 2 (1)		n/a		1 (46) ≥3 (46)	Bone (23) Liver (23)	Sunitinib 21 (20.4) Sorafenib 39 (37.4) Everolimus 35 (34.0) Temsirolimus 5 (4.9) Other 9 (8.7)
Trask (2011) [31]	Sorafenib (62)	n/a	n/a	7.4 (6.7–11.0)	n/a	0 (21) 1 (41)		n/a		n/a	Lung (44) Node (30) Liver (20) Soft Tissue (11) Bone (8) Other (30)	Axitinib 62 (100)
Rini (2011) (a) [32]	Sunitinib (194) Cytokines (126) Bevacizumab (29) Temsirolimus (12)	n/a	n/a	n/a	n/a	0 (195) 1 (162) ≥1 (1)	100 (28.0) °	134 (37.0) °	118 (33.0) °	n/a	n/a	Axitinib 361 (100)
Rini (2011) (b) [32]	Sunitinib (195) Cytokines (125) Bevacizumab (30) Temsirolimus (12)					0 (200) 1 (160) ≥1 (0)	101 (28.0) °	130 (36.0) °	120 (33.0) °			Sorafenib 362 (100)

Table 2. *Cont.*

Author (Year)	First Line Regimen (*n*)	Reason for Discontinuation *n* (%)		First-line PFS (Months) Mean (Range)	First-Line Response Rate (%)	ECOG PS Score (*n*)	Prognostic Category *n* (%)			Metastatic Sites (*n*)	Involved Metastatic Sites (*n*)	Second Line Regimen (%)
		Toxicity	Progression				Favorable /Good	Intermediate	Poor			
Zimmerman (2009) [33]	Sorafenib (22)	n/a	n/a	12.5 (n/a)	PR 7 (31.8%) SD 15 (68.2%)	n/a	10 (45.5) °	12 (54.5) °	0 (0) °	1 (3) 2 (1) ≥ 3 (18)	Lung (16) Liver (11) Lymph nodes (11) Bone (10) Brain (5)	Sunitinib 22 (100)
Di Lorenzo (2009) [34]	Interferon- alfa (5) IL-2 (4) Sunitinib (50) Sunitinib + Interferon (2)	n/a	n/a	n/a	CR 1 (1.9) PR 21 (40.4) SD 7 (13.5) PD 23 (44.2)	0 (33) 1 (15) 2 (4)	40 (76.9) °	9 (17.3) °	3 (5.78) °	1 (24) 2 (18) ≥3 (10)	Lung (38) Liver (12) Lymph nodes (12) Adrenal (5) Bone (4) Kidney (3) Soft tissue (2)	Sorafenib 52 (100)
Tamaskar (2008) [35]	Thalidomide (6) Lenalidomide (5) Volociximab (6) Bevacizumab (7) AG13736 (2) Sunitinib (5) Sorafenib (4)	n/a	n/a	n/a	n/a	n/a		n/a		n/a	Lung (21) Lymph node (18) Bone (13) Liver (11) Soft tissue (22) Brain (5)	Sunitinib and/or Sorafenib (n/a)
Motzer (2006) [36]	Interferon–apha (35) IL-2 (19) Interferon-alpha + IL-2 (9)	n/a	n/a	n/a	6%	0 (34) 1(29)	34 (54.0) °	29 (46.0) °	0 (0) °	1 (8) ≥ 2 (55)	Lung (52) Liver (10) Bone (32)	Sunitinib 63 (100)

Table 2. *Cont.*

Author (Year)	First Line Regimen (n)	Reason for Discontinuation n (%)		First-line PFS (Months) Mean (Range)	First-Line Response Rate (%)	ECOG PS Score (n)	Prognostic Category n (%)			Metastatic Sites (n)	Involved Metastatic Sites (n)	Second Line Regimen (%)
		Toxicity	Progression				Favorable /Good	Intermediate	Poor			
Escudier (2004) (a) [37]	Cytokine-based (374) IL (191) Interferon (307) Both IL-2 and interferon (124)	n/a	n/a	n/a	n/a	0 (219) 1 (223) 2 (7) Unknown (2)	233 (52.0) °	218 (48.0) °	0 (0) °	1 (62) 2 (131) >2 (256) Unknown (2)	Lung (348) Liver (116)	Sorafenib 451 (100)
Escudier (2004) (b) [37]	Cytokine-based (368) IL (189) Interferon (314) Both IL-2 and interferon (135)					0 (210) 1 (236) 2 (4) Unknown (2)	228 (50.0) °	223 (50) °	0 (0) °	1 (63) 2 (129) >2 (258)	Lung (348) Liver (117)	Placebo 452 (100)

CR: Complete Response; ECOG PS: Eastern Cooperative Oncology Group Performance Status; L: Interleukin; PD: progressive disease; PD-1: programmed death-1; PFS: Progression-free survival; PR: Partial response; R: Retrospective; RCT: Randomized Controlled Trial; SD: Stable disease; EGFR-TKI: vascular endothelial growth factor receptor tyrosine kinase inhibitor; n/a: not available; #: International Metastatic Renal Cell Carcinoma Database Consortium score; °: Memorial Sloan–Kettering Cancer Centre score; PFS: Progression Free Survival; n/a: not available.

3.3.1. Eastern Cooperative Oncology Group Performance Status (ECOG PS) Score

ECOG PS score at initiation of second-line therapy was reported in 15 studies enrolling a total of 4303 patients. Of those, 2092 patients (48.6%) showed an ECOG PS score of 0 whereas 2211 (52.4%) showed the ECOG PS score at progression ≥1.

3.3.2. Prognostic Scores

Prognostic score before starting second-line therapy was reported in 23 studies enrolling 6583 patients. In details, MSKCC and the IMDC were used in 18 and 5 studies, respectively. The percentage of patients showing a favorable, intermediate, and poor prognostic score according to the MSKCC and IMDC scores were 31.8%, 53.9%, 14.3% and 8.7%, 65.3%, and 26%, respectively.

3.3.3. Number of Metastasis and Metastatic Sites

The number of metastatic sites at progression was reported in 14 studies enrolling 1680 patients. One metastatic site was recorded in 372 (22.1%) patients. Conversely, in 1308 patients (77.8%) ≥2 sites were involved. Eighteen studies involving 4726 patients described the number of specific metastatic sites. The most frequent metastatic sites were lung, bones, lymph nodes and liver. Specifically, the number of patients harbouring lung, bone, lymph node and liver metastases were 1976 (41.8%), 763 (16.1%), 751 (15.9%) and 748 (15.8%), respectively. Less frequent metastatic sites were adrenal gland (n = 186, 3.9%), soft tissue (n = 133, 2.8%), central nervous system (n = 29, 0.6%), brain (n = 25, 0.5%), kidney (n = 12, 0.2%), mediastinum (n = 4, 0.1%) and chest wall (n = 1, 0.01%).

3.4. *Second Line Therapy*

Details about the type of second-line therapy were reported in 26 studies involving 5634 patients. Specifically, 2793 patients (49.6%) received mTOR inhibitors (Everolimus: 2107 (76.4%), Temsirolimus: 644 (23.0%), not specified: 42 (1.5%)). Tyrosin kinase inhibitors were administrated in 2170 patients (38.5%) (Axitinib: 739 (34.0%), Sunitinib: 664 (30.6%), Cabozanitinib: 423 (19.5%), Pazopanib: 193 (8.9%), Lenvatinib:110 (5.0%), not specified: 41 (1.9%)). Immunotherapy was given to 53 patients (0.9%) (Interleukin and/or Interferon (14, 26.4%), ICIs (39, 73.6%)). Moreover, 29 patients (0.5%) received Bevacizumab. Unspecified clinical trial drugs were administrated in 93 patients (1.6%) and 452 patients (8.0%) received placebo. Finally, 9 patients received Carfilzomib (0.1%) and 35 patients (0.6%) received Trebabanib. Detailed clinical and pathological prophile of mRCC patients according to second-line therapy was only possible in 18 studies [10–13,16,17,22–26,31–34,36,37]. Table 3 describes the available clinical and pathological features of mRCC patients stratified according the following second-line therapies: axitinib, cabozantinib, nivolumab, everolimus plus levatinib. The features of patients undergoing therapy with VEGF-targeted therapy in combination with immunotherapy could not be extracted. Mean age of patients when entering these second-line therapies was <65 years in all cases. The percentage of patients who underwent prior nephrectomy was lower among patients receiving axitinib (29.3%) and higher among those receiving nivolumab (87.2%). The percentage of patients with a good/intermediate prognostic profile was hugher among patients receiving cabozantinib (86.8%) and lower among those breceiving everolimus plus levatinib (60.4%).

Table 3. Clinical and pathological characteristics according to second line treatment regimens.

Characteristic	Axitinib (n = 532)	Cabozantinib (n = 365)	Nivolumab (n = 39)	Everolimus + Levatinib (n = 58)
Male:Female	400:132	277:88	29:10	42:16
Age at progression, years (mean)	64.5	63.0	63.0	59.0
Histology of Primary Tumor, *n* (%)				
Clear cell carcinoma	510 (95.9)	35 (9.5)	29 (74.4)	58 (100)
Non-Clear cell carcinoma	22 (4.1)	0 (0)	10 (25.6)	-
Not specified	0 (0)	330 (90.6)	0 (0)	-
T-Stage, *n* (%)				
T1	1 (0.2)	n/a	n/a	n/a
T2	1 (0.2)	n/a	n/a	n/a
T3	4 (0.7)	n/a	n/a	n/a
T4	59 (11.1)	n/a	n/a	n/a
Not specified	467 (87.8)	n/a	n/a	n/a
Fuhrman or WHO/ISUP Grade, *n* (%)	n/a	n/a	n/a	n/a
Prior nephrectomy, *n* (%)	156 (29.3)	268 (73.4)	34 (87.2)	50 (86.2)
Reason for Discontinuation, *n* (%)				
Progression	21 (3.9)	n/a	28 (71.8)	n/a
Toxicity	20 (3.7)	n/a	11 (28.2)	n/a
Not specified	491 (92.2)	n/a	0 (0)	n/a
ECOG PS Score, *n* (%)				
0	258 (48.5)	226 (61.9)	n/a	27 (46.5)
1	221 (41.5)	104 (28.5)	n/a	24 (41.4)
2	3 (0.6)	0 (0)	n/a	0 (0)
Not specified	50 (9.4)	35 (9.6)	n/a	7 (12.1)
Prognostic Category, *n* (%)				
Favorable/Good	118 (22.2)	161 (44.1)	2 (5.1)	12 (20.8)
Intermediate	207 (38.9)	156 (42.7)	23 (59.0)	23 (39.6)
Poor	136 (25.6)	48 (13.2)	14 (35.9)	23 (39.6)
Not specified	71 (13.3)	0 (0)	0 (0)	-
Metastatic sites, *n* (%)				
1	25 (4.7)	6 (1.6)	21 (53.8)	18 (31.0)
≥2	22 (4.1)	14 (3.8)	18 (46.2)	33 (56.9)
Not specified	485 (91.2)	345 (94.6)	0 (0)	7 (12.1)
Involved Metastatic Sites, *n* (%)				
Lung	73 (13.7)	21 (5.7)	n/a	33 (56.9)
Liver	24 (4.5)	9 (2.5)	n/a	11 (18.9)
Lymph node	39 (7.3)	11 (3.0)	n/a	25 (43.1)
Bone	16 (3.0)	8 (2.2)	n/a	15 (25.9)
Other	53 (9.9)	15 (4.1)	n/a	4 (6.9)
Not specified	408 (77.7)	330 (90.4)	n/a	0 (0)

Percentage are calculated on the total number of patients treated with the specific second-line regimen.

4. Discussion

RCC incidence is rising at an average of 1.1% each year with 16% of the cases being metastatic at the time of presentation [5,38]. mRCC poses one of the great therapeutic challenges in oncology. Indeed, it is typically refractory to traditional cytotoxic chemotherapies, and until recently management options were limited to immunotherapy or palliative options. The paradigm of treatment and the prognosis of patients with mRCC has significantly changed in recent years thanks to the development and widespread use of molecular targeted agents, including VEGF pathway inhibitors, mammalian target of rapamycin pathway inhibitors, immune checkpoint inhibitors (ICIs). Since 2005, new'first-line regimens have significantly improved the survival of mRCC patients. However, treatment discontinuation is often necessary due to disease progression, therapy-limiting toxicity, or patient request [9]. Thanks to recent improvements in targeted therapies clinicians have the opportunity to offer patients several lines of therapy. Nowadays, near half of patients with mRCC receive a second-line therapy [5]. The current European Association of Urology guidelines strongly recommend offering either nivolumab or cabozantinib for ICIs-naive VEGFr-refractory clear-cell mRCC and to offer any VEGF-targeted therapy that has not been previously used in combination with immunotherapy as second-line therapy for patients refractory to ICIs (strength of rating: weak) [39]. The National Comprehensive Cancer Network Guidelines recommend Cabozantinib, Nivolumab, Axitinib, and Lenvatinib plus Everolimus as category 1 after TKI treatment [40].

Nivolumab is an ICI antibody that disrupts the interaction of the PD-1 receptor with its ligands PD-L1 and PD-L2 [41]. It suppresses tumor growth by inducing the proliferation of cancer antigen-specific T cells and enhancing cytotoxic activity [41]. Axitinib is a potent, selective, second-generation inhibitor of vascular endothelial growth factor receptor (VEGFR)1, 2 and 3 [42]. Cabozantinib is a multitargeted receptor tyrosine kinase inhibitor with activity against hepatocyte growth factor receptor (tyrosine-protein kinase Met), vascular endothelial growth factor receptor 2 (VEGFR-2) and protoncogene tyrosine-protein kinase receptor Ret [43]. Lenvatinib is a small-molecule TKI that inhibits VEGFR1-3, fibroblast growth factor receptor (FGFR1-4), platelet-derived growth factor receptor α (PDGFRα), stem cell factor receptor (KIT), and rearranged during transfection (RET) [44]. Novel second-line treatment strategies have shown overall survival benefit up to 25 months compared to everolimus. However, the field of RCC treatments is evolving at a rapid and unprecedented pace that makes it difficult for researcher and clinicians to keep up with the latest evidence and derive the best recommendations and decisions. In the era of personalized medicine, we face the concrete difficulty of "targeting" available target therapies mainly due to the lack of reliable predictive factors, that are urgently needed. Beside molecular predictive factors, a detailed clinical-pathological picture of specific subsets of patients to treat is often required. Indeed, although guidelines are useful in the general population setting, clinicians are challenged with selecting treatments for individual patients. In this context, they have to consider a range of factors from the clinical-pathological profile, and prior therapy to less obvious but central issues in the daily life of patients [3]. To our knowledge, this is the first systematic review summarizing the demographic and clinicopathologic profile of mRCC patients who enter a second-line therapy. Our results provide the basis for many hypotheses that need to be tested in future investigations. Demographic features have relevant clinical implications for mRCC patients. Racial/ethnic and gender disparities have been described in terms of RCC incidence and survival. Black patients have been reported to have a significantly higher incidence rate and lower relative survival rate than all other races/ethnicities, whereas Asians/Pacific Islanders show an opposite trend [45].

A higher predominance in men over women has been described (1.5:1), together with a slightly lower relative survival rate [45]. Our results demonstrate that the majority of mRCC patients who receive a second-line therapy enrolled in clinical studies of captured in real-world databases have a Caucasian/White ethnic origin and are male. The relevance of ethnicity in terms of mRCC response to first-line therapies is widely under-investigated and deserves future evaluations. Rose et al. demonstrated that both Caucasian and African American patients with mRCC had a significant increase in rates of systemic treatment with an accompanying improvement in survival since the introduction of targeted therapies [46]. However, African American patients showed a survival disadvantage compared to Caucasians independent of treatment received, probably due to tumour biology, comorbidities, or disease burden [46]. The authors hypothesized that the racial disparity in survival may be related to factors unaffected by the implementation of therapies and that treatment bias does not explain the survival disparity [46]. Although gene polymorphism may explain the disparity of response and tolerability in mRCC patients receiving targeted therapy, further studies about the exact mechanism are required. Interestingly, the male to female ratio we observed when describing the population of mRCC is higher than the 1.5:1 incidence ratio. This finding leads to hypothesize a gender difference in terms of tumor progression and/or drug toxicity. Gender influences epidemiology, histology, surgical treatment, complications, response to medical therapy, and long-term oncological and functional outcomes in RCC [47,48]. In detail, the male gender has been associated with worse RCC clinical features and prognosis. The reason of such discrepancy should be further evaluated, as it could be related either to the immune-related genes of the X chromosome or to the hormonal sex influences on cancer susceptibility or both [47]. Furthermore, a gender selection bias should also be considered as a potential explanation for this observation. Indeed, as recently reported by Mancini et al., men are included in clinical trials and prospective studies on genitourinary cancers more often than women [48,49]. A better clarification of gender-related mechanisms can lead to the possibility of including gender factors in risk-predictive nomograms and allow the possibility for personalized gender-oriented treatment options [48,49].

Mean patient ages range from 57 to 70 years. Currently, uncertainties exist about the prognostic effect of age on RCC. Some authors have pointed out that older age is correlated with a higher stage and pathological grade, suggesting an adverse association with prognosis [50]. In their study, Zhang et al. found that younger patients with mRCC receiving targeted therapy had a poorer prognosis compared with older patients [50]. Interestingly, the mean age of patients receiving axitinib, cabozantinib, nivolumab, and the combination of everolimus plus levatinib was < 65 years. Of note, younger patients also have theoretically a low comorbidity status and can better tolerate further lines of treatment. The age profile emphasizes the need to improve the accessibility to second lines of treatment. Moreover, this evidence points out the need for further studies assessing the outcomes of second-line therapies in older patients.

Each kidney cancer histology has unique genomic and clinical features that should be taken into account when planning appropriate targeted therapies [51]. Clear cell RCC represents approximately 75% of renal cancers. As expected, clear-cell histology is highly prevalent among the mRCC population captured by our review. However, non-clear cell histology is reported in up to 25.6% of these patients. Unfortunately, non-clear cell kidney cancer still represents an unmet need from a therapeutic point of view and available treatments have demonstrated limited efficacy in this subset of patients [51].

The majority of patients entering a second-line therapy discontinued first-line drugs due to disease progression. However, a non-negligible percentage of them (up to 48.8%) discontinued it due to toxicity. This finding has relevant clinical implications. Although demonstrated only for mRCC patients who discontinue VEGF-targeted therapies, it has been reported that patients who discontinue first-line therapy because of toxicity have better outcomes than patients who stop it because of disease progression [51]. Whether the former subset of patients should receive different consideration when starting next line of therapy still remains a controversial issue [52].

The number and typology of metastatic sites have a relevant prognostic role in mRCC patients. Patients with only one metastatic site have been reported to have a better prognosis when compared to patients with multiple sites involved [53]. Although most patients entering a second line therapy have more than one metastatic site, there is a considerable percentage of patients with only one site involved. Several authors demonstrated variable outcomes depending on the patterns of metastasis. Although the lung is the most frequently involved metastatic site in patients undergoing a second-line therapy, our analysis points out a heterogeneous distribution of metastatic sites. Typically, bone and brain metastases represent significant therapeutic dilemmas as they are poorly responsive to medical therapy [2]. Bone is involved in a significant number of mRCC patients entering a second-line therapy. Published data have pointed to the potential utility of cabozantinib in patients with bone metastasis, thus providing a potential rationale to personalize second-line therapies according to the metastatic sites [2].

Although most mRCC patients receiving second-line therapy had a prior nephrectomy, a significant percentage of them (up to 83.3% in some series) did not receive surgery. The role of cytoreductive nephrectomy (CN) has profoundly changed in recent years along with the evolution of medical therapy [53]. The theoretical benefits of CN include facilitation of spontaneous regression, reduction of de novo metastases, and palliation of symptoms [54]. However, these potential benefits must be considered in the context of perioperative morbidity and the delayed receipt of systemic treatments. In the cytokine era, CN provided a crystal-clear benefit in terms of overall survival and it was considered the standard of care [54]. More recently, based on the results of the CARMENA and SURTIME trials, patients with MSKCC intermediate- and poor-risk are deemed not suitable for upfront CN as this will delay the beginning of target therapy thus potentially decreasing the overall survival [54]. Therefore, although CN still remains an important tool in the multimodality management of mRCC, careful patient selection is of paramount importance and discussion in multidisciplinary teams is required. To date, the role of CN in the setting of ICI remains largely undefined and future trials are required to provide insight on patient selection and optimal timing of CN in this clinical scenario [54]. Stratification of mRCC according to prognostic models has relevant clinical implications and guidelines recommend tailoring first-line therapies accordingly. Most patients receiving a second-line therapy belong to the favorable/intermediate prognostic categories with the latter being the most represented in most series. Future investigations are required to explore the role of second-line agents' selection according to the prognostic risk category.

The potential limitations of this review must be acknowledged: available studies often provide incomplete and heterogeneously reported clinicopathologic data. In most cases, patients enrolled in the included studies are selected on the basis of predefined inclusion and exclusion criteria thus being not completely representative of patients found in everyday clinical practice. Finally, this study simply describes the characteristics of patients who receive a second-line regimen while future studies are needed to depict the profile of the entire population of patients who discontinue a first line regimen.

5. Conclusions

Based on data from both clinical trials and real-life observational registries, patients who are submitted to second-line therapy represent a heterogeneous group. Most of the reported cases, however, show a good performance status, are younger than 70 years and have a good/intermediate prognostic profile. Future studies are needed to better characterize profiles and subtypes of patients submitted to second-line treatments.

Author Contributions: M.C. (Massimiliano Creta), V.M., G.C. (Giuseppe Celentano), C.B. and N.L. conceived and designed the study; F.F., F.E. and R.L.R. collected the data; C.C.R., F.M., G.C. (Gianluigi Califano), and L.N. analyzed the data; M.C. (Massimiliano Creta), M.C. (Marco Capece), G.C. (Giuseppe Celentano) and N.L. wrote the paper. All authors have read and agreed to the published version of the manuscript.

References

1. Flanigan, R.C.; Campbell, S.C.; Clark, J.I.; Picken, M.M. Metastatic renal cell carcinoma. *Curr. Treat. Options Oncol.* **2003**, *4*, 385–390. [CrossRef] [PubMed]
2. Gong, J.; Maia, M.C.; Dizman, N.; Govindarajan, A.; Pal, S.K. Metastasis in renal cell carcinoma: Biology and implications for therapy. *Asian J. Urol.* **2016**, *3*, 286–292. [CrossRef] [PubMed]

3. Tannir, N.M.; Pal, S.K.; Atkins, M.B. Second-Line Treatment Landscape for Renal Cell Carcinoma: A Comprehensive Review. *Oncologist* **2018**, *23*, 540–555. [CrossRef] [PubMed]
4. Schwab, M.; Hofmann, R.; Heers, H.; Hegele, A. mRCC Outcome in the Treatment of Metastatic Renal Cell Carcinoma—A German Single-center Real-world Experience. *Vivo* **2018**, *32*, 1617–1622. [CrossRef]
5. Jain, R.K.; Gandhi, S.; George, S. Second-line systemic therapy in metastatic renal-cell carcinoma: A review. *Urol. Oncol.* **2017**, *35*, 640–646. [CrossRef]
6. Liberati, A.; Altman, D.G.; Tetzlaff, J.; Mulrow, C.; Gøtzsche, P.C.; Ioannidis, J.P.; Clarke, M.; Devereaux, P.J.; Kleijnen, J.; Moher, D. The PRISMA statement for reporting systematic reviews and meta-analyses of studies that evaluate health care interventions: Explanation and elaboration. *Ann. Intern. Med.* **2009**, *151*, W65–W94. [CrossRef]
7. Jadad, A.R. *Randomised Controlled Trials*; BMJ Publishing Group: London, UK, 1998.
8. Slim, K.; Nini, E.; Forestier, D.; Kwiatkowski, F.; Panis, Y.; Chipponi, J. Methodological index for non-randomized studies (minors): Development and validation of a new instrument. *Anz. J. Surg.* **2003**, *73*, 712–716. [CrossRef]
9. Eggers, H.; Ivanyi, P.; Hornig, M.; Grünwald, V. Predictive Factors for Second-Line Therapy in Metastatic Renal Cell Carcinoma: A Retrospective Analysis. *J. Kidney Cancer Vhl.* **2017**, *4*, 8–15. [CrossRef]
10. Suzuki, K.; Terakawa, T.; Furukawa, J.; Harada, K.; Hinata, N.; Nakano, Y.; Fujisawa, M. Clinical outcomes of second-line treatment following prior targeted therapy in patients with metastatic renal cell carcinoma: A comparison of axitinib and nivolumab. *Int. J. Clin. Oncol.* **2020**, *25*, 1678–1686. [CrossRef]
11. Tomita, Y.; Tatsugami, K.; Nakaigawa, N.; Osawa, T.; Oya, M.; Kanayama, H.; Nakayama Kondoh, C.; Sassa, N.; Nishimura, K.; Nozawa, M.; et al. Cabozantinib in advanced renal cell carcinoma: A phase II, open-label, single-arm study of Japanese patients. *Int. J. Urol.* **2020**, *27*, 952–959. [CrossRef]
12. Hamieh, L.; Beck, R.L.; Le, V.H.; Hsieh, J.J. The Efficacy of Lenvatinib Plus Everolimus in Patients with Metastatic Renal Cell Carcinoma Exhibiting Primary Resistance to Front-Line Targeted Therapy or Immunotherapy. *Clin. Genitourin. Cancer* **2020**, *18*, 252–257.e2. [CrossRef] [PubMed]
13. Yoshida, K.; Takagi, T.; Kondo, T.; Kobayashi, H.; Iizuka, J.; Fukuda, H.; Ishihara, H.; Okumi, M.; Ishida, H.; Tanabe, K. Efficacy of axitinib in patients with metastatic renal cell carcinoma refractory to nivolumab therapy. *Jpn. J. Clin. Oncol.* **2019**, *49*, 576–580. [CrossRef] [PubMed]
14. Shah, A.Y.; Kotecha, R.R.; Lemke, E.A.; Chandramohan, A.; Chaim, J.L.; Msaouel, P.; Xiao, L.; Gao, J.; Campbell, M.T.; Zurita, A.J.; et al. Outcomes of patients with metastatic clear-cell renal cell carcinoma treated with second-line VEGFR-TKI after first-line immune checkpoint inhibitors. *Eur. J. Cancer* **2019**, *114*, 67–75. [CrossRef] [PubMed]
15. Bersanelli, M.; Iacovelli, R.; Buti, S.; Houede, N.; Laguerre, B.; Procopio, G.; Lheureux, S.; Fischer, R.; Negrier, S.; Ravaud, A.; et al. Metastatic Renal Cell Carcinoma Rapidly Progressive to Sunitinib: What to Do Next? *Eur. Urol. Oncol.* **2019**, *19*, S2588. [CrossRef]
16. Hasanov, E.; Tidwell, R.S.S.; Fernandez, P.; Park, L.; McMichael, C.; Tannir, N.M.; Jonasch, E. Phase II Study of Carfilzomib in Patients With Refractory Renal Cell Carcinoma. *Clin. Genitourin. Cancer* **2019**, *17*, 451–456. [CrossRef]
17. Semrad, T.J.; Groshen, S.; Luo, C.; Pal, S.; Vaishampayan, U.; Joshi, M.; Quinn, D.I.; Mack, P.C.; Gandara, D.R.; Lara, P.N. Randomized Phase 2 Study of Trebananib (AMG 386) with or without Continued Anti-Vascular Endothelial Growth Factor Therapy in Patients with Renal Cell Carcinoma Who Have Progressed on Bevacizumab, Pazopanib, Sorafenib, or Sunitinib—Results of NCI/CTEP Protocol 9048. *Kidney Cancer* **2019**, *3*, 51–61.
18. Auvray, M.; Auclin, E.; Barthelemy, P.; Bono, P.; Kellokumpu-Lehtinen, P.; Gross-Goupil, M.; De Velasco, G.; Powles, T.; Mouillet, G.; Vano, Y.A.; et al. Second-line targeted therapies after nivolumab-ipilimumab failure in metastatic renal cell carcinoma. *Eur. J. Cancer* **2019**, *108*, 33–40. [CrossRef]
19. Ishihara, H.; Kondo, T.; Yoshida, K.; Omae, K.; Takagi, T.; Iizuka, J.; Tanabe, K. Time to progression after first-line tyrosine kinase inhibitor predicts survival in patients with metastatic renal cell carcinoma receiving second-line molecular-targeted therapy. *Urol. Oncol.* **2017**, *35*, e1–e542. [CrossRef]
20. Lakomy, R.; Poprach, A.; Bortlicek, Z.; Melichar, B.; Chloupkova, R.; Vyzula, R.; Zemanova, M.; Kopeckova, K.; Svoboda, M.; Slaby, O.; et al. Utilization and efficacy of second-line targeted therapy in metastatic renal cell carcinoma: Data from a national registry. *BMC Cancer* **2017**, *17*, 880. [CrossRef]

21. Davis, I.D.; Xie, W.; Pezaro, C.; Donskov, F.; Wells, J.C.; Agarwal, N.; Srinivas, S.; Yuasa, T.; Beuselinck, B.; Wood, L.A.; et al. Efficacy of Second-line Targeted Therapy for Renal Cell Carcinoma According to Change from Baseline in International Metastatic Renal Cell Carcinoma Database Consortium Prognostic Category. *Eur. Urol.* **2017**, *71*, 970–978. [CrossRef]
22. D'Aniello, C.; Vitale, M.G.; Farnesi, A.; Calvetti, L.; Laterza, M.M.; Cavaliere, C.; Della Pepa, C.; Conteduca, V.; Crispo, A.; De Vita, F.; et al. Axitinib after Sunitinib in Metastatic Renal Cancer: Preliminary Results from Italian "Real-World" SAX Study. *Front. Pharmacol.* **2016**, *7*, 331. [CrossRef] [PubMed]
23. Motzer, R.J.; Hutson, T.E.; Glen, H.; Michaelson, M.D.; Molina, A.; Eisen, T.; Jassem, J.; Zolnierek, J.; Maroto, J.P.; Mellado, B.; et al. Lenvatinib, everolimus, and the combination in patients with metastatic renal cell carcinoma: A randomised, phase 2, open-label, multicentre trial. *Lancet Oncol.* **2015**, *16*, 1473–1482. [CrossRef]
24. Choueiri, T.K.; Escudier, B.; Powles, T.; Mainwaring, P.N.; Rini, B.I.; Donskov, F.; Hammers, H.; Hutson, T.E.; Lee, J.L.; Peltola, K.; et al. METEOR Investigators. Cabozantinib versus Everolimus in Advanced Renal-Cell Carcinoma. *N. Engl. J. Med.* **2015**, *373*, 1814–1823. [CrossRef] [PubMed]
25. Bergmann, L.; Kube, U.; Doehn, C.; Steiner, T.; Goebell, P.J.; Kindler, M.; Herrmann, E.; Janssen, J.; Weikert, S.; Scheffler, M.T.; et al. Everolimus in metastatic renal cell carcinoma after failure of initial anti-VEGF therapy: Final results of a noninterventional study. *BMC Cancer* **2015**, *15*, 303. [CrossRef] [PubMed]
26. Hutson, T.E.; Escudier, B.; Esteban, E.; Bjarnason, G.A.; Lim, H.Y.; Pittman, K.B.; Senico, P.; Niethammer, A.; Lu, D.R.; Hariharan, S.; et al. Randomized phase III trial of temsirolimus versus sorafenib as second-line therapy after sunitinib in patients with metastatic renal cell carcinoma. *J. Clin. Oncol.* **2014**, *32*, 760–767. [CrossRef] [PubMed]
27. Signorovitch, J.E.; Vogelzang, N.J.; Pal, S.K.; Lin, P.L.; George, D.J.; Wong, M.K.; Liu, Z.; Wang, X.; Culver, K.; Scott, J.A.; et al. Comparative effectiveness of second-line targeted therapies for metastatic renal cell carcinoma: Synthesis of findings from two multi-practice chart reviews in the United States. *Curr. Med. Res. Opin.* **2014**, *30*, 2343–2353. [CrossRef] [PubMed]
28. Wong, M.K.; Yang, H.; Signorovitch, J.E.; Wang, X.; Liu, Z.; Liu, N.S.; Qi, C.Z.; George, D.J. Comparative outcomes of everolimus, temsirolimus and sorafenib as second targeted therapies for metastatic renal cell carcinoma: A US medical record review. *Curr. Med. Res. Opin.* **2014**, *30*, 537–545. [CrossRef] [PubMed]
29. Park, K.; Lee, J.L.; Park, I.; Park, S.; Ahn, Y.; Ahn, J.H.; Ahn, S.; Song, C.; Hong, J.H.; Kim, C.S.; et al. Comparative efficacy of vascular endothelial growth factor (VEGF) tyrosine kinase inhibitor (TKI) and mammalian target of rapamycin (mTOR) inhibitor as second-line therapy in patients with metastatic renal cell carcinoma after the failure of first-line VEGF TKI. *Med. Oncol.* **2012**, *29*, 3291–3297.
30. Busch, J.; Seidel, C.; Erber, B.; Issever, A.S.; Hinz, S.; Kempkensteffen, C.; Magheli, A.; Miller, K.; Grünwald, V.; Weikert, S. Retrospective comparison of triple-sequence therapies in metastatic renal cell carcinoma. *Eur. Urol.* **2013**, *64*, 62–70. [CrossRef]
31. Trask, P.C.; Bushmakin, A.G.; Cappelleri, J.C.; Tarazi, J.; Rosbrook, B.; Bycott, P.; Kim, S.; Stadler, W.M.; Rini, B. Baseline patient-reported kidney cancer-specific symptoms as an indicator for median survival in sorafenib-refractory metastatic renal cell carcinoma. *J. Cancer Surviv.* **2011**, *5*, 255–262. [CrossRef]
32. Rini, B.I.; Escudier, B.; Tomczak, P.; Kaprin, A.; Szczylik, C.; Hutson, T.E.; Michaelson, M.D.; Gorbunova, V.A.; Gore, M.E.; Rusakov, I.G.; et al. Comparative effectiveness of axitinib versus sorafenib in advanced renal cell carcinoma (AXIS): A randomised phase 3 trial. *Lancet* **2011**, *378*, 1931–1939. [CrossRef]
33. Zimmermann, K.; Schmittel, A.; Steiner, U.; Asemissen, A.M.; Knoedler, M.; Thiel, E.; Miller, K.; Keilholz, U. Sunitinib treatment for patients with advanced clear-cell renal-cell carcinoma after progression on sorafenib. *Oncology* **2009**, *76*, 350–354. [CrossRef] [PubMed]
34. Di Lorenzo, G.; Cartenì, G.; Autorino, R.; Bruni, G.; Tudini, M.; Rizzo, M.; Aieta, M.; Gonnella, A.; Rescigno, P.; Perdonà, S.; et al. Phase II study of sorafenib in patients with sunitinib-refractory metastatic renal cell cancer. *J. Clin. Oncol.* **2009**, *27*, 4469–4474. [CrossRef] [PubMed]
35. Tamaskar, I.; Garcia, J.A.; Elson, P.; Wood, L.; Mekhail, T.; Dreicer, R.; Rini, B.I.; Bukowski, R.M. Antitumor effects of sunitinib or sorafenib in patients with metastatic renal cell carcinoma who received prior antiangiogenic therapy. *J. Urol.* **2008**, *179*, 81–86. [CrossRef] [PubMed]
36. Motzer, R.J.; Michaelson, M.D.; Redman, B.G.; Hudes, G.R.; Wilding, G.; Figlin, R.A.; Ginsberg, M.S.; Kim, S.T.; Baum, C.M.; DePrimo, S.E.; et al. Activity of SU11248, a multitargeted inhibitor of vascular endothelial growth factor receptor and platelet-derived growth factor receptor, in patients with metastatic renal cell carcinoma. *J. Clin. Oncol.* **2006**, *24*, 16–24. [CrossRef]

37. Escudier, B.; Eisen, T.; Stadler, W.M.; Szczylik, C.; Oudard, S.; Siebels, M.; Negrier, S.; Chevreau, C.; Solska, E.; Desai, A.A.; et al. Sorafenib in advanced clear-cell renal-cell carcinoma. *N. Engl. J. Med.* **2007**, *356*, 125–134. [CrossRef]
38. Schiavina, R.; Mari, A.; Antonelli, A.; Bertolo, R.; Bianchi, G.; Borghesi, M.; Brunocilla, E.; Fiori, C.; Longo, N.; Martorana, G.; et al. A snapshot of nephron-sparing surgery in Italy: A prospective, multicenter report on clinical and perioperative outcomes (the RECORd 1 project). *Eur. J. Surg. Oncol.* **2015**, *41*, 346–352. [CrossRef]
39. Ljungberg, B.; Albiges, L.; Bensalah, K.; Bex, A.; Giles, R.H.; Hora, M.; Kuczyk, M.A.; Lam, T.; Marconi, L.; Merseburger, A.S.; et al. *EAU Guidelines on Renal Cell Carcinoma;* European Association of Urology: Arnhem, The Netherlands, 2020.
40. Motzer, R.J.; Jonasch, E.; Agarwal, N.; Bhayani, S.; Bro, W.P.; Chang, S.S.; Choueiri, T.K.; Costello, B.A.; Derweesh, I.H.; Fishman, M.; et al. Kidney cancer, version 2.2017, NCCN clinical practice guidelines in oncology. *J. Natl. Compr. Canc. Netw.* **2017**, *15*, 804–834. [CrossRef]
41. Guo, L.; Zhang, H.; Chen, B. Nivolumab as Programmed Death-1 (PD-1) Inhibitor for Targeted Immunotherapy in Tumor. *J. Cancer* **2017**, *8*, 410–416. [CrossRef]
42. Kimura, M.; Usami, E.; Teramachi, H.; Yoshimura, T. A comparative study of nivolumab and axitinib in terms of overall survival, treatment continuation, and cost for patients with metastatic renal cell carcinoma. *Mol. Clin. Oncol.* **2020**, *12*, 284–289. [CrossRef]
43. Bowles, D.W.; Kessler, E.R.; Jimeno, A. Multi-targeted tyrosine kinase inhibitors in clinical development: Focus on XL-184 (cabozantinib). *Drugs Today* **2011**, *47*, 857–868. [CrossRef] [PubMed]
44. Suyama, K.; Iwase, H. Lenvatinib: A Promising Molecular Targeted Agent for Multiple Cancers. *Cancer Control.* **2018**, *25*, 1073274818789361. [CrossRef] [PubMed]
45. Stafford, H.S.; Saltzstein, S.L.; Shimasaki, S.; Sanders, C.; Downs, T.M.; Sadler, G.R. Racial/ethnic and gender disparities in renal cell carcinoma incidence and survival. *J. Urol.* **2008**, *179*, 1704–1708. [CrossRef] [PubMed]
46. Rose, T.L.; Deal, A.M.; Krishnan, B.; Nielsen, M.E.; Smith, A.B.; Kim, W.Y.; Milowsky, M.I. Racial disparities in survival among patients with advanced renal cell carcinoma in the targeted therapy era. *Cancer* **2016**, *122*, 2988–2995. [CrossRef] [PubMed]
47. Clocchiatti, A.; Cora, E.; Zhang, Y.; Dotto, G.P. Sexual dimorphism in cancer. *Nat. Rev. Cancer* **2016**, *16*, 330–339. [CrossRef]
48. Mancini, M.; Righetto, M.; Baggio, G. Gender-Related Approach to Kidney Cancer Management: Moving Forward. *Int. J. Mol. Sci.* **2020**, *21*, 3378. [CrossRef]
49. Mancini, M.; Righetto, M.; Baggio, G. Spotlight on gender-specific disparities in bladder cancer. *Urologia* **2020**, *87*, 103–114. [CrossRef]
50. Zhang, G.; Zhu, Y.; Dong, D.; Gu, W.; Zhang, H.; Sun, L.; Ye, D. Clinical outcome of advanced and metastatic renal cell carcinoma treated with targeted therapy: Is there a difference between young and old patients? *Onco Targets Ther.* **2014**, *7*, 2043–2052. [CrossRef]
51. Vaishampayan, U. Evolving Treatment Paradigms in Non-clear Cell Kidney Cancer. *Curr. Treat. Options Oncol.* **2018**, *19*, 5. [CrossRef]
52. De Velasco, G.; Xie, W.; Donskov, F.; Albiges, L.; Beuselinck, B.; Srinivas, S.; Agarwal, N.; Lee, J.L.; Brugarolas, J.; Wood, L.A.; et al. Discontinuing VEGF-targeted Therapy for Progression Versus Toxicity Affects Outcomes of Second-line Therapies in Metastatic Renal Cell Carcinoma. *Clin. Genitourin. Cancer* **2017**, *15*, 403–410.e2. [CrossRef]
53. Shimizu, Y.; Iguchi, T.; Tamada, S.; Yasuda, S.; Kato, M.; Ninomiya, N.; Yamasaki, T.; Nakatani, T. Oncological outcomes classified according to metastatic lesions in the era of molecular targeted drugs for metastatic renal cancer. *Mol. Clin. Oncol.* **2018**, *8*, 791–796. [CrossRef] [PubMed]
54. Singla, N.; Ghandour, R.A.; Margulis, V. Is cytoreductive nephrectomy relevant in the immunotherapy era? *Curr. Opin. Urol.* **2019**, *29*, 526–530. [CrossRef] [PubMed]

10

Exploratory Pilot Study of Circulating Biomarkers in Metastatic Renal Cell Carcinoma

Ilaria Grazia Zizzari [1], Chiara Napoletano [1,*], Alessandra Di Filippo [1], Andrea Botticelli [2], Alain Gelibter [2], Fabio Calabrò [3], Ernesto Rossi [4], Giovanni Schinzari [4], Federica Urbano [2], Giulia Pomati [2], Simone Scagnoli [2], Aurelia Rughetti [1], Salvatore Caponnetto [2], Paolo Marchetti [2,5] and Marianna Nuti [1]

1 Laboratory of Tumor Immunology and Cell Therapy, Department of Experimental Medicine, Policlinico Umberto I, "Sapienza" University of Rome, 00161 Rome, Italy; ilaria.zizzari@uniroma1.it (I.G.Z.); alessandra.difilippo@uniroma1.it (A.D.F.); aurelia.rughetti@uniroma1.it (A.R.); marianna.nuti@uniroma1.it (M.N.)

2 Division of Oncology, Department of Radiological, Oncological and Pathological Science, Policlinico Umberto I, "Sapienza" University of Rome, 00161 Rome, Italy; andrea.botticelli@uniroma1.it (A.B.); alain.gelibter@uniroma1.it (A.G.); federica.urbano@uniroma1.it (F.U.); giuliapomati@tiscali.it (G.P.); simone.scagnoli@uniroma1.it (S.S.); salvo.caponnetto@uniroma1.it (S.C.); paolo.marchetti@uniroma1.it (P.M.)

3 Division of Medical Oncology B, San Camillo Forlanini Hospital Rome, 00149 Rome, Italy; fabiocalabro1@alice.it

4 Department of Medical Oncology, Fondazione Policlinico A.Gemelli Rome, 00168 Rome, Italy; Ernesto.rossi@guest.policlinicogemelli.it (E.R.); giovanni.schinzari@policlinicogemelli.it (G.S.)

5 Division of Oncology, Department of Clinical and Molecular Medicine, Ospedale Sant'Andrea, "Sapienza" University of Rome, 00189 Rome, Italy

* Correspondence: chiara.napoletano@uniroma1.it

Simple Summary: The identification of biomarkers in response to therapeutic treatment is one of the main objectives of personalized oncology. Predictive biomarkers are particularly relevant for oncologists challenged by the busy scenario of possible therapeutic options in mRCC patients, including immunotherapy and TKIs. In fact the activation of the immune system can determine the outcome and success of the different therapeutic strategies. In this study we evaluated changes in the immune system of TKI mRCC-treated patients defining immunological profiles related to response characterized by specific biomarkers. The validation of the proposed immune portrait to an extended number of patients could allow characterization and selection of responsive and non-responsive patients from the beginning of the therapeutic process.

Abstract: With the introduction of immune checkpoint inhibitors (ICIs) and next-generation vascular endothelial growth factor receptor–tyrosine kinase inhibitors (VEGFR–TKIs), the survival of patients with advanced renal cell carcinoma (RCC) has improved remarkably. However, not all patients have benefited from treatments, and to date, there are still no validated biomarkers that can be included in the therapeutic algorithm. Thus, the identification of predictive biomarkers is necessary to increase the number of responsive patients and to understand the underlying immunity. The clinical outcome of RCC patients is, in fact, associated with immune response. In this exploratory pilot study, we assessed the immune effect of TKI therapy in order to evaluate the immune status of metastatic renal cell carcinoma (mRCC) patients so that we could define a combination of immunological biomarkers relevant to improving patient outcomes. We profiled the circulating levels in 20 mRCC patients of exhausted/activated/regulatory T cell subsets through flow cytometry and of 14 immune checkpoint-related proteins and 20 inflammation cytokines/chemokines using multiplex Luminex assay, both at baseline and during TKI therapy. We identified the $CD3^+CD8^+CD137^+$ and

$CD3^+CD137^+PD1^+$ T cell populations, as well as seven soluble immune molecules (i.e., IFNγ, sPDL2, sHVEM, sPD1, sGITR, sPDL1, and sCTLA4) associated with the clinical responses of mRCC patients, either modulated by TKI therapy or not. These results suggest an immunological profile of mRCC patients, which will help to improve clinical decision-making for RCC patients in terms of the best combination of strategies, as well as the optimal timing and therapeutic sequence.

Keywords: TKIs; mRCC; biomarkers; soluble factors

---

1. Introduction

Renal cell carcinoma (RCC) represents 2–3% of cancer diagnoses in adults [1]. To date, nephrectomy remains the main therapeutic choice for most patients with localized disease; however, one-third of patients present metastatic disease at diagnosis and one-quarter of all patients could ultimately experience disease relapse. In the past decade, the prognosis of metastatic renal carcinoma (mRCC) has considerably improved due to the recent introduction of the vascular endothelial growth factor receptor–tyrosine kinase inhibitors (VEGFR–TKIs) and immune checkpoint inhibitors (ICIs). New synergistic combinations between TKIs and ICIs could increase the first line of therapeutic strategies in RCC. Although the recent improvements and advances in genomic sequencing and molecular characterizations have allowed an accurate definition of prognosis, predictive biomarkers are still needed to select the patients beneficiaries of the different therapeutic approaches. Diagnostic tools that pool biomarker data could help to tailor treatment strategies based on the biological and immunological parameters of the patient [2].

Indeed, it is well-known that immunological features can affect the prognosis of patients, but it has also been described in depth that target therapy presents several immunological effects. From this perspective, a dynamic immunological portrait of patients and cancer can influence not only the response to immunotherapy, but also the response to target therapy.

The question is how to increase the number of responsive patients to target and immunotherapy; therefore, it is necessary to understand the immunity underlying patients. The immune system represents, in fact, a key point for the clinical outcome of RCC patients, taking into account the potential prognostic values such as the tumor-infiltrating immune cells that create a microenvironment regulating cancer progression [3]. Furthermore, several immunosuppressive molecules, such as vascular endothelial growth factor (VEGF), characterize the microenvironment of this tumor with the ability to promote neo-angiogenesis and tumor growth as well as negatively impact immune response. VEGF signaling modulates T cell biology and function. Indeed, VEGF decreases T-cell progenitors in the thymus and differentiated T cells in the lymphoid organs and dampens their effector function. Furthermore, VEGF fosters immune-suppression by accumulation of regulatory T cells (Tregs) and contributing to T-cells exhaustion. Thus, while the neoangiogenic hallmark always represents a crucial pathway in RCC, making this tumor sensible to antiangiogenic therapies [4,5], also the immune system can be considered an off target for these therapies [6,7]. Indeed bevacizumab and sorafenib reverse the immunosuppressive effects of VEGF and restore the maturation of dendritic cells (DCs) [8,9]. Pazopanib improves DC differentiation and maturation and seems to modulate the $CD137^+$ (4-1BB, a member of the TNF-receptor family) T-cell population [10]. Other TKIs, such as sunitinib, modulate immunosuppressive cells such as MDSC and Tregs [11,12].

Moreover, recent evidence demonstrates that several soluble immune molecules involved in immune regulation, such as soluble immune checkpoint-related proteins (sICs; i.e., es.sCTLA-4 and sPD1), can influence the development, prognosis and treatment of cancer [13]. These are functional proteins released by immune cells as alternative splice variants or by cleavage of membrane-bound proteins and can diffuse in serum [14,15]. However, only a few studies have evaluated the role of sICs in in the outcome of renal cancer.

The aim of our study was to evaluate the immunological effect of TKIs and the impact of the immune profile of patients in response to TKI therapy.

2. Results

2.1. Patient Characteristics

Study Population

The characteristics of patients are listed in Table 1. Twenty mRCC patients were enrolled. The median age at diagnosis was 56.5 years (range: 36–78 years); 15 (75%) patients were males and nine (45%) had a previous history of smoking. Clear cell RCC was the most represented histology (16 patients; 80%), followed by one case of clear cell carcinoma with sarcomatoid features, one case of chromophobe, and two cases with another histology. According to Fuhrman grading, nine patients (45%) were defined as G3, seven (35%) as G2, and four (20%) cases as unknown. Almost all patients in the study underwent nephrectomy (18 patients; 90%); 11 patients (55%) had metastatic disease at the first diagnosis of renal cancer. At diagnosis of metastatic disease, liver metastases occurred in four patients (20% of cases), whereas nodal, lung, bone, brain, and adrenal metastases occurred in eight patients (40%), 12 patients (60%), five patients (25%), three patients (15%), and one patient (5%), respectively. Overall, five patients were classified as poor risk according to their Metastatic Renal Cell Cancer Database Consortium (IMDC) scores, 10 patients as intermediate risk, and five patients as good risk. With regard to first-line treatment, eight (40%) and 12 (60%) patients received sunitinib and pazopanib, respectively. The toxicities to first-line therapy were in line with the treatment received. Most patients discontinued the first-line therapy due to progressive disease (16 patients; 80%); one patient (5%) stopped the treatment because of toxicity, while three patients (15%) remained on treatment. The first-line median progression-free survival (PFS) was 11 months (range: 1–31 months). Ten patients (50%) underwent second-line treatment with Nivolumab. Globally, second-line treatment was well tolerated; however, five patients (50%) stopped second-line treatment due to progressive disease and one patient due to toxicity, while in four patients, the treatment was ongoing at the last follow-up visit. The second-line median PFS was 4 months (range: 1–22 months). Of these patients, two received third-line therapy with cabozantinib. In one patient, the PFS was 8 months and treatment was discontinued for progressive disease, while in one patient, treatment remained ongoing. Responsive and non-responsive patients were considered on the basis of the first clinical revaluation and 3–4 months after beginning TKI treatment. Clinical and radiological outcomes were assessed as parameters to differentiate responsive and non-responsive patients. Tumor response was assessed every 3–4 months using immune-related Response Evaluation Criteria in Solid Tumors (i-RECIST). According to i-RECIST, responsive patients (R) were considered those who achieved complete or partial radiological response or a stable disease at the first radiological evaluation. Conversely, patients who experienced a radiological progression of disease or a clinically significant worsening of cancer-related symptoms were considered as non-responders (NR).

Table 1. Clinical and pathological characteristics and treatment.

Characteristic	All Patients (N = 20) (100%)
Age (years) Median Age (range)	56.5 (36–78)
Gender	
Male	15 (75)
Female	5 (25)
Risk Factors Smoking history (SH)	9 (45)

Table 1. *Cont.*

Characteristic	All Patients (N = 20) (100%)
Histology	
Clear cell carcinoma	16 (80)
Other	4 (20)
Fuhrman grading	
G2	7 (35)
G3	9 (45)
Unknown	4 (20)
Metastatic site at diagnosis	
Liver	4 (20)
Nodal	8 (40)
Lung	12 (60)
Bone	5 (25)
Brain	3 (15)
Adrenal	1 (5)
IMDC score	
Poor risk	5 (25)
Intermediate	10 (50)
Good risk	5 (25)
I-line treatment	20
Sunitinib	8 (40)
Pazopanib	12 (60)
II-line treatment	10 (50)
Nivolumab	10 (100)
III-line treatment	2
Cabozantinib	2

2.2. *$CD137^+$ T Cells Are Associated with the Response to TKIs in mRCC Patients*

CD137 is a co-stimulatory molecule expressed on activated T cells, and the engagement with its ligand contributes to enhancing the proliferation and effector functions of lymphocytes, preventing apoptosis [16]. It is considered a bonafide marker of recently activated tumor-reactive T cells.

Figure 1A shows the expression of CD137 molecule on $CD3^+$, $CD8^+$, and $CD4^+$ T cells in responsive and non-responsive patients before treatment (T0) and during treatment (>T0). At T0, responsive patients had a significantly higher percentage of $CD3^+CD137^+$ T cells (2.7% ± 0.92%) compared to non-responsive (0.9% ± 0.87%) (p = 0.003), which was also maintained during TKI treatment (%$CD3^+CD137^+$: 2.6% ± 0.78% in responsive patients vs. 0.67% ± 0.4% in non-responsive patients; p = 0.0001). In particular, CD137 expression was associated with the $CD8^+$ T cell subpopulation. In fact, at T0, the expression of CD137 on $CD8^+$ T cells was significantly higher in responsive patients (2.02% ± 0.7%) compared to non-responsive patients (0.6% ± 0.5%) (p = 0.001). The same significant trend was observed during TKI treatment ($CD8^+CD137^+$ subpopulation was 1.91% ± 0.75% in responsive patients vs. 0.43% ± 0.25% in non-responsive; p = 0.0008). Instead, no significant differences were obtained for $CD4^+$ T-cell subpopulation (%$CD4^+CD137^+$ at T0: 0.6% ± 0.2% in responsive patients vs. 0.27% ± 0.18% in non-responsive, p = 0.28; at >T0: 0.87% ± 0.28% in responsive vs. 0.23% ± 0.08% in non-responsive, p = 0.18).

These results show that $CD137^+$ T cells could represent a possible biomarker that is able to identify patients that could clinically benefit from TKI treatment.

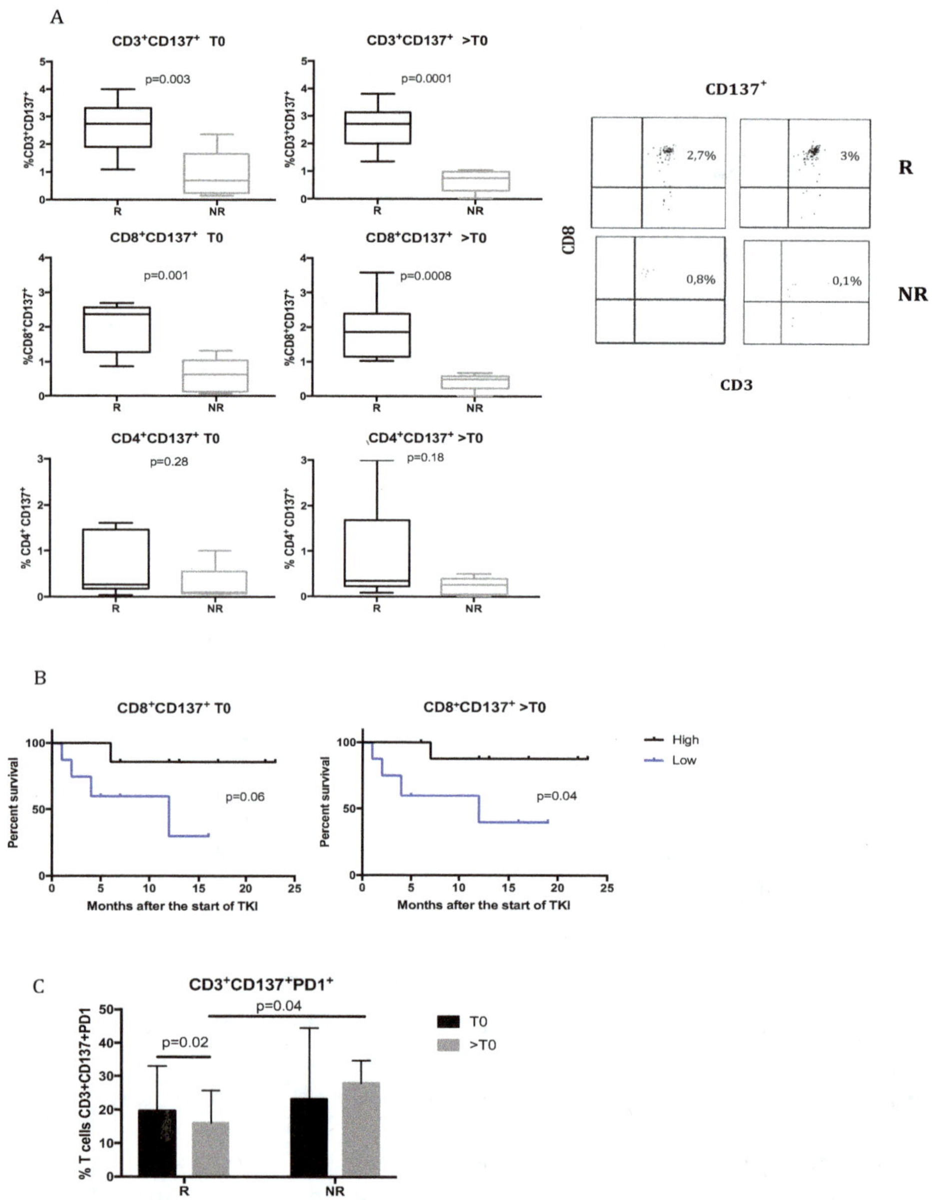

Figure 1. (**A**) Immune cell subpopulations were evaluated using flow cytometry and analyzed by FACSDiva Software. To analyze the CD137$^+$ T cells, lymphocytes were first gated on FSC-A and SSC-A, and then the CD3$^+$ T-cell subpopulation was selected from the lymphocytes. CD3$^+$CD137$^+$ T cells were then selected and analyzed for CD4 and CD8. The results are shown as percentages of CD3$^+$CD137$^+$, CD8$^+$CD137$^+$ and CD4$^+$CD137$^+$ T cells in responsive (R) and non-responsive (NR) patients at baseline (T0) and during tyrosine kinase inhibitor (TKI) treatment (>T0). The dot plot analysis of the CD3$^+$CD8$^+$CD137$^+$ T lymphocytes is shown in the right of panel A. The results are representative of one R patient and one NR metastatic renal carcinoma (mRCC) patient. (**B**) Survival analysis at baseline and during treatment of mRCC patients treated with TKI. At T0, survival analysis of the mRCC patients was conducted, comparing those with greater than 1.4% of CD8$^+$CD137$^+$ T cells to those with less or equal to 1.4%. During TKI therapy (>T0), a survival curve was calculated using the value of 1.3% to distinguish high and low percentages of CD8$^+$CD137$^+$ T cells. Log-rank tests were used to compare the survival between two groups. (**C**) Expression of PD1 molecules on the CD3$^+$CD137$^+$ T lymphocytes. The results are reported as percentages of PD1 normalized on CD3$^+$CD137$^+$ T cells in R and NR patients a T0 and during TKI therapy (>T0). Statistical significance was determined by a Student's unpaired *t*-test. A *p*-value of <0.05 was considered statistically significant.

The Kaplan–Meier survival curves for patients with high and low concentrations of $CD8^{+}CD137^{+}$ T cells are shown in Figure 1B. During treatment with TKI, the median survival times were 12 months in the group with a low concentration of $CD8^{+}CD137^{+}$ T cells and undefined in the group with a high concentration $CD8^{+}CD137^{+}$ T cells ($p = 0.04$, log-rank test). The same trend was observed at baseline, despite the fact that the difference between high and low concentrations of CD137 T cells was not statistically significant. These data suggest that the maintenance of $CD8^{+}$ $CD137^{+}$ T cells in circulation is associated with the duration of the response to TKIs.

The expression of PD1 molecules on the $CD3^{+}CD137^{+}$ T-cell population was also analyzed (Figure 1C). It was observed that during TKI treatment, responsive patients experienced a significant downregulation of PD1 expression ($p = 0.02$). Moreover, at >T0, PD1 resulted significantly higher in non-responsive compared to responsive patients (27.9 ± 3.4 vs. 16 ± 3.2, respectively; $p = 0.04$).

The higher percentage of $PD1^{+}$ on $CD3^{+}CD137^{+}$ T cells in non-responsive patients could suggest that these patients could possibly benefit from an anti-PD1 therapy already at the time of evaluation.

Regulatory T cells and other exhaustion markers were analyzed, but no difference was observed between patients.

2.3. *TKI Treatment Modulates Soluble Immune Molecules*

In order to evaluate the impact of TKI treatment in the release of soluble immune molecules in mRCC patients, the levels of immune checkpoint-related proteins and inflammatory cytokines were evaluated in the sera of mRCC patients before (T0) and during TKI therapy (>T0). It was recently demonstrated that the soluble isoforms of the checkpoint receptors can contribute to immune regulation, representing putative biomarkers for tumor outcome and patient stratification [17]. Moreover, much evidence has demonstrated that these molecules are involved in positive or negative immune regulation and that changes in their plasma levels affect the development, prognosis, and treatment of cancer [13].

Figure 2A shows that TKI treatment in mRCC patients modulates several sICs. In particular, the concentration of sPDL2 significantly decreased during TKI therapy (7842.5 ± 2865 pg/mL for T0 vs. 4989 ± 4462 pg/mL for >T0; $p = 0.02$). Similar results were observed for sHVEM (4085.5 ± 3388 pg/mL for T0 vs. 1777 ± 1578 pg/mL for >T0; $p = 0.01$). It was shown that the high concentration of sHVEM seems to contribute to tumor development and progression [18]. Moreover, the results indicate that TKI treatment also affects the release of sPD1 and sGITR, decreasing the concentration of both molecules between T0 and >T0 (sPD1: 561.5 ± 431 pg/mL for T0 vs. 238 ± 176 pg/mL for >T0, $p = 0.02$; sGITR: 548 ± 425 pg/mL for T0 vs. 214 ± 212 pg/mL for >T0, $p = 0.01$).

The correlations between the fold-changes (>T0/T0) of soluble immune checkpoint molecules were also calculated and are shown in Figure S1. The fold-change of sPD1 was positively correlated with that of sGITR ($p = 0.009$, $r = 0.65$) and sHVEM ($p = 0.002$, $r = 0.59$). Additionally, a positive correlation between the fold-change of sHVEM and sGITR ($p = 0.0009$, $r = 0.76$) was also found, while no correlation was obtained for sPDL2.

When the association between these soluble molecules and clinical responses was evaluated (Figure 2B), sPD-L2 resulted in the significant modulation of unique soluble immune checkpoint-related proteins in mRCC responsive patients (R) during TKI treatment (sPDL2: 8855 ± 3985 pg/mL for T0 vs. 5057 ± 4243 pg/mL for >T0, $p = 0.01$). No significant modulation was obtained in non-responsive patients (NR). On the other hand, it was recently demonstrated that sPDL2 is the strongest predictor of recurrence in ccRCC; patients with a high level of sPDL2 had, in fact, a significantly increased risk of recurrence [19].

These data demonstrate that TKIs impact the release of immune molecules, suggesting their possible role in the clinical outcome of mRCC patients.

The results were independent of the TKI administered and no significant data were obtained for other soluble factors tested (cytokine and checkpoint related proteins; Table S2).

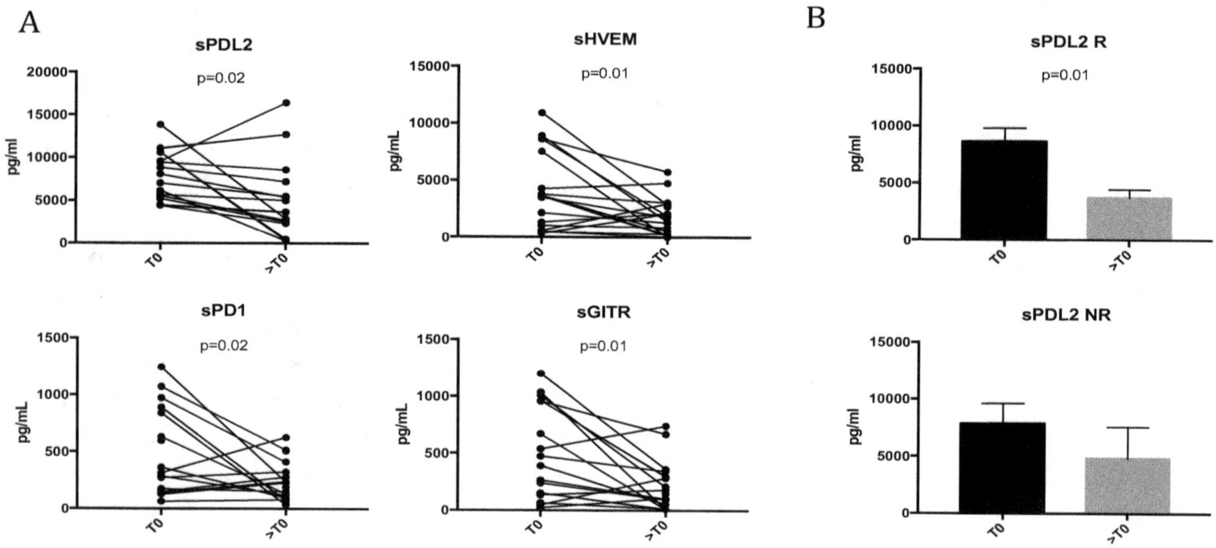

Figure 2. Changes in the soluble immune checkpoint-related proteins during TKI therapy in mRCC patients. (**A**) Analysis of soluble immune checkpoint-related proteins levels (i.e., sPDL2, sHVEM, sPD1, and sGITR) in patients with mRCC at baseline (T0) and after 3–4 months of TKI treatment (>T0). The proteins were analyzed by Luminex multiplex assay and the results are reported as the concentration (pg/mL) of soluble checkpoint inhibitors present in the serum of mRCC patients. (**B**) sPDL2 levels in the serum of mRCC responsive (R) and non-responsive (NR) patients analyzed at T0 and >T0. sPDL2 resulted in the only significantly modulated molecule associated with response to TKI treatment. Statistical significance was determined by a Student's paired *t*-test, and a *p*-value < 0.05 was considered statistically significant.

2.4. TKI Responsive Patients Have Low Levels of Serum IFNγ

To analyze the contribution of immune cytokines to the response to treatment, the sera of mRCC responsive and non-responsive patients were analyzed at T0 and during TKI therapy. Figure 3A shows that before beginning TKI therapy, those mRCC patients that would benefit from treatment had a significantly lower concentration of IFNγ compared to non-responsive patients (27.47 ± 8.5 pg/mL for R vs. 515.8 ± 210.6 pg/mL for NR; $p = 0.007$). The same significant trend was found for >T0 (48.74 ± 21.24 for R patients vs. 267.8 ± 77.12 for NR; $p = 0.002$). These data show that low levels of IFNγ correlates with response to TKI treatment. IFNγ plays a key role in antitumor immune responses in the elimination stage of the immunoediting paradigm. However, recent evidence suggests that IFNγ may also play a significant role in promoting tumorigenesis [20].

To determine whether mRCC patients treated with TKIs derive survival benefit based on IFNγ levels, survival rates were examined. Figure 3B shows that IFNγ predicts, at baseline, the duration of the response to TKI treatment in mRCC patients. Patients with low levels of IFNγ (<65 pg/mL) had a longer duration of response to TKI therapy compared to patients with higher levels (>65 pg/mL). The average time of the duration of the response was undefined vs. 7 months ($p = 0.04$), and no significant correlation was observed during treatment (>T0).

2.5. Upregulation of sPDL1 and sCTLA4 in Non-Responsive Patients During TKI Treatment

The serum levels of other cytokines and soluble checkpoint-related proteins were evaluated according to the response to therapy at T0 and >T0. Among the molecules analyzed, sPDL1 and sCTLA4 resulted statistically significant. In particular, as shown in Figure 3C, the average concentration values in the serum obtained at T0 for sPDL1 and sCTLA4 highlighted a trend of a higher release of these molecules in non-responsive patients. This difference was statistically significant during TKI treatment: sPDL1 levels in responsive patients were 56.25 ± 36.5 pg/mL vs. 146.5 ± 122.3 pg/mL for non-responsive patients ($p = 0.03$); sCTL4 levels were 281.6 ± 133 pg/mL for responsive patients compared to 616.4 ± 330.3 pg/mL for non-responsive patients (p = 0.008). These data suggest a possible higher circulating immunosuppressive status in mRCC patients that would not benefit from TKI therapy.

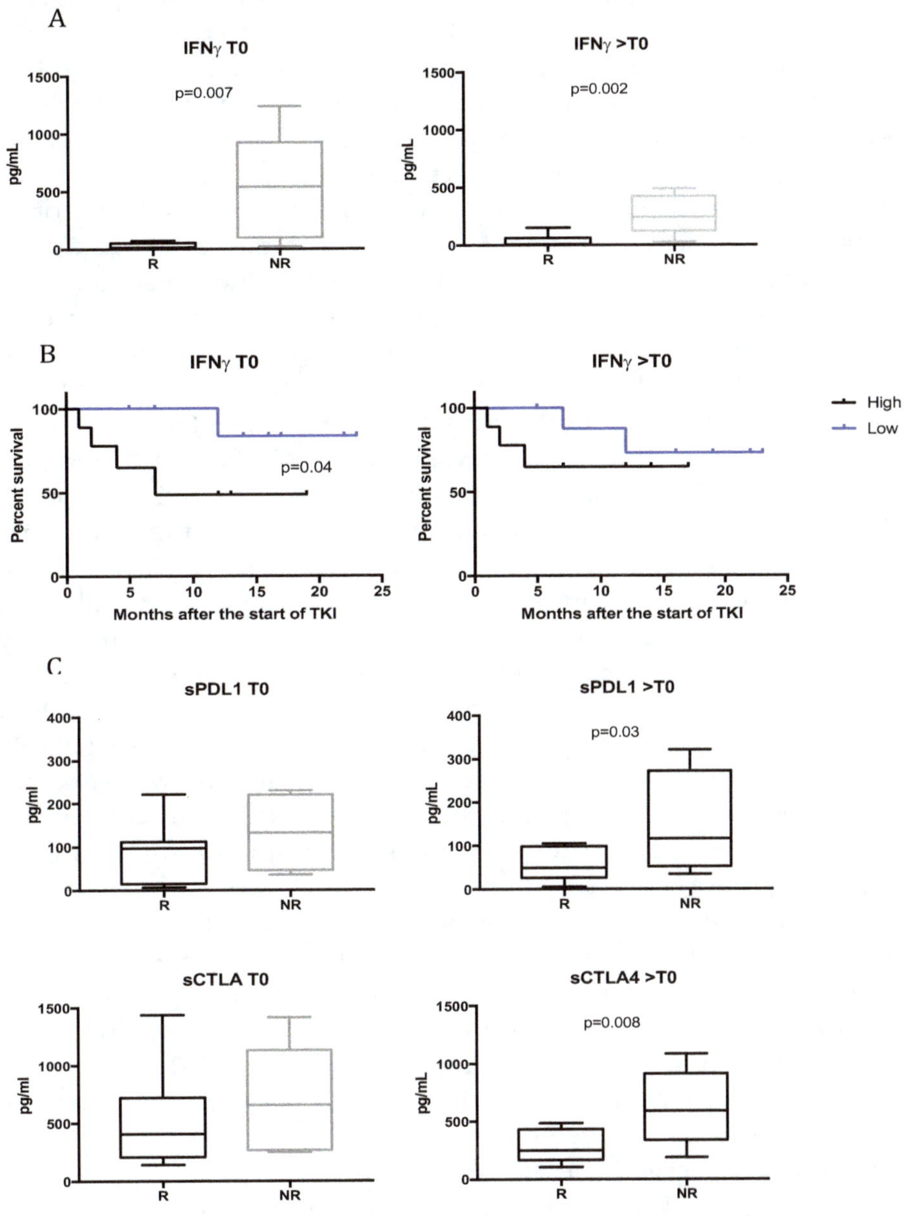

Figure 3. Profiling of levels of immune molecules at baseline and during TKI treatment in responsive (R) and non-responsive (NR) patients. (**A**) Box plots of IFNγ levels in R and NR mRCC patients at T0 and >T0. The lines in the boxes show the median values. The error bars show the minimum and maximum values. (**B**) Survival curve analysis of the mRCC patients at baseline and during TKI treatment according to the levels of IFNγ. For T0, the median value considered for patients belonging to the high-concentration group was >65 pg/mL, while for those belonging to the low-concentration group was ≤65 pg/mL. For the analysis of survival during TKI treatment, the median value of IFNγ levels used to dichotomize patients was >59 pg/mL for the high-concentration group and ≤59 pg/mL for the low-concentration group. A log-rank test was used to compare the survival between two groups. (**C**) Box plots of sPDL1 and sCTLA4 at baseline and 3–4 months after the start of TKI therapy (>T0). A Student's unpaired t-test was used to compare R vs. NR patients and a p-value < 0.05 was considered statistically significant.

3. Discussion

Angiogenesis plays a key role in RCC tumorigenesis and progression, directing the immune system through the abnormal formation of tumor vessels and the promotion of an immunosuppressive tumor microenvironment. Therefore, antiangiogenic treatments remain a valid therapeutic option in selected patients, since they modulate immune responses [10,21,22]. This activity is essential to enhancing the performance of immunotherapy agents, which have shown promising treatment outcomes also for advanced RCC [23]. Immune checkpoint inhibitors combined with TKIs will become a new standard of care in treatment-naive patients with advanced RCC [6]. However, not all patients benefit from immune checkpoint therapy and, at present, no effective biomarkers can be included in the therapeutic algorithm, despite large research efforts. Thus, the identification of reliable predictive factors is necessary. Only a few studies have investigated the role of immune cells and circulating immune molecules in RCC, especially in metastatic cancer patients. In this study, we observed, for the first time, that TKIs are able to modulate soluble immune checkpoint-related proteins. Moreover, we identified an association between circulating biomarkers and the response to TKI treatment. In particular, we identified that $CD3^{+}CD8^{+}CD137^{+}$ T cells are a population of activated T lymphocytes significantly more expressed in responsive patients, both at baseline than during TKI treatment, suggesting that CD137 could represent a predictive biomarker of response to TKI. The CD137 receptor is considered a biomarker of tumor-reactive cells. It has been demonstrated that signaling through CD137 induces the activation of $CD8^{+}$ T cells in a CD28-independent manner, enhancing T-cell survival, promoting their effector function, and favoring memory differentiation [24,25]. The results obtained in our study are in line with that observed in a previous study conducted on a limited number of mRCC patients, where we identified modulations occurring in the immune T cell repertoire of mRCC during TKI treatment. Among the different biomarkers tested, we were able to detect a $CD137^{+}$ T-cell subset in mRCC arising during pazopanib treatment [10]. In this study, we further observed that this population correlates with the response to TKI therapy. In fact, we obtained an increase in $CD3^{+}CD137^{+}$ T cells at baseline in those mRCC patients who benefited from TKI treatment. Moreover, we observed that $CD3^{+}CD137^{+}$ T lymphocytes are mainly cytotoxic T cells and that the maintenance of $CD8^{+}CD137^{+}$ in circulation is associated with the duration of response to treatment, suggesting that CD137 could represent a promising target for antitumor immune activation strategies. Numerous studies have demonstrated that although both activated $CD4^{+}$ and $CD8^{+}$ T cells express CD137, signals through CD137 are more biased toward $CD8^{+}$ T cells, both in vitro and in vivo [26–28]. Interestingly, the in vivo administration of agonistic anti-CD137 antibody promotes $CD8^{+}$ T-cell expansion, providing protection against several diseases, including cancer [29,30]. In fact, CD137 has previously been shown to be important in positively regulating effector T-cell responses in cancer [31,32]. Freeman et al. recently observed that, in tumor types heavily infiltrated with $CD8^{+}$ T cells, CD137 is associated with increased $CD8^{+}$ T-cell effector function and improved patient survival [33].

In this study, we also observed the expression of PD1 on $CD137^{+}$ T cells, particularly in non-responsive patients during TKI therapy. A previous report showed the presence of a rare population of a $CD8^{+}CD137^{+}PD1^{+}$ T cell subset in lung cancer patients [24]. Moreover, it was demonstrated that the co-expression of PD-1 and CD137 on tumor-infiltrating lymphocytes (TILs) contributes to the synergistic effects of the combination of anti-PD-1-blocking agents and CD137 agonists [34]. These data suggest that a subpopulation may potentially exert a critical antitumor effect through combination immunotherapy with anti-PD1-blocking agents and CD137 agonists, opening up possible new therapeutic strategies in the management of advanced RCC patients. On the other hand, immune checkpoints play important roles in immune regulation, and blocking immune checkpoints on the cell membrane has proven to be an effective strategy in the treatment of cancer [13]. However, the influence of soluble receptors and ligands on immune modulation and cancer outcome has not been studied. To date, only few studies have investigated the contribution of soluble factors to the clinical efficacy provided by ICIs; this has led to the incorrect assumption that these antibodies act only at the level of membrane-based interactions [17]. Soluble receptors and ligands, which are part of a family that includes full-length receptors and ligands, are produced by mRNA expression or by the cleavage of membrane-bound proteins and are found free in the plasma. Recent studies indicate that soluble isoforms of immune checkpoint receptors are centrally involved in immune regulation and, to date, only few studies have examined the association between soluble immune checkpoint-related proteins and cancer outcomes [35].

Here, we identified soluble immune checkpoint-related proteins and inflammatory cytokines modulated by TKI therapy and associated with the clinical outcomes of mRCC patients. It is well-known that TKIs affect the immune system [6]. Antiangiogenic therapies contrast the immunosuppressive effects induced by angiogenic factors, increasing the tumor infiltration of mature DCs and effector T cells and decreasing the infiltration of immunosuppressive cells, mainly regulatory T cells and myeloid-derived suppressor cells [8,11,12,36–38]. Nevertheless, the impact of TKI treatment on soluble immune checkpoint-related inhibitors and the possible role induced by these factors in response or resistance to treatment has not yet been elucidated in mRCC. Recently, it was demonstrated that sorafenib induces changes in soluble checkpoint protein levels in patients with advanced hepatocellular carcinoma [15]. Here, we demonstrated that TKIs modulate soluble ICs (i.e., sPDL2, sHVEM, sPD1, and sGITR) and we identified sPDL2 as a unique biomarker significantly downregulated in responsive patients during TKI treatment. This finding is supported by previous work describing sPDL2 as the most significant predictive biomarker of recurrence risk in ccRCC [19]. The high expression of PDL2 in tumors is also correlated with decreased cancer-free survival in RCC patients [39]. Moreover, high levels of sPDL2 are correlated with poor survival post-CAR T cells infusion in relapsed and refractory B-cell lymphoma and leukemia patients [40]. Therefore, we speculate that sPDL2 represents a biomarker correlated in response to TKI treatment, although these findings warrant further confirmation. Moreover, our results indicate that changes in soluble ICI during TKI treatment are positively correlated to one another, in contrast to sPDL2, which seems to be an independent factor. According to several studies that have reported the role of soluble checkpoint molecules in the promotion and progression of cancer, downregulating immune activation [18], here we demonstrated that IFNγ, sPDL1 and sCTLA4 play important roles in regulating the response to TKI treatment. Interestingly, we observed that low levels of IFNγ correlated with the response to TKI therapy, both at baseline and after 3–4 months after starting treatment. Moreover, the low levels of IFNγ at baseline seems to be associated with a better response to TKI treatment in terms of the duration of the response. Indeed, early studies on IFNγ and cancer biology established its role as an antitumor cytokine; however, now it is known that this cytokine can have a dual role in shaping the outcome of cancer [41]. A lot of genes induced by IFNγ are, in fact, involved in cancer cell immune evasion, such as PDL1, PDL2, CTLA4, and IDO [42,43]. It was shown that IFNγ promotes the expression of PDL1 and PDL2, both on tumor cells and on immune infiltrating cells, and suppresses the effector function of tumor-specific T cells or NK cells through interaction with the immune inhibitory receptor PD1 [44,45]. Moreover, our data show that sPDL1 is associated with poor response to TKI treatment, confirming the predictive role of this molecule for poor prognosis and increased risk of death in mRCC [46–48]. sCTLA4 was the other soluble protein that showed a significant correlation with failure to response during TKI treatment. It is possible that the increase in sPDL1 and sCTLA is linked to the high levels of IFNγ, but this is a mechanism that needs to be evaluated in a larger number of patients. Recently, IFNγ-induced PD-L1/2 expression was also referred to as a mechanism of adaptive immune resistance to immune checkpoint therapy [49].

4. Materials and Methods

4.1. Patient Selection

This was a multicenter, prospective, observational study. Twenty consecutive patients affected by metastatic renal carcinoma, referred to three Italian oncology units (i.e., Policlinico Umberto I Hospital, Sapienza University; A. Gemelli Hospital, Cattolica University; San Camillo Forlanini Hospital) and treated with at least one line of treatment, were enrolled. Blood samples were collected at different time points: before starting and during therapy (i.e., at the first clinical revaluation and 3–4 months after beginning treatment). The clinical and survival data of identified patients were retrieved from clinical records. A specific database, including the following clinical and pathological features for each patient, was built: age, sex, smoking status, histology, Fuhrman grading, date of diagnosis of metastatic disease, date of nephrectomy, IMDC score, first-line treatment, date of progression to first-line treatment, toxicities related to first-line treatment, second-line treatment, date of progression to second-line treatment, toxicities related to second-line treatment, and third-line treatment. Written informed consent was obtained from all patients. The study was approved by the Ethics Committee of Policlinico Umberto I (Ethical Committee Protocol, RIF.CE: 4181).

4.2. *PBMC (Peripheral Blood Mononuclear Cells) Purification and Sera Collection*

PBMCs were isolated from the peripheral blood (40 mL) of mRCC patients before (T0) and during TKI therapy (>T0, at first clinical revaluation) using Ficoll–Hypaque gradient (1077 g/mL; Pharmacia LKB). At the same time, sera were collected and stored at −80 °C until use.

4.3. *Immune Phenotype*

A multi-parametric analysis by flow cytometry was conducted to evaluate various T-cell subsets and function as the combined expression of the following markers:

- T cell exhaustion/activation: Anti-CD3-APC-H7/CD8-PerCp-Cy5.5/CD137-PeCy7/PD1-PE/CTLA4-APC/Tim3-BB515;
- T regulatory cells: Anti-CD4-APC-H7/CD25-PE/CD45RA-BB515/FoxP3-Alexa647.

Flow cytometric analysis was performed using a FACSCanto flow cytometer running FACS Diva data acquisition and analysis software (version 8.0.2, BD Biosciences, San Diego, CA, USA). In Table S1 are listed the catalog numbers and clones of the antibodies used in this study.

4.4. *Inflammatory Cytokine, Chemokine and Soluble Checkpoint Inhibitor Detection*

The sera from mRCC patients were assayed to quantify cytokines and soluble checkpoint molecules using the ProcartaPlex Human Inflammation Panel (20 Plex, catalog number EPX200-12185-901; sE-Selectin; GM-CSF; ICAM-1/CD54; IFN alpha; IFN gamma; IL-1 alpha; IL-1 beta; IL-4; IL-6; IL-8; IL-10; IL-12p70; IL-13; IL-17A/CTLA-8; IP-10/CXCL10; MCP-1/CCL2; MIP-1alpha/CCL3; MIP-1 beta/CCL4; sP-Selectin; TNF alpha) (eBioscence, Vienna, Austria) and the Human Immuno-Oncology Checkpoint 14-Plex ProcartaPlex Panel 1 (catalog number EPX14A-15803-901; BTLA; GITR; HVEM; IDO; LAG-3: 47; PD1; PD-L1; PD-L2; TIM-3; CD28; CD80; CD137; CD27; CD152) (eBioscence). Samples were measured using Luminex 200 platform (BioPlex; Bio-Rad, Bio-Rad, Hercules, CA, USA) and data, expressed in pg/mL of protein, were analyzed using Bio-Plex Manager Software (version 6.1, Bio-Rad).

4.5. *Statistical Analysis*

Descriptive statistics (i.e., average and standard deviation) were used to describe the various data. Student's paired and unpaired *t*-tests were used to compare two groups. Statistical significance was indicated when the *p*-value was less than 0.05.

Keplan–Meier analysis and log-rank test were used to evaluate the percentage of survival related to the duration of response. Correlations of fold-changes in levels of two proteins were assessed through Spearman's rank correlation test. A *p*-value of <0.05 was considered statistically significant.

5. Conclusions

Our data identified new circulating biomarkers, both cells and molecules, that are associated with TKI treatment/response in mRCC and that allow to characterize responsive and non-responsive patients (Table 2). Subsequent validation studies will be performed to validate these markers in a network medicine framework and to test their predictive value for treatment outcomes both in TKI- and immunotherapy-treated patients. These new developments in the research of biomarkers could considerably improve clinical decision-making for RCC patients. Defining the best combination for each patient, as well as the optimal therapeutic sequence, will be essential to guide treatment decisions in clinical practice. In conclusion, the immune-modulating effects of TKI open the way to new therapeutic strategies for mRCC and other cancers, suggesting variations in the administration timing of treatment and new possible combinations with other TKIs, ICIs, or of immune agents, including cancer vaccines and immunostimulatory agents.

Table 2. Circulating biomarkers modulated in mRCC patients.

mRCC Patients	Baseline	During TKI Treatment
Responsive patients	High $CD3^+CD8^+CD137^+$ Low PD1 on $CD137^+$ T cells Low IFNγ	High $CD3^+CD8^+CD137^+$ Low IFNγ Low sPDL2
Non-responsive patients	Low $CD3^+CD8^+CD137^+$ High IFNγ	Low $CD3^+CD8^+CD137^+$ High PD1 on CD137 T cells High IFNγ High sPDL1 High sCTLA4
sICs modulated by TKI	sPDL2, sHVEM, sPD1, sGITR	

Author Contributions: Conceptualization: I.G.Z., C.N., P.M., and M.N.; methodology: I.G.Z., C.N., A.D.F., A.R.; formal analysis: I.G.Z. and A.D.F; data curation: I.G.Z., A.D.F and A.B.; validation: I.G.Z., C.N. and A.R.; investigation resources: A.B., F.C., A.G., E.R., G.S., F.U., G.P., S.S, S.C.; writing—original draft preparation, I.G.Z., C.N., and M.N.; writing—review and editing: A.B., A.G., F.C., E.R., G.S., F.U., G.P., S.S., A.R., S.C., P.M; supervision: C.N. and M.N. Project administration: M.N. All authors read and agreed to the published version of the manuscript.

Acknowledgments: The authors would like to thank L. Grato for his helpful collaboration.

References

1. Motzer, R.J.; Escudier, B.; Tomczak, P.; Hutson, T.E.; Michaelson, M.D.; Negrier, S.; Oudard, S.; Gore, M.E.; Tarazi, J.; Hariharan, S.; et al. Axitinib versus sorafenib as second-line treatment for advanced renal cell carcinoma: Overall survival analysis and updated results from a randomised phase 3 trial. *Lancet Oncol.* **2013**, *14*, 552–562. [CrossRef]
2. Kotecha, R.R.; Motzer, R.J.; Voss, M.H. Towards individualized therapy for metastatic renal cell carcinoma. *Nat. Rev. Clin. Oncol.* **2019**, *16*, 621–633. [CrossRef] [PubMed]
3. Grivennikov, S.I.; Greten, F.R.; Karin, M. Immunity, inflammation, and cancer. *Cell* **2010**, *140*, 883–899. [CrossRef] [PubMed]
4. Santoni, M.; Pantano, F.; Amantini, C.; Nabissi, M.; Conti, A.; Burattini, L.; Zoccoli, A.; Berardi, R.; Santoni, G.; Tonini, G.; et al. Emerging strategies to overcome the resistance to current mTOR inhibitors in renal cell carcinoma. *Biochim. Biophys. Acta Rev. Cancer* **2014**, *1845*, 221–231. [CrossRef]
5. Gustafson, M.P.; Lin, Y.; Bleeker, J.S.; Warad, D.; Tollefson, M.K.; Crispen, P.L.; Bulur, P.A.; Harrington, S.M.; Laborde, R.R.; Gastineau, D.A.; et al. Intratumoral CD14+ cells and circulating CD14+HLA-DRlo/neg monocytes correlate with decreased survival in patients with clear cell renal cell carcinoma. *Clin. Cancer Res.* **2015**, *21*, 4224–4233. [CrossRef] [PubMed]
6. Hirsch, L.; Flippot, R.; Escudier, B.; Albiges, L. Immunomodulatory Roles of VEGF Pathway Inhibitors in Renal Cell Carcinoma. *Drugs* **2020**, *80*, 1169–1181. [CrossRef]
7. Rassy, E.; Flippot, R.; Albiges, L. Tyrosine kinase inhibitors and immunotherapy combinations in renal cell carcinoma. *Ther. Adv. Med. Oncol.* **2020**, *12*. [CrossRef]

8. Alfaro, C.; Suarez, N.; Gonzalez, A.; Solano, S.; Erro, L.; Dubrot, J.; Palazon, A.; Hervas-Stubbs, S.; Gurpide, A.; Lopez-Picazo, J.M.; et al. Influence of bevacizumab, sunitinib and sorafenib as single agents or in combination on the inhibitory effects of VEGF on human dendritic cell differentiation from monocytes. *Br. J. Cancer* **2009**, *100*, 1111–1119. [CrossRef]
9. Napoletano, C.; Ruscito, I.; Bellati, F.; Zizzari, I.G.; Rahimi, H.; Gasparri, M.L.; Antonilli, M.; Panici, P.B.; Rughetti, A.; Nuti, M. Bevacizumab-based chemotherapy triggers immunological effects in responding multi-treated recurrent ovarian cancer patients by favoring the recruitment of effector T cell subsets. *J. Clin. Med.* **2019**, *8*, 380. [CrossRef]
10. Zizzari, I.G.; Napoletano, C.; Botticelli, A.; Caponnetto, S.; Calabrò, F.; Gelibter, A.; Rughetti, A.; Ruscito, I.; Rahimi, H.; Rossi, E.; et al. TK inhibitor pazopanib primes DCs by downregulation of the β-catenin pathway. *Cancer Immunol. Res.* **2018**, *6*, 711–722. [CrossRef]
11. Draghiciu, O.; Nijman, H.W.; Hoogeboom, B.N.; Meijerhof, T.; Daemen, T. Sunitinib depletes myeloid-derived suppressor cells and synergizes with a cancer vaccine to enhance antigen-specific immune responses and tumor eradication. *Oncoimmunology* **2015**, *4*, e989764. [CrossRef] [PubMed]
12. Adotevi, O.; Pere, H.; Ravel, P.; Haicheur, N.; Badoual, C.; Merillon, N.; Medioni, J.; Peyrard, S.; Roncelin, S.; Verkarre, V.; et al. A decrease of regulatory T cells correlates with overall survival after sunitinib-based antiangiogenic therapy in metastatic renal cancer patients. *J. Immunother.* **2010**, *33*, 991–998. [CrossRef] [PubMed]
13. Gu, D.; Ao, X.; Yang, Y.; Chen, Z.; Xu, X. Soluble immune checkpoints in cancer: Production, function and biological significance. *J. Immunotherap. Cancer* **2018**, *6*, 132. [CrossRef] [PubMed]
14. Daassi, D.; Mahoney, K.M.; Freeman, G.J. The importance of exosomal PDL1 in tumour immune evasion. *Nat. Rev. Immunol.* **2020**, *20*, 209–215. [CrossRef] [PubMed]
15. Dong, M.P.; Enomoto, M.; Thuy, L.T.T.; Hai, H.; Hieu, V.N.; Hoang, D.V.; Iida-Ueno, A.; Odagiri, N.; Amano-Teranishi, Y.; Hagihara, A.; et al. Clinical significance of circulating soluble immune checkpoint proteins in sorafenib-treated patients with advanced hepatocellular carcinoma. *Sci. Rep.* **2020**, *10*, 1–10. [CrossRef]
16. Melero, I.; Murillo, O.; Dubrot, J.; Hervás-Stubbs, S.; Perez-Gracia, J.L. Multi-layered action mechanisms of CD137 (4-1BB)-targeted immunotherapies. *Trends Pharmacol. Sci.* **2008**, *29*, 383–390. [CrossRef]
17. Dahal, L.N.; Schwarz, H.; Ward, F.J. Hiding in plain sight: Soluble immunomodulatory receptors. *Trends Immunol.* **2018**, *39*, 771–774. [CrossRef]
18. Heo, S.K.; Ju, S.A.; Kim, G.Y.; Park, S.M.; Back, S.H.; Park, N.H.; Min, Y.J.; An, W.G.; Thi Nguyen, T.H.; Kim, S.M.; et al. The presence of high level soluble herpes virus entry mediator in sera of gastric cancer patients. *Exp. Mol. Med.* **2012**, *44*, 149–158. [CrossRef]
19. Wang, Q.; Zhang, J.; Tu, H.; Liang, D.; Chang, D.W.; Ye, Y.; Wu, X. Soluble immune checkpoint-related proteins as predictors of tumor recurrence, survival, and T cell phenotypes in clear cell renal cell carcinoma patients. *J. Immunotherap. Cancer* **2019**, *7*, 334. [CrossRef]
20. Zaidi, M.R. The interferon-gamma paradox in cancer. *J. Interferon Cytokine Res.* **2019**, *39*, 30–38. [CrossRef]
21. D'Aniello, C.; Berretta, M.; Cavaliere, C.; Rossetti, S.; Facchini, B.A.; Iovane, G.; Mollo, G.; Capasso, M.; Della Pepa, C.; Pesce, L.; et al. Biomarkers of prognosis and efficacy of anti-angiogenic therapy in metastatic clear cell renal cancer. *Front. Oncol.* **2019**, *9*, 1400. [CrossRef] [PubMed]
22. Nuti, M.; Zizzari, I.G.; Botticelli, A.; Rughetti, A.; Marchetti, P. The ambitious role of anti angiogenesis molecules: Turning a cold tumor into a hot one. *Cancer Treat. Rev.* **2018**, *70*, 41–46. [CrossRef] [PubMed]
23. Rijnders, M.; de Wit, R.; Boormans, J.L.; Lolkema, M.P.J.; van der Veldt, A.A.M. Systematic review of immune checkpoint inhibition in urological cancers. *Eur. Urol.* **2017**, *72*, 411–423. [CrossRef]
24. Nong, J.; Wang, J.; Gao, X.; Zhang, Q.; Yang, B.; Yan, Z.; Wang, X.; Yi, L.; Wang, Q.; Gao, Y.; et al. Circulating CD137 $^{+}$ CD8 $^{+}$ T cells accumulate along with increased functional regulatory T cells and thoracic tumour burden in lung cancer patients. *Scand. J. Immunol.* **2019**, *89*, e12765. [CrossRef]
25. Perez-Ruiz, E.; Etxeberria, I.; Rodriguez-Ruiz, M.E.; Melero, I. Anti-CD137 and PD1/PD-L1 antibodies en route toward clinical synergy. *Clin. Cancer Res.* **2017**, *23*, 5326–5328. [CrossRef] [PubMed]
26. Shuford, W.W.; Klussman, K.; Tritchler, D.D.; Loo, D.T.; Chalupny, J.; Siadak, A.W.; Brown, T.J.; Emswiler, J.; Raecho, H.; Larsen, C.P.; et al. 4-1BB costimulatory signals preferentially induce CD8+ T cell proliferation and lead to the amplification in vivo of cytotoxic T cell responses. *J. Exp. Med.* **1997**, *186*, 47–55. [CrossRef]

27. Seo, S.K.; Choi, J.H.; Kim, Y.H.; Kang, W.J.; Park, H.Y.; Suh, J.H.; Choi, B.K.; Vinay, D.S.; Kwon, B.S. 4-1BB-mediated immunotherapy of rheumatoid arthritis. *Nat. Med.* **2004**, *10*, 1088–1094. [CrossRef] [PubMed]
28. Takahashi, C.; Mittler, R.S.; Vella, A.T. Cutting edge: 4-1BB is a bona fide CD8 T cell survival signal. *J. Immunol.* **1999**, *162*, 5037–5040.
29. Agarwal, A.; Newell, K.A. The role of positive costimulatory molecules in transplantation and tolerance. *Curr. Opin. Organ Transplant.* **2008**, *13*, 366–372. [CrossRef]
30. Vinay, D.S.; Kwon, B.S. 4-1BB (CD137), an inducible costimulatory receptor, as a specific target for cancer therapy. *BMB Rep.* **2014**, *47*, 122–129. [CrossRef]
31. Choi, B.K.; Lee, S.C.; Lee, M.J.; Kim, Y.H.; Kim, Y.W.; Ryu, K.W.; Lee, J.H.; Shin, S.M.; Lee, S.H.; Suzuki, S.; et al. 4-1BB-based isolation and expansion of CD8+ T cells specific for self-tumor and non-self-tumor antigens for adoptive T-cell therapy. *J. Immunother.* **2014**, *37*, 225–236. [CrossRef]
32. Wolfl, M.; Kuball, J.; Ho, W.Y.; Nguyen, H.; Manley, T.J.; Bleakley, M.; Greenberg, P.D. Activation-induced expression of CD137 permits detection, isolation, and expansion of the full repertoire of CD8+ T cells responding to antigen without requiring knowledge of epitope specificities. *Blood* **2007**, *110*, 201–210. [CrossRef] [PubMed]
33. Freeman, Z.T.; Nirschl, T.R.; Hovelson, D.H.; Johnston, R.J.; Engelhardt, J.J.; Selby, M.J.; Kochel, C.M.; Lan, R.Y.; Zhai, J.Y.; Ghasemzadeh, A.; et al. A conserved intratumoral regulatory T cell signature identifies 4-1BB as a pan-cancer target. *J. Clin. Investig.* **2020**, *130*, 1405–1416. [CrossRef]
34. Azpilikueta, A.; Agorreta, J.; Labiano, S.; Pérez-Gracia, J.L.; Sánchez-Paulete, A.R.; Aznar, M.A.; Ajona, D.; Gil-Bazo, I.; Larrayoz, M.; Teijeira, A.; et al. Successful immunotherapy against a transplantable mouse squamous lung carcinoma with anti-PD1 and anti-CD137 monoclonal antibodies. *J. Thorac. Oncol.* **2016**, *11*, 524–536. [CrossRef] [PubMed]
35. Bian, B.; Fanale, D.; Dusetti, N.; Roque, J.; Pastor, S.; Chretien, A.S.; Incorvaia, L.; Russo, A.; Olive, D.; Iovanna, J. Prognostic significance of circulating PD1, PD-L1, pan-BTN3As, BTN3A1 and BTLA in patients with pancreatic adenocarcinoma. *Oncoimmunology* **2019**, *8*, e1561120. [CrossRef]
36. Finke, J.H.; Rini, B.; Ireland, J.; Rayman, P.; Richmond, A.; Golshayan, A.; Wood, L.; Elson, P.; Garcia, J.; Dreicer, R.; et al. Sunitinib reverses type-1 immune suppression and decreases T-regulatory cells in renal cell carcinoma patients. *Clin. Cancer Res.* **2008**, *14*, 6674–6682. [CrossRef]
37. Yuan, H.; Cai, P.; Li, Q.; Wang, W.; Sun, Y.; Xu, Q.; Gu, Y. Axitinib augments antitumor activity in renal cell carcinoma via STAT3-dependent reversal of myeloid-derived suppressor cell accumulation. *Biomed. Pharmacother.* **2014**, *68*, 751–756. [CrossRef]
38. Hipp, M.M.; Hilf, N.; Walter, S.; Werth, D.; Brauer, K.M.; Radsak, M.P.; Weinschenk, T.; Singh-Jasuja, H.; Brossart, P. Sorafenib, but not sunitinib, affects function of dendritic cells and induction of primary immune responses. *Blood* **2008**, *111*, 5610–5620. [CrossRef]
39. Shin, S.J.; Jeon, Y.K.; Kim, P.J.; Cho, Y.M.; Koh, J.; Chung, D.H.; Go, H. Clinicopathologic analysis of PD-L1 and PD-L2 expression in renal cell carcinoma: Association with oncogenic proteins status. *Ann. Surg. Oncol.* **2016**, *23*, 694–702. [CrossRef]
40. Enblad, G.; Karlsson, H.; Gammelgård, G.; Wenthe, J.; Lövgren, T.; Amini, R.M.; Wikstrom, K.I.; Essand, M.; Savoldo, B.; Hallböök, H.; et al. A phase I/IIa trial using CD19-targeted third-generation CAR T cells for lymphoma and leukemia. *Clin. Cancer Res.* **2018**, *24*, 6185–6194. [CrossRef]
41. Mojic, M.; Takeda, K.; Hayakawa, Y. The dark side of IFN-γ: Its role in promoting cancer immunoevasion. *Int. J. Mol. Sci.* **2018**, *19*, 89. [CrossRef] [PubMed]
42. Garcia-Diaz, A.; Shin, D.S.; Moreno, B.H.; Saco, J.; Escuin-Ordinas, H.; Rodriguez, G.A.; Zaretsky, J.M.; Sun, L.; Hugo, W.; Wang, X.; et al. Interferon receptor signaling pathways regulating PD-L1 and PD-L2 expression. *Cell Rep.* **2017**, *19*, 1189–1201. [CrossRef] [PubMed]
43. Ayers, M.; Ribas, A.; Mcclanahan, T.K. IFN-g g-related mRNA profile predicts clinical response to PD1 blockade The Journal of Clinical Investigation. *J. Clin. Investig.* **2017**, *127*, 2930–2940. [CrossRef] [PubMed]
44. Abiko, K.; Matsumura, N.; Hamanishi, J.; Horikawa, N.; Murakami, R.; Yamaguchi, K.; Yoshioka, Y.; Baba, T.; Konishi, I.; Mandai, M. IFN-γ from lymphocytes induces PD-L1 expression and promotes progression of ovarian cancer. *Br. J. Cancer* **2015**, *112*, 1501–1509. [CrossRef] [PubMed]

45. Bellucci, R.; Martin, A.; Bommarito, D.; Wang, K.; Hansen, S.H.; Freeman, G.J.; Ritz, J. Interferon-γ-induced activation of JAK1 and JAK2 suppresses tumor cell susceptibility to NK cells through upregulation of PD-L1 expression. *Oncoimmunology* **2015**, *4*. [CrossRef] [PubMed]
46. Chen, G.; Huang, A.C.; Zhang, W.; Zhang, G.; Wu, M.; Xu, W.; Yu, Z.; Yang, J.; Wang, B.; Sun, H.; et al. Exosomal PD-L1 contributes to immunosuppression and is associated with anti-PD1 response. *Nature* **2018**, *560*, 382–386. [CrossRef]
47. Chen, Y.; Li, M.; Liu, J.; Pan, T.; Zhou, T.; Liu, Z.; Tan, R.; Wang, X.; Tian, L.; Chen, E.; et al. sPD-L1 expression is associated with immunosuppression and infectious complications in patients with acute pancreatitis. *Scand. J. Immunol.* **2017**, *86*, 100–106. [CrossRef]
48. Fukuda, T.; Kamai, T.; Masuda, A.; Nukui, A.; Abe, H.; Arai, K.; Yoshida, K.I. Higher preoperative serum levels of PD-L1 and B7-H4 are associated with invasive and metastatic potential and predictable for poor response to VEGF-targeted therapy and unfavorable prognosis of renal cell carcinoma. *Cancer Med.* **2016**, *5*, 1810–1820. [CrossRef]
49. Sharma, P.; Hu-Lieskovan, S.; Wargo, J.A.; Ribas, A. Primary, adaptive, and acquired resistance to cancer immunotherapy. *Cell* **2017**, *168*, 707–723. [CrossRef]

11

Artesunate Inhibits Growth of Sunitinib-Resistant Renal Cell Carcinoma Cells through Cell Cycle Arrest and Induction of Ferroptosis

Sascha D. Markowitsch [1], Patricia Schupp [1], Julia Lauckner [1], Olesya Vakhrusheva [1], Kimberly S. Slade [1], René Mager [1], Thomas Efferth [2], Axel Haferkamp [1] and Eva Juengel [1,*]

1 Department of Urology and Pediatric Urology, University Medical Center Mainz, Langenbeckstraße 1, 55131 Mainz, Germany; sascha.markowitsch@unimedizin-mainz.de (S.D.M.); pschupp@students.uni-mainz.de (P.S.); jlauckne@students.uni-mainz.de (J.L.); olesya.vakhrusheva@unimedizin-mainz.de (O.V.); kimberlysue.slade@unimedizin-mainz.de (K.S.S.); rene.mager@unimedizin-mainz.de (R.M.); axel.haferkamp@unimedizin-mainz.de (A.H.)

2 Institute of Pharmaceutical and Biomedical Sciences, Johannes Gutenberg University Mainz, Staudingerweg 5, 55128 Mainz, Germany; efferth@uni-mainz.de

* Correspondence: eva.juengel@unimedizin-mainz.de

Simple Summary: Renal cell carcinoma (RCC) is the most common kidney malignancy. Due to development of therapy resistance, efficacy of conventional drugs such as sunitinib is limited. Artesunate (ART), a drug originating from Traditional Chinese Medicine, has exhibited anti-tumor effects in several non-urologic tumors. ART inhibited growth, reduced metastatic properties, and curtailed metabolism in sunitinib-sensitive and sunitinib–resistant RCC cells. In three of four tested cell lines, ART's growth inhibitory effects were accompanied by cell cycle arrest and modulation of cell cycle regulating proteins. In a fourth cell line, KTCTL-26, ART evoked ferroptosis, an iron-dependent cell death, and exhibited stronger anti-tumor effects than in the other cell lines. The regulatory protein, p53, was only detectable in the KTCTL-26 cells, possibly making p53 a predictive marker of cancer that may respond better to ART. ART, therefore, may hold promise as an additive therapy option for selected patients with advanced or therapy-resistant RCC.

Abstract: Although innovative therapeutic concepts have led to better treatment of advanced renal cell carcinoma (RCC), efficacy is still limited due to the tumor developing resistance to applied drugs. Artesunate (ART) has demonstrated anti-tumor effects in different tumor entities. This study was designed to investigate the impact of ART (1–100 μM) on the sunitinib-resistant RCC cell lines, Caki-1, 786-O, KTCTL26, and A-498. Therapy-sensitive (parental) and untreated cells served as controls. ART's impact on tumor cell growth, proliferation, clonogenic growth, apoptosis, necrosis, ferroptosis, and metabolic activity was evaluated. Cell cycle distribution, the expression of cell cycle regulating proteins, p53, and the occurrence of reactive oxygen species (ROS) were investigated. ART significantly increased cytotoxicity and inhibited proliferation and clonogenic growth in both parental and sunitinib-resistant RCC cells. In Caki-1, 786-O, and A-498 cell lines growth inhibition was associated with G0/G1 phase arrest and distinct modulation of cell cycle regulating proteins. KTCTL-26 cells were mainly affected by ART through ROS generation, ferroptosis, and decreased metabolism. p53 exclusively appeared in the KTCTL-26 cells, indicating that p53 might be predictive for ART-dependent ferroptosis. Thus, ART may hold promise for treating selected patients with advanced and even therapy-resistant RCC.

Keywords: renal cell carcinoma (RCC); sunitib resistance; artesunate (ART); Traditional Chinese Medicine (TCM); growth inhibition; ferroptosis; reactive oxygen species (ROS)

1. Introduction

Accounting for ~85% of cases, renal cell carcinoma (RCC) is the most common kidney cancer and one of the most aggressive urologic cancers [1]. At initial diagnosis, RCC patients often present at an advanced stage with an accordingly poor prognosis [2]. Better understanding of the molecular modes of action underlying RCC led to the development of targeted therapies affecting angiogenic activity and immune checkpoint inhibitors. However, due to the development of resistance, the efficacy of even these targeted treatments is limited. Since RCC is an angiogenic disease, a promising avenue of treatment is to block angiogenesis, thereby suppressing the supply of oxygen and nutrients to the tumor. Initially, the anti-angiogenic activity of the tyrosine kinase inhibitor (TKI) sunitinib extends the progression-free survival of patients [3], but resistance occurs during treatment [4]. Thus, therapy resistance is one, if not the main, problem, in treating advanced RCC. Novel treatment strategies combining targeted therapy and immunotherapy have been introduced [5–7]. However, even with combined drug application resistance occurs and adverse side effects are common [5,8,9].

Certainly, in part due to the long-term curative failure of conventional therapy, the demand for traditional and alternative medicine is growing worldwide [10,11]. Patients hope that complementary therapeutic approaches would increase effectiveness and/or reduce side effects [12,13], and 40–50% of European cancer patients indeed use complementary and alternative therapies [14–16]. However, solid and reliable studies with regard to natural substances and their derivatives are sparse and the lack of proven efficacy coupled with uncoordinated self-treatment is perilous. Contraindications as well as adverse side effects of herbal compounds combined with conventional therapy also cannot be ignored [17].

Some studies have been carried out indicating anti-tumor effects of natural compounds and their derivatives, especially if applied together with established therapies or by counteracting therapy resistance [18–21]. Artemisinin from the annual mugwort (*Artemisia annua*) has been used in Traditional Chinese Medicine for over 2000 years, particularly in treating malaria [22] and is still in use. An anti-tumor effect of the artemisinin derivative, artesunate (ART), was reported in 2001 [23]. Subsequently, anti-tumor effects of ART in vitro and in vivo were reported in different tumor entities, including therapy-resistant tumors, with fewer side effects in combination with conventional therapy [23–27]. ART, a semi-synthetic water-soluble derivative of artemisinin, exhibits hydrophilic properties in contrast to the natural substance, and has better bioavailability and anti-tumor activity than artemisinin [28,29]. In therapy-sensitive and doxorubicin-resistant T-leukemia cells, ART induced apoptosis and displayed a synergistic effect in combination with doxorubicin [30]. ART's anti-tumor effect had also been demonstrated in gastrointestinal [31] and breast cancer [32]. Here, ART specifically affected neoplastic tissue and spares healthy tissue [33].

The mode of action of ART is not yet fully understood. Both in the malaria pathogen and in tumor cells, high cellular iron content seems to play a role in the response to ART (and artemisinin) [34]. A high iron content facilitates ferroptosis, an iron-dependent cell death caused by reactive oxygen species (ROS) formation [34–38]. Iron has been identified as central player in cancer progression [39]. This could explain why artemisinin and ART specifically affect tumor cells but not normal cells with lower iron content [33]. Correspondingly, RCC cells express significantly more iron-regulated genes [40]. Furthermore, RCC tissue, particularly clear cell RCC tissue, compared to healthy tissue, exhibits significant higher transferrin receptor 1 (TfR1) expression, which is responsible for iron uptake and associated with worse survival outcomes [41]. Moreover, artemisinin and its derivatives inhibit angiogenesis [42–45]. ART reduced the expression of angiogenic proteins in hemangioendothelioma cells, and thus has been postulated to be a therapeutic option for angiogenic cancers [46], including RCC. Indeed, ART exerted potent, selective cytotoxicity in therapy-sensitive RCC [47] and inhibited invasiveness in vitro and in vivo. It induced ferroptosis in therapy-sensitive RCC cells [48] and enhanced the anti-tumor effect of the TKI sorafenib [47].

Investigations exploring the effect of ART on therapy-sensitive RCC are scant and unavailable in regard to therapy-resistant RCC. Thus, the present study was designed to evaluate ART's impact on sensitive and more importantly sunitinib-resistant RCC cells, by evaluating the effect of this drug on tumor growth and underlying molecular mechanisms. The intent of this study was to implement rationale for a founded treatment option with a compound of natural origin for patients with advanced and/or therapy-resistant RCC.

2. Results

2.1. Confirmation of Sunitinib Resistance in RCC Cells

Sunitinib-sensitive and sunitinib-resistant RCC cell lines, Caki-1, 786-O, KTCTL-26, and A-498, were employed with the sunitinib-sensitive (parental) RCC sub-lines serving as controls. Cells were designated sunitinib-resistant if the IC50 under escalating sunitinib dosage (0.1–100 μM) was approximately twice as high as the IC50 of the sunitinib-sensitive counterpart. Even though the A-498 cells barely reached the designated IC50 (IC50 of 19.30 μM in the resistant cells compared to 10.43 μM in their parental counterparts), all four cell lines fulfilled this specification (Table 1). Here, with an IC50 of 10.43 μM, parental A-498 revealed the weakest sunitinib response, compared to the other three RCC cell lines. The most prominent difference in IC50 was found in Caki-1 cells with an IC50 of 2.58 μM in parental and 19.13 μM in resistant cells, indicating that initial high sensitivity may lead to stronger resistance development in RCC cells. The differences in IC50 for the parental and resistant 786-O and KTCTL-26 cell lines lay between those of the A-498 and Caki-1cells. The IC50 of parental 786-O of 3.97 μM elevated in the resistant 786-O to an IC50 of 11.16 μM. In KTCTL-26 cells, IC50 of 6.37 μM in the parental cells increased to an IC50 of 13.31 μM in the resistant counterparts.

Table 1. Verification of sunitinib resistance: IC50 values of parental and sunitinib-resistant renal cell carcinoma (RCC) cells following 72 h application of 0.1–100 μM sunitinib $n = 5$.

Cell Line	Parental	Resistant	Unit
Caki-1	2.58	19.13	μM
786-O	3.97	11.16	μM
KTCTL-26	6.37	13.31	μM
A-498	10.43	19.30	μM

2.2. Artesunate Inhibits Cell Growth of Parental and Sunitinib-Resistant RCC Cells

ART induced a dose- and time-dependent growth inhibition in all parental and resistant RCC cell lines, compared to the untreated controls (Figure 1), with comparable IC50 values for corresponding parental and resistant sub-lines. A significant growth reduction of parental Caki-1 cells with an IC50 of 10.41 μM ART after 72 h was apparent (Figure 1a). The sunitinib-resistant Caki-1 cells were similarly inhibited with an IC50 of 11.69 μM ART after 72 h treatment (Figure 1b). In both parental and sunitinib-resistant Caki-1 cells, significant growth inhibition was first reached with 5 μM ART (Figure 1a,b). Parental and sunitinib-resistant A-498 cells also first showed significant growth inhibition at a concentration of 5 μM ART, with an IC50 of 12.51 μM ART for the parental and 12.08 μM ART for the sunitinib-resistant cells (Figure 1g,h). The most prominent growth inhibition was found in the 786-O cell lines, with an IC50 of 1.62 μM ART in the parental and an IC50 of 1.99 μM ART in the resistant 786-O cells (Figure 1c,d). In 786-O cells, exposure to 1 μM ART already resulted in significant growth inhibition that further increased with ascending concentration (Figure 1c,d). In all three of the abovementioned RCC cell lines, tumor cell growth was arrested but not reduced below the initially seeded basal cell count, even at the highest concentration of 100 μM ART (Figure 1a–d,g,h). In KTCTL-26 a significant decrease in parental and sunitinib-resistant cells, below the initial seeding cell count (Figure 1e,f), did take place. ART's IC50 values for the KTCTL-26 cell lines were higher (parental: IC50 = 17.02 μM, sunitinib-resistant: IC50 = 17.79 μM) than those of the other cell lines. Comparable to Caki-1 and A-498 cells, the first significant inhibitory response in regard to KTCTL-26 growth was detected after exposure to 5 μM ART (Figure 1e,f). In summary, ART treatment significantly suppressed tumor cell growth in all four RCC cell lines, but only in the KTCTL-26 cell line did growth reduction result in a decrease of cell counts below the number of initially seeded cells.

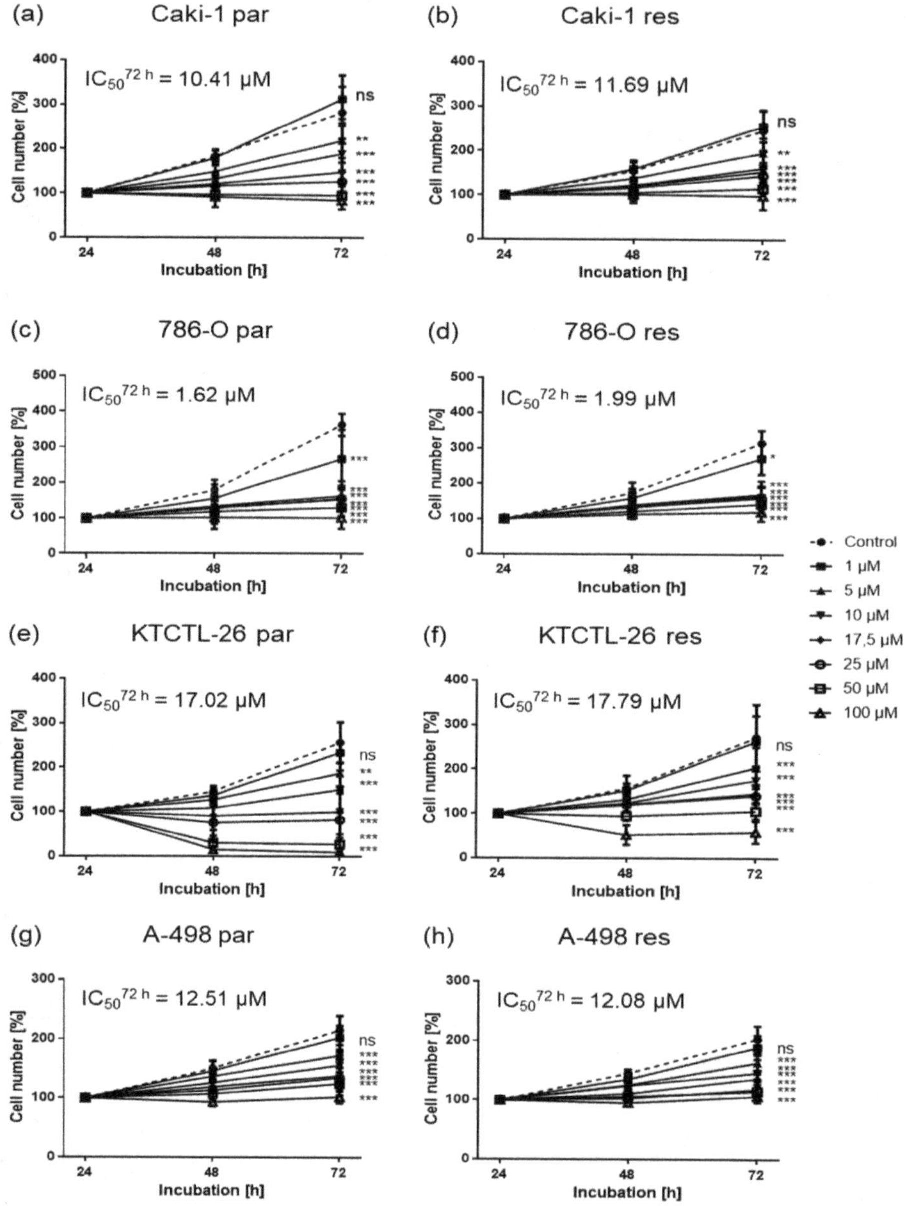

Figure 1. Tumor cell growth after exposure to artesunate (ART): Tumor cell growth of parental (par) and sunitinib-resistant (res) Caki-1 (**a**,**b**), 786-O (**c**,**d**), KTCTL-26 (**e**,**f**), A-498 (**g**,**h**) cells after 24, 48, and 72 h treatment with ascending ART concentrations (1–100 µM). Cell number set to 100% after 24 h incubation. The IC50 of ART after 72 h treatment is specified. Error bars indicate standard deviation (*SD*). Significant difference to untreated control: * $p \leq 0.05$, ** $p \leq 0.01$, *** $p \leq 0.001$, ns = not significant. $n = 5$.

2.3. *Artesunate Impairs RCC Cell Proliferation*

Exposure to ART for 72 h contributed to significant dose-dependent inhibition of RCC cell proliferation (Figure 2). The proliferation of parental and sunitinib-resistant Caki-1 and 786-O cells was already significantly reduced after treatment with 10 µM ART, compared to the untreated controls (Figure 2a,b). Parental KTCTL-26 cells revealed a significant proliferation inhibition after exposure to 20 µM ART, while resistant KTCTL-26 cells were significantly inhibited at 30 µM ART (Figure 2c).

A-498 cells behaved differently in respect to the inhibiting concentration of ART. Proliferation of the resistant A-498 cells was already significantly reduced after treatment with 20 μM ART, whereas a concentration of 30 μM ART was necessary to significantly decrease proliferation in parental A-498 cells (Figure 2d).

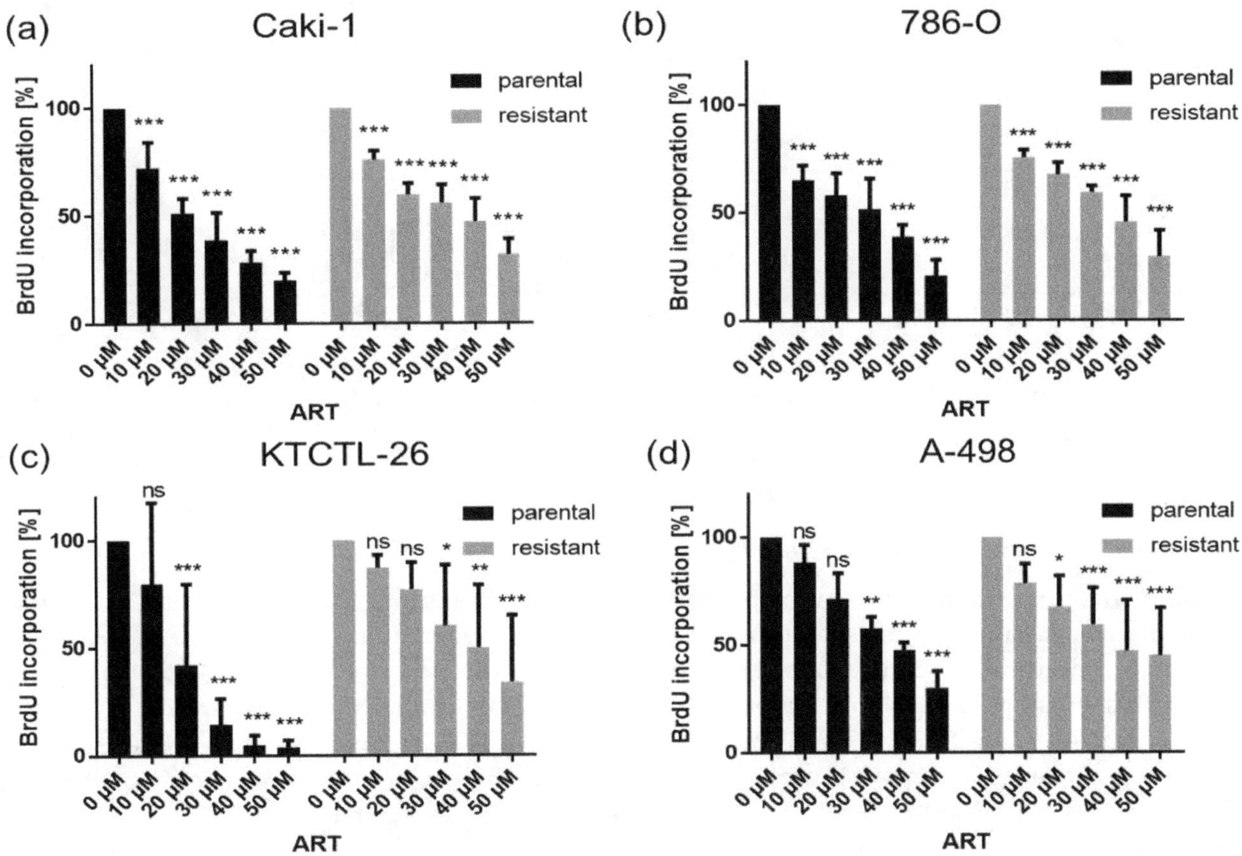

Figure 2. Cell proliferation: Tumor cell proliferation of parental (par) and sunitinib-resistant Caki-1 (**a**), 786-O (**b**), KTCTL-26 (**c**), and A-498 (**d**) RCC cells incubated for 72 h with ART (10–50 μM). Untreated controls were set to 100%. Error bars indicate standard deviation (*SD*). Significant difference to untreated control: * $p \leq 0.05$, ** $p \leq 0.01$, *** $p \leq 0.001$, ns = not significant. $n = 5$.

2.4. *Artesunate Reduces Clonogenic Growth of the RCC Cell Lines*

In all RCC cell lines, ART induced a significant dose-dependent reduction in clone colonies after 10 days incubation (Figure 3). Ten μM ART contributed to significant inhibition of the clonogenic growth of the RCC cells, compared to the untreated controls. In parental and resistant Caki-1 cells, the administration of 50 μM ART diminished the clonogenic growth by more than 90% (Figure 3a). Microscopically, parental Caki-1 cells formed larger colonies, compared to the sunitinib-resistant Caki-1 cells (Figure 3a). Treatment of 786-O cells with 10 μM ART resulted in an approximately 50% decrease in clone colonies (Figure 3b). 786-O cells exposed to 50 μM ART completely inhibited colony formation in the parental and resulted in only a few colonies in the resistant cell line. In parental and sunitinib-resistant KTCTL-26 and A-498 cells, 10 μM ART significantly diminished the clonogenic growth by more than 50% (Figure 3c,d). KTCTL-26 colonies were no longer formed after exposure to 30 μM ART in parental and exposure to 50 μM ART in resistant cells (Figure 3c). Neither parental nor resistant A-498 colonies were detectable after exposure to 40 and 50 μM ART (Figure 3d). Microscopic comparison showed that both parental and resistant A-498 cells exhibited a lower potential to develop colonies, compared to the other RCC cell lines (Figure 3d).

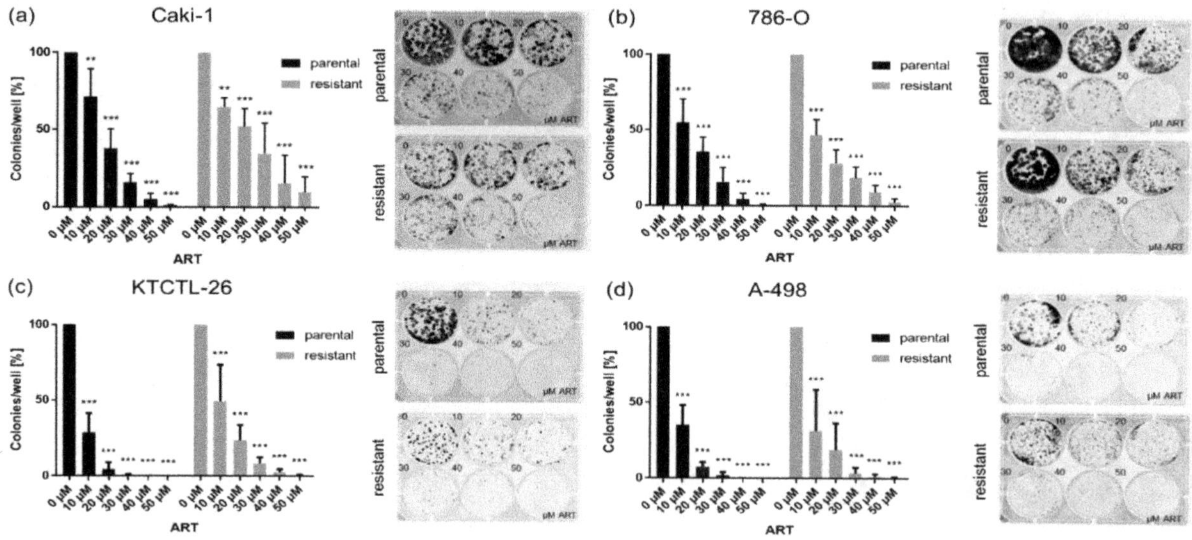

Figure 3. Clonogenic growth of RCC cells: Clonogenic growth of parental and resistant Caki-1 (**a**), 786-O (**b**), KTCTL-26 (**c**), and A-498 (**d**) cells treated with ART (10–50 µM) for 10 days. Untreated cells served as controls (set to 100%). Error bars indicate standard deviation (*SD*). Significant difference to untreated control: ** $p \leq 0.01$, *** $p \leq 0.001$. $n = 5$.

2.5. *Artesunate Induces Cell Cycle Arrest in Both Parental and Sunitinib-Resistant RCC Cells*

Diminished growth behavior in the parental and sunitinib-resistant RCC cell lines Caki-1, 786-O, and A-498 was accompanied by a significant G0/G1 phase arrest after exposure to ART, compared to the untreated controls (Figure 4a,b,d). Concomitantly, the number of S and G2/M phase cells significantly decreased, except in the parental 786-O cells, exhibiting only a significant reduction in the S phase (Figure 4b). In KTCTL-26 ART induced a significant G0/G1 phase arrest in the resistant cells, but no changes were apparent in the parental counterpart (Figure 4c). Overall, the effect of ART on KTCTL-26 regarding induction of cell cycle arrest was less pronounced than in the other RCC cell lines. To explore the influence of ART on cell cycle regulating protein levels, Caki-1 and 786-O were utilized as exemplary cell lines.

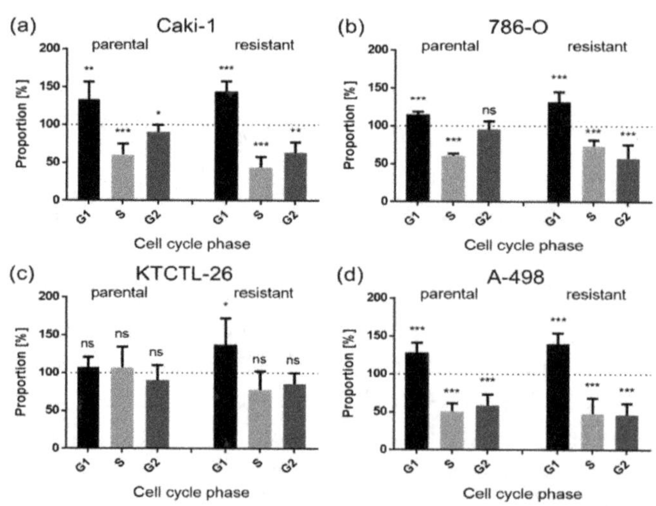

Figure 4. Distribution of cell cycle phases: Proportion of parental and sunitinib-resistant RCC cells, Caki-1 (**a**), 786-O (**b**), KTCTL-26 (**c**), and A-498 (**d**), in the G0/G1, S, and G2/M phases after 48 h treatment with ART (20 µM). Untreated cells served as controls (dotted line; set to 100%). Error bars indicate standard deviation (*SD*). Significant difference to untreated control: * $p \leq 0.05$, ** $p \leq 0.01$, *** $p \leq 0.001$, ns = not significant. $n = 5$.

2.6. Artesunate-Induced Cell Cycle Arrest was Accompanied by Alterations in the Expression and Activity of Cell Cycle Regulating Proteins

Alterations in the cell cycle phases of Caki-1 and 786-O after administration of ART were associated with distinct modulation in cell cycle regulating proteins (Figure 5, Figure 6, Figure 7). The treatment of parental and sunitinib-resistant Caki-1 and 786-O cells with 20 μM ART led to a significant reduction of the cell cycle activating proteins cyclin A, cyclin B, and CDK1, as well as to deactivation of CDK1 (pCDK1), all of which are proteins involved in S and G2/M phase progression. In addition, CDK2, which associates with cyclin A during the S phase, significantly decreased in parental Caki-1 cells after exposure to ART, compared to the untreated controls (Figures 5 and 6g, Figure S1g). The expression of the tumor suppressor p27 significantly increased in parental and resistant Caki-1 cells with ART application (Figures 5 and 6b, Figure S1b). However, in 786-O cells, p27 expression significantly decreased after ART application (Figures 5 and 7b, Figure S2b). Protein expression of p21 was not significantly altered in Caki-1 cells (Figures 5 and 6a, Figure S1a) but tended to increase in parental 786-O cells and was significantly increased in resistant 786-O cells (Figures 5 and 7a, Figure S2a). Activity of CDK2 (pCDK2) was not detectable in Caki-1 and 786-O cells.

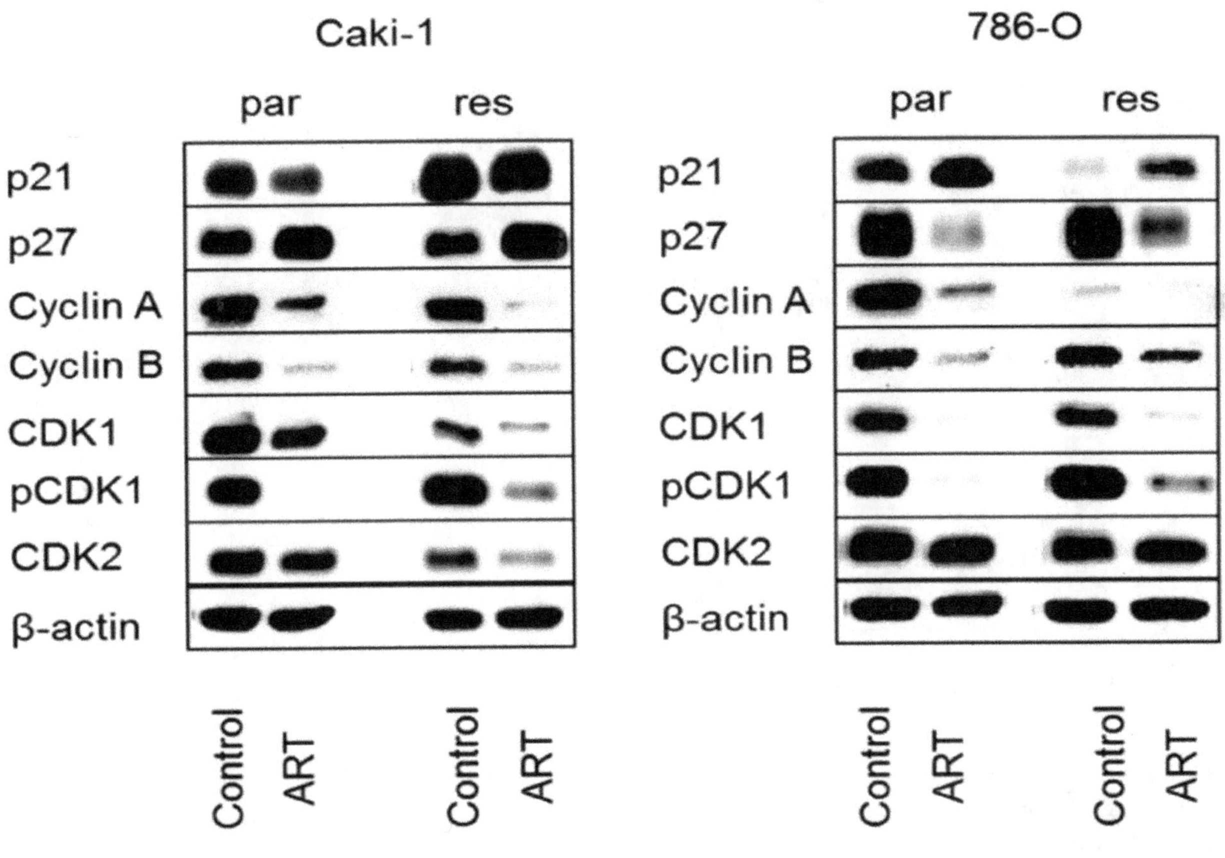

Figure 5. Protein expression profile of cell cycle regulating proteins: Representative Western blot analysis of cell cycle regulating proteins in parental (par) and sunitinib-resistant (res) Caki-1 (**left** panel) and 786-O (**right** panel) cells after 48 h exposure to ART (20 μM).

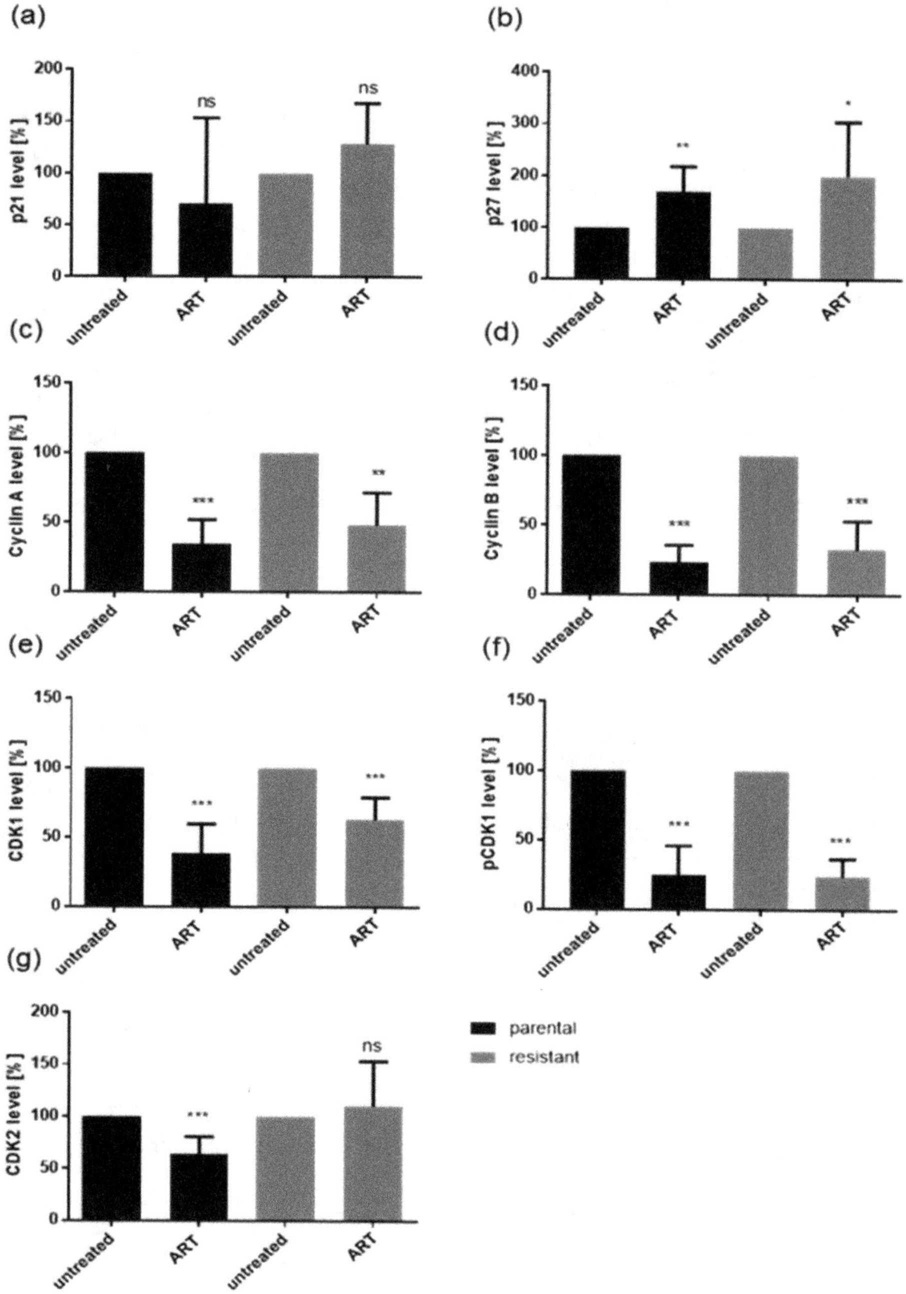

Figure 6. Protein expression profile of cell cycle regulating proteins: Pixel density analysis (Western blot) of the cell cycle regulating proteins p21 (**a**), p27 (**b**), cyclin A (**c**), cyclin B (**d**), CDK1 (**e**), pCDK1 (**f**), and CDK2 (**g**) in parental and resistant Caki-1 cells after 48 h exposure to ART (20 μM), compared to untreated controls (set to 100%). Each protein analysis was accompanied and normalized by a housekeeping protein. Error bars indicate standard deviation (*SD*). Significant difference to untreated control: * $p \leq 0.05$, ** $p \leq 0.01$, *** $p \leq 0.001$, ns = not significant. $n = 4$. For detailed information regarding the Western blots see Figure S1a–g.

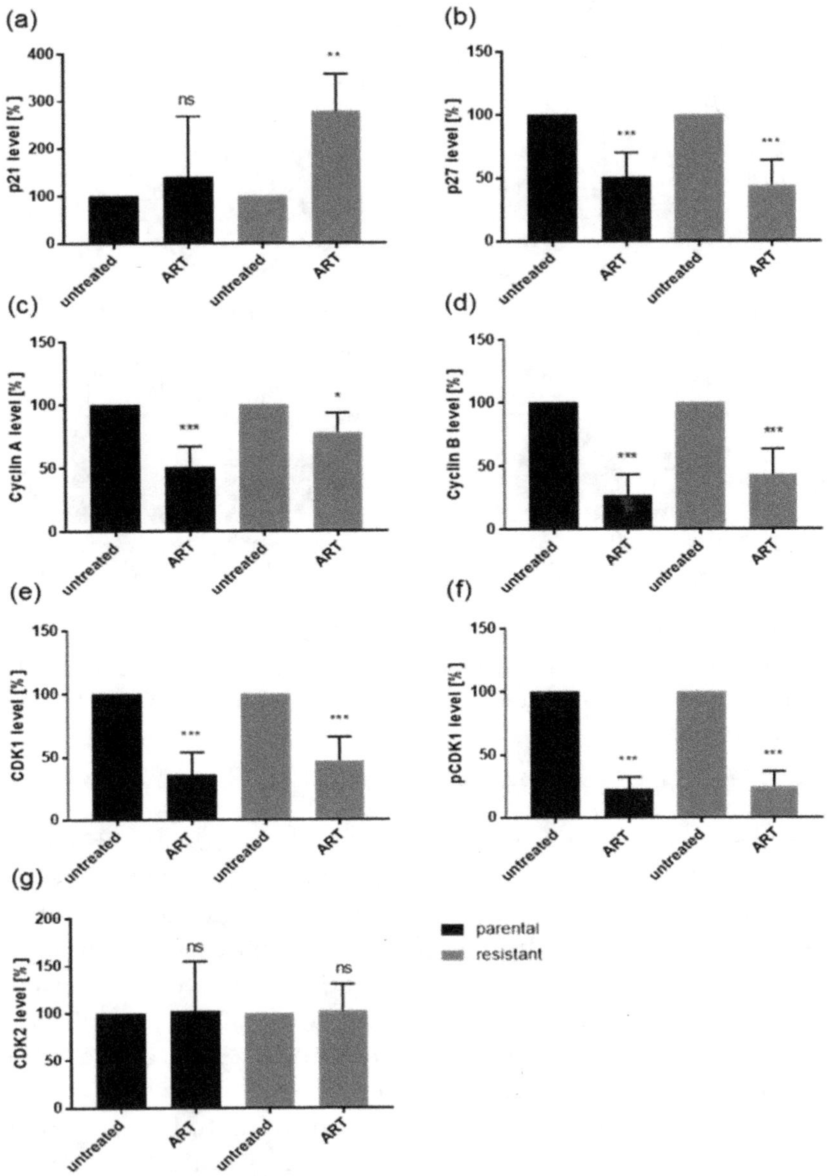

Figure 7. Protein expression profile of cell cycle regulating proteins: Pixel density analysis (Western blot) of the cell cycle regulating proteins p21 (**a**), p27 (**b**), cyclin A (**c**), cyclin B (**d**), CDK1 (**e**), pCDK1 (**f**), and CDK2 (**g**) in parental and resistant 786-O cells after 48 h exposure to ART (20 μM), compared to untreated controls (set to 100%). Each protein analysis was accompanied and normalized by a housekeeping protein. Error bars indicate standard deviation (*SD*). Significant difference to untreated control: * $p \leq 0.05$, ** $p \leq 0.01$, *** $p \leq 0.001$, ns = not significant. $n = 4$. For detailed information regarding the Western blots see Figure S2a–g.

2.7. *Artesunate Only Slightly Contributes to Apoptosis*

To investigate whether the growth inhibitory effect of ART was associated with cell death events, apoptosis was assessed (Figure 8). The only significant increase in apoptotic cells in parental or sunitinib-resistant RCC cells after exposure to ART occurred in resistant Caki-1 cells (Figure 8a).

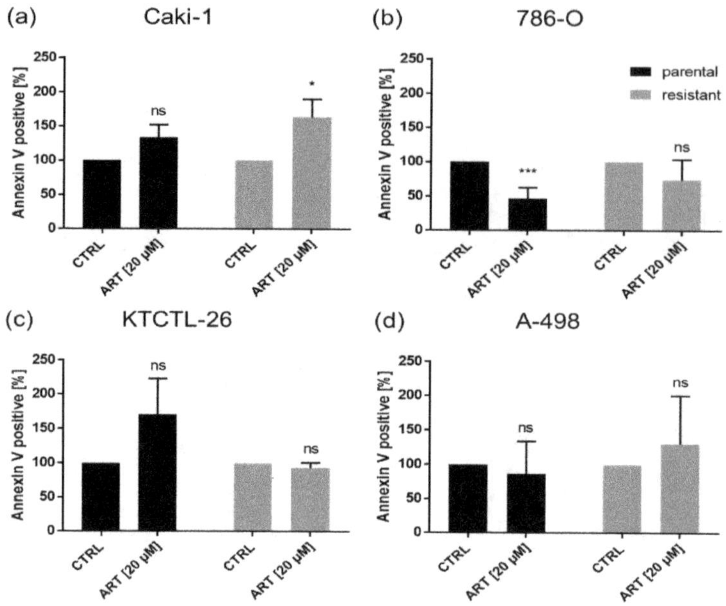

Figure 8. Apoptotic events: Parental and resistant Caki-1 (**a**), 786-O (**b**), KTCTL-26 (**c**), and A-498 (**d**) cells treated for 48 h with ART (20 μM). Untreated cells served as controls (set to 100%). Error bars indicate standard deviation (*SD*). Significant difference to untreated control: * $p \leq 0.05$, *** $p \leq 0.001$, ns = not significant. $n = 5$.

2.8. Artesunate Results in Ferroptosis Induction in KTCTL-26 Cells

Since ART has been shown to induce the iron-dependent cell death termed ferroptosis [35,36,38], this type of cell death was investigated by utilizing ferrostatin-1, a ferroptosis inhibitor. Proliferation inhibition observed under ART exposure in parental and sunitinib-resistant KTCTL-26 cells was significantly reversed following the combined administration of ART with the ferroptosis inhibitor ferrostatin-1 (Figure 9a,b). This cancellation of ART's inhibitory effect caused proliferation rates to return to those of the untreated control cells. Application of ferrostatin-1 did not cancel ART's proliferation inhibition in parental or sunitinib-resistant Caki-1, 786-O, and A-498 cells. Thus, only the KTCTL-26 cell lines were investigated in further detail.

An essential process during ferroptosis is ROS generation. To investigate whether ART in fact generates ROS, Trolox, an antioxidant was used to intercept free radicals and thus prevent ferroptosis. ART in combination with Trolox significantly abrogated the proliferation inhibition observed with ART treatment alone, so that the proliferation rate of the KTCTL-26 cells was comparable to that of the untreated controls (Figure 9c,d). To further corroborate the results of the aforementioned experiments, glutathione (GSH) expression, a part of the anti-oxidative protective system of the cells, was evaluated. GSH significantly decreased in KTCTL-26 cells after treatment with 50 μM ART, compared to the untreated controls (Figure 9e), indicating ROS generation and GSH consumption. The GSH content was more strongly reduced in parental than in resistant KTCTL-26 cells. In both parental and sunitinib-resistant KTCTL-26 cells, the inhibitory effect significantly increased when ART was combined with iron (Figure 9e). Since GPX4 is essential for anti-oxidative protection and designated as a ferroptosis related protein, GPX4 expression was also assessed. Application of 50 μM ART resulted in a significant reduction of GPX4 in both parental and resistant KTCTL-26 cells (Figures 9f,g and S3).

p53 has been described as a ferroptosis indicator [49,50]. Thus, the expression of p53 in parental and sunitinib-resistant RCC cells was investigated. Expression of p53 was not detectable in the parental and sunitinib-resistant Caki-1, 786-O, and A-498 cells (Figures 9h and S4). Notably, in KTCTL-26 cells, the only cells where ART did induce ferroptosis, distinct p53 expression in parental and even stronger p53 expression in the resistant cells was detected (Figures 9h,i and S4).

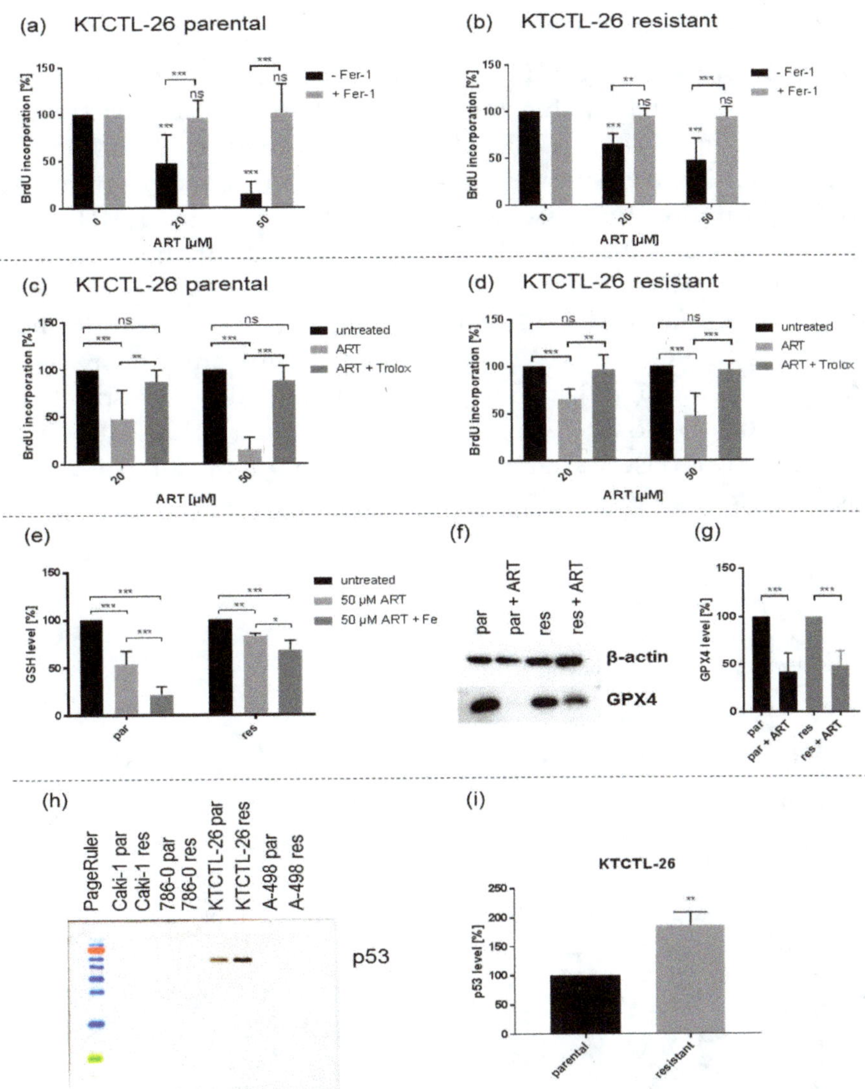

Figure 9. Artesunate induced ferroptosis by reactive oxygen species (ROS) formation in p53-positive KTCTL-26 cells: Ferroptosis induction (**a**,**b**) Proliferation of parental (**a**) and sunitinib-resistant KTCTL-26 cells (**b**) treated for 48 h with ART (20, 50 µM) and ferrostatin-1 (Fer-1) (20 µM). Untreated (100%) and ART mono-treated cells served as controls. Error bars indicate standard deviation (*SD*). Significant difference compared to untreated controls, except for asterisk brackets indicating significant difference between ferrostatin-1 untreated and treated cells: * = $p \leq 0.05$, ** = $p \leq 0.01$, *** = $p \leq 0.001$, ns = not significant. $n = 5$. Indications of ROS generation (**c**–**g**): Proliferation of parental (**c**) and sunitinib-resistant KTCTL-26 cells (**d**) treated for 48 h with ART (20, 50 µM) and Trolox (0.5 mM). Untreated cells served as controls (100%). $n = 5$. GSH level (%) of parental (par) and resistant (res) KTCTL-26 cells after 24 h incubation with ART (50 µM) and holo-transferrin (Fe) (**e**). Untreated controls served as controls (100%). $n = 5$. GPX4 expression: Representative Western blot of GPX4 expression in parental (par) and sunitinib-resistant (res) KTCTL-26 cells after 48 h exposure to ART (50 µM) (**f**). Pixel density analysis of GPX4 level (%) after 48 h exposure to ART (50 µM) in parental (par) and resistant (res) KTCTL-26 cells (**g**). Untreated cells served as controls (100%). β-actin served as internal control. $n = 5$. Protein expression of p53 (**h**,**i**) Representative Western blot analysis of p53 in parental (par) and resistant (res) Caki-1, 786-O, KTCTL-26, and A-498 cells (**h**). Pixel density analysis of p53 expression in parental (100%) and resistant KTCTL-26 cells (**i**) p53 protein analysis was accompanied and normalized by a total protein control. $n = 3$. Error bars indicate standard deviation (*SD*). Significant difference indicated by: * $p \leq 0.05$, ** $p \leq 0.01$, *** $p \leq 0.001$, ns = not significant. For detailed information regarding the Western blots of (**f**) and (**h**) see Figures S3 and S4.

2.9. Artesunate Influences the Metabolism of RCC Cells

The ART-induced ferroptosis in KTCTL-26 cells was accompanied by a significant increase in ROS. Since ferroptosis is associated with a high iron content and accelerated metabolism, ART's impact on the oxygen consumption rate (OCR) of the KTCTL-26 cells, expressed by basal respiration, adenosine triphosphate (ATP) production-coupled respiration, maximum and reserve capacities, and non-mitochondrial respiration, was assessed (Figure 10). Exposure to ART significantly inhibited the spare respiratory capacity, representing the ability of cells to enhance respiration in response to physiological or pharmacological stress, in resistant KTCTL-26 cells (Figure 10e). Decreased spare respiration capacity in the resistant KTCTL-26 cells was accompanied by diminished ATP production (Figure 10f). Also, in parental RCC cells, ATP production significantly decreased after exposure to ART (Figure 10f). ART exerted no significant effect on basal or maximum respiration in either parental or resistant cells (Figure 10c,d). No alteration in the extracellular acidification rate connected with anaerobic glycolytic activity was observed after exposure to ART in the KTCTL-26 cells, thus indicating no shift towards compensatory glycolysis.

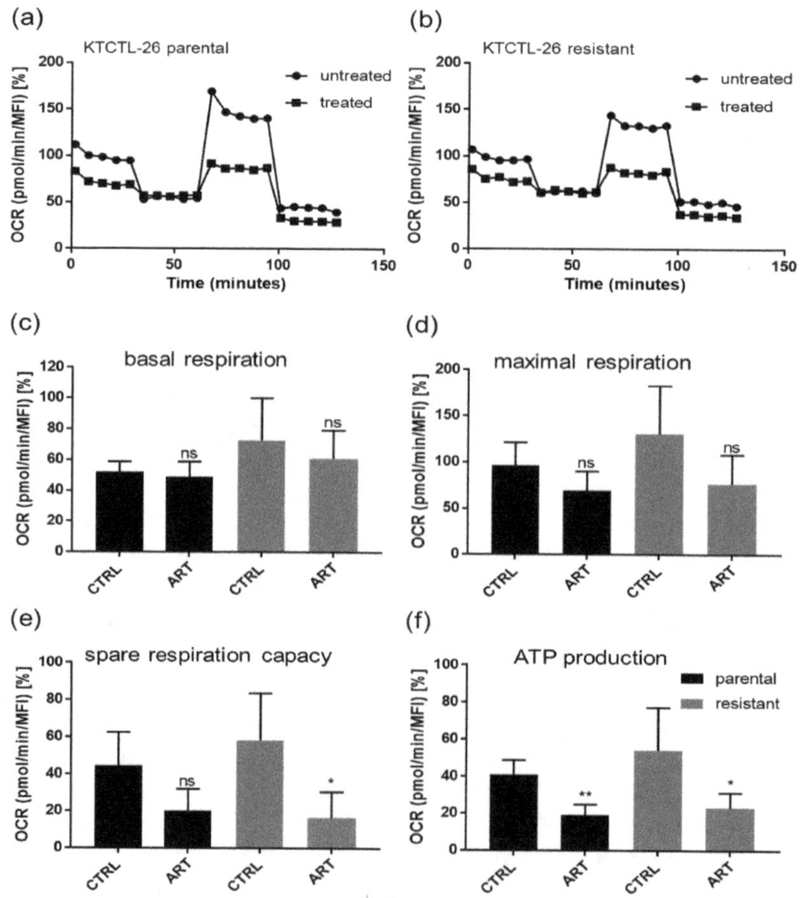

Figure 10. Mitochondrial respiration: Representative mitochondrial respiration in parental (**a**) and resistant (**b**) KTCTL-26 cells after 24 h treatment with 20 µM ART (=treated). Untreated cells served as controls. Data pertaining to the oxygen consumption rate (OCR) were normalized to total basal respiration (set to 100%) consisting of mitochondrial and non-mitochondrial respiration. Extracted values for mitochondrial basal oxygen consumption rate (OCR) (**c**), maximal OCR (**d**), respiratory reserve capacity (**e**), and adenosine triphosphate (ATP) production (**f**) after 24 h ART application (ART). MFI = mean fluorescence intensity. Error bars indicate standard deviation (*SD*). Significant difference to untreated control: * $p \leq 0.05$, ** $p \leq 0.01$, ns = not significant. $n = 4$.

3. Discussion

Although current therapeutic approaches have improved progression-free survival of advanced RCC patients, the disease at this stage ultimately remains incurable due to the inevitable development of resistance to treatment. Interestingly, in the current study RCC cells exhibiting a more sensitive initial response to sunitinib developed strong resistance in the course of chronic treatment. Sunitinib-resistant Caki-1 cells were nearly 10-fold less sensitive than their parental counterparts, which initially could be held in check by a relatively low sunitinib dose. Overcoming this resistance is therefore of primary importance. Since adding ART to conventional anti-cancer therapy has been shown to overcome resistance during treatment of other tumor entities, the impact of ART on a panel of sunitinib-sensitive and sunitinib-resistant RCC cell lines was investigated.

Exposure to ART resulted in a significant inhibition of tumor cell growth and proliferation in all tested parental and sunitinib-resistant RCC cells, indicating an anti-tumor potential in highly heterogenic types of cancer. KTCTL-26 cells displayed the highest sensitivity to ART. The IC50 for ART in the RCC cells was in the lower one- to two-digit μM range (2 to 18 μM). In good accordance with other investigators, ART has been shown to inhibit cell growth of therapy-sensitive RCC cells in the two-digit μM range, up to 50 μM [47]. Combined administration of ART with sorafenib, a first-generation TKI akin to sunitinib, even further reduced cell growth [47]. Several studies on non-urological tumor entities have also demonstrated growth inhibition after ART application. In hemangioendothelioma cells, ART time- and dose-dependently reduced tumor cell growth, concomitantly decreasing the expression of VEGF-A, VEGFR1, VEGFR2, and HIF-1α [46]. Thus, it has been postulated that ART may hold promise in treating vascular tumors, of which RCC is a member. Moreover, significant growth inhibition was observed in a mouse model of hemangioendothelioma carcinoma cells following ART treatment, with significantly reduced tumor size [46]. In different gastric cancer cell lines, ART exposure has also resulted in a significant growth reduction [51]. In bone tumor cell lines, ART also impacted tumor cell growth [52]. In the present investigation, the growth of KTCTL-26 cells, a bone tumor cell line, was even diminished to below zero after ART treatment. This was accompanied by an increased number of annexin V positive cells, indicating apoptosis induction by ART. Other investigators have reported an anti-proliferative effect of ART in ovarian carcinoma cells in vitro [53] as well as in chemotherapy-sensitive and -resistant thyroid cancer cells [54]. In patients with colorectal cancer, ART application reduced disease progression through anti-proliferative action [31]. Artemisinin, the native lead compound, also inhibited proliferation in gastric cancer cell lines by up-regulating p53 [55]. Nevertheless, ART inhibits tumor cells by both p53-dependent and also -independent mechanisms [56,57].

Clonogenic growth provides information about the growth of single tumor cells at metastatic sites and advanced RCC is characterized by its ability to spread and survive at these sites. A prolonged 10 μM ART exposure of up to 10 days contributed to a significant reduction of clone colonies in all parental and respective sunitinib-resistant RCC cell lines. KTCTL-26, but also A-498 cells displayed a high sensitivity towards ART with regard to clone colony formation, followed by 786-O and Caki-1. In good accordance with Jeong et al., a significant decrease in clonogenic growth in therapy-sensitive Caki-1 and 786-O cells has been shown [47]. Not only ART, but also artemisinin significantly diminished clonogenic growth in therapy-sensitive RCC cells by down-regulating AKT, a survival protein, and up-regulating E-cadherin, an epithelial differentiation marker [58]. E-cadherin loss is associated with poor prognosis and continued spread of disease [59]. Since AKT up-regulation and loss of E-cadherin have previously been demonstrated in therapy-resistant RCC cells [60–64], it is conceivable that these proteins are also affected by ART in the sunitinib-resistant RCC cells.

Reduced cell growth and proliferation in response to ART were associated with impaired cell cycle progression. Parental and resistant Caki-1, 786-O, and A-498 cells displayed a significant G0/G1 phase arrest after exposure to 20 μM ART. Accumulation of the cells in G0/G1 correlated with a significant reduction of the cells in the S and G2/M phase. However, parental KTCTL-26 cells were not affected, and their sunitinib-resistant counterparts were only moderately affected. Concordant with the present investigation, ART and other derivatives of artemisinin have been shown to promote cell cycle arrest in the G0/G1 phase in several tumor entities [65,66]. Application of ART in epidermoid carcinoma cells has been shown to halt cells in the G0/G1 phase [65]. Artemisinin application has resulted in a similar effect in cell cultures from endometrial tumors [66]. In therapy-sensitive RCC cells, Caki-1, and 786-O, 50 μM ART has been shown to induce a G2/M phase arrest [47], whereas the G0/G1 cell cycle arrest observed in the present investigation was induced with 20 μM ART. These differences in cell cycle arrest could be due to the different ART concentrations. Depending on dose, other investigators have demonstrated a ROS-dependent cell cycle arrest induced by ART in both the G0/G1 and G2/M phases in breast cancer cells [67].

Cell cycle progression is controlled by alternating CDK-cyclin complexes. In good accordance with the G0/G1 cell cycle arrest induced by ART, the cell cycle activating proteins CDK 1/2 and cyclin A/B, responsible for S and G2/M phase progression, were down-regulated, whereas the cell cycle inhibiting proteins, p21 in 786-O cells, and p27 in Caki-1 cells, were elevated. The CDK2-cyclin A complex mediates DNA replication in the S phase [68]. The CDK1-cyclin A complex promotes S phase transition, and CDK1-cyclin B complex drives transition from the G2 to M phase [69]. Hence, there is strong evidence that CDK1, CDK2, cyclin A, and B down-regulation by ART evokes the G0/G1 phase arrest, inhibiting growth of the RCC cells. Indeed, blocking CDK1/2 or cyclin A/B by small interfering RNA has been shown to significantly reduce cell growth in Caki-1, KTCTL-26, and A-498 cells [18,19]. Increased p21 and p27 after ART application are also indicative of cell cycle arrest, as both proteins mediate cell cycle arrest in the G0/G1 phase [70,71]. In epidermoid cancer cells, administration of ART resulted in a G0/G1 phase arrest and concomitant p27 increase [65]. Consistent with the current investigation, cell cycle arrest of the epidermoid cancer cells after ART treatment correlated with down-regulation of cyclin A1, cyclin B, and CDK2 [65]. However, in 786-O cells the expression of p27 was already high and significantly diminished after ART exposure. Studies on bone cancer have demonstrated that p27 in addition to its anti-tumor function can play a role in oncogenesis [72]. In line with this, for some renal cell carcinomas, increased p27 expression was associated with worse prognosis [73]. This may hold true for the 786-O cell lines but remains speculative and requires further investigation. Thus, ART seems to act cell type-dependently, attributable to the initial protein content and/or stage of disease. This might also be clinically important with regard to the intra-tumor heterogeneity of RCC [74], since RCC is a tumor entity harboring varying molecular signatures with different sensitivity to treatment [75].

Evidence has been presented showing that cell death may also be responsible for growth inhibition by ART [47,51]. However, in the current study, only in sunitinib-resistant Caki-1 cells were significant apoptotic effects apparent after ART treatment. Based on the dose–response curves and the fact that KTCTL-26 cells reveal no or just slight effects on cell cycle progression, it might be assumed that ART enables cell death in the KTCTL-26 cell line. However, ART did not induce apoptosis in the KTCTL-26 cells. Furthermore, 786-O and A-498 cell lines also displayed no apoptosis induction under ART treatment. Other investigators have shown that ART induced apoptosis in tumor cells, but often only after application of higher ART concentrations than used in the current study. In stomach tumors, apoptotic events were detected in vitro with concentrations upwards of 50 μM ART [51]. Similarly, induction of apoptosis was apparent after 48 h exposure to 50 μM ART in therapy-sensitive Caki-1 and 786-O cells [47]. Since the tumor cell growth of Caki-1, 786-O, and A-498 cell lines was also not reduced below the initial cell count at seeding, even with the higher 50 μM ART concentration, apoptosis induction by ART can only play a minor role in controlling RCC. This leaves the question open as to how to explain the reduction in the KTCTL-26 cells below that of the initial seeding count after exposure to ART.

One explanation of the magnitude of this ART-induced growth inhibitory effect might be induction of ferroptosis. Indeed, parental and sunitinib-resistant KTCTL-26 demonstrated a significant reversion in ART's growth inhibitory effect after additional application of the ferroptosis inhibitor ferrostatin-1, indicating that ART does induce ferroptosis. Accordingly, ferroptotic effects have been demonstrated in cell cultures of head and neck cancer after ART treatment [25]. In pancreatic cancer cells, ART also triggered ferroptosis [36], and sorafenib combined with ART induced ferroptosis in liver cancer cells [76].

Caki-1, 786-O, and A-498 cells did not show any response to ferrostatin-1, indicating that ferroptosis does not take place in these cell lines. The ART-induced growth inhibition in these cells must therefore mainly act through cell cycle arrest.

Since ART induced ROS generation during ferroptosis [48], Trolox, a vitamin E derivative and anti-oxidant that neutralizes ROS [32], was applied to investigate whether the inhibitory effect of ART could be canceled. In both parental and sunitinib-resistant KTCTL-26 cells, the inhibitory effect of ART was significantly reversed, showing that ART can act through ROS generation. Glutathione (GSH), a key regulator of excessive ROS levels [77], was also significantly reduced after ART administration. ART evoked a stronger GSH reduction in parental KTCTL-26 cells than in resistant cells, which might mean that these resistant RCC cells have a higher basal ROS tolerance. Support for this thesis is provided by a proteomic study, showing that glutathione metabolism in sunitinib-resistant 786-O RCC cells was increased 4–5 times compared to parental cells [78]. Hence, adding ART to sunitinib treatment might counteract ROS tolerance in therapy-resistant cells, and facilitate ferroptosis. In the current investigation, combining ART with iron further potentiated the decrease of GSH in both parental and sunitinib-resistant KTCTL-26 cell lines. ART in combination with lysosomal iron led to the development of ROS and ultimately induces apoptosis via the intrinsic pathway [32]. Increased efficacy of ART in the presence of iron has been shown in pancreatic [36] and in breast cancer cell lines [32]. A high iron content within the tumor cells therefore seems to augment ART's efficacy, and tumor cells with increased iron metabolism could be selectively targeted, including RCC [79].

Phospholipid-hydroxy peroxide-glutathione peroxidase (PHGPx, gene: GPX4) is another key protein involved in augmented ROS generation. Substances containing an endoperoxid group, such as ART, directly inhibit GPX4, first sensitizing "GPX4 tumors" to ferroptosis [80] and ultimately leading to ferroptosis [81]. GPX4 was significantly reduced in parental and resistant KTCTL-26 cells after ART treatment. Over-expression of GPX4 prevented ferroptosis in colorectal cancer in in vitro studies [82]. Consequently, this might also be the case for the KTCTL-26 cell lines.

p53 has been described as a possible ferroptosis enhancer [49,50]. Interestingly, p53 was exclusively expressed in the parental and sunitinib-resistant KTCTL-26 cell lines, the only RCC cell lines demonstrating ferroptosis induction after exposure to ART. p53 inhibited cysteine influx and thus disrupted GSH metabolism [83]. Furthermore, and consistent with our results, ferroptosis could not be induced in p53-defective cells. Hence, p53 expression may impact GSH metabolism and might be a predictor for ferroptosis induction in parental and sunitinib-resistant RCC cells. Still, this is speculative and requires further investigation. In tumor cells inducing apoptosis, cell death is regulated by both p53-dependent and -independent pathways [56,57].

Along with induction of ferroptosis, ART exposure resulted in significantly diminished ATP production and spare reserve capacity in both parental and sunitinib-resistant KTCTL-26 cells, throttling the energy supply necessary for tumor cell progression. Consistent with this, ART administration in B-cell lymphoma cells and prolactinoma cells led to reduced ATP production [84,85].

The results presented here show that ART induced significant growth inhibitory effects in parental and, more importantly, sunitinib-resistant RCC cells. Although all four RCC cell lines responded to ART, cell type-specific responses were evident. This might give an insight on how ART may act in heterogeneous tumors. In parental and resistant Caki-1, 786-O, and A-498 cells, growth inhibitory effects were accompanied by cell cycle arrest in the G0/G1 phase and respective modulation of the cell cycle regulating proteins. It may therefore be assumed that ART led to growth and proliferation inhibition, but not to tumor cell death. In contrast, parental and sunitinib-resistant KTCTL-26 cells were mainly affected by ART through ferroptosis and decreased metabolism, leading to both growth inhibition and tumor cell death. Notably, p53 was only evident in the KTCTL-26 cells, indicating that p53 might be predicative for ART-dependent ferroptosis and induce a more effective drug response, which could be clinically relevant. The in vitro data give a first insight into the anti-tumor activity of ART in RCC cells that might in its strength and the respective mechanism depend on the initial protein profile of the tumor cells and therewith aspects of the intra-tumor heterogeneity. However, since in vitro data reveal an isolated tumor cell system, further investigations are necessary to verify our postulates and in vivo studies need to clarify whether ART shows similar anti-tumor effects under physical conditions in parental and sunitinib-resistant RCC.

4. Materials and Methods

4.1. Cell Cultures

Renal cell carcinoma cell lines Caki-1, 786-O, KTCTL-26, and A-498 were kindly provided by Prof. Dr. Roman Blaheta (Department of Urology, University Hospital Frankfurt, Goethe-University, GER), initially purchased from Promocell (LGC Promochem, Wesel, Germany). Caki-1 cells were grown and sub-cultured in Iscove Basal medium (Biochrom GmbH, Berlin, Germany), 786-O, KTCTL-26, and A-498 were grown in RPMI-1640 medium (Gibco, Thermo Fisher Scientific, Darmstadt, Germany). Media were supplemented with 10% fetal calf serum (FCS) (Gibco, Thermo Fisher Scientific, Darmstadt, Germany), 1% glutamax (Gibco, Thermo Fisher Scientific, Darmstadt, Germany), and 1% Anti/Anti (Gibco, Thermo Fisher Scientific, Darmstadt, Germany). Twenty mM HEPES-buffer (Sigma-Aldrich, Darmstadt, Germany) was added to the RPMI-1640 medium. Tumor cells were cultivated in a humidified, 5% CO_2 incubator.

4.2. Resistance Induction and Application of Sunitinib and Artesunate

Resistance to sunitinib was induced by chronic exposure to ascending sunitinib (free Base, Massachusetts LC Laboratories, Woburn, MA, USA) concentrations from 0.1–1 µM until the cells survived and adapted to the highest dosage. Sunitinib resistance in the RCC cells occurred in average 10 weeks after starting application. Thereafter, they were maintained with 1 µM sunitinib applied three times a week. The IC50 (half-maximal inhibitory concentration) of sunitinib was investigated to verify drug resistance. After starving chronically sunitinib-treated RCC cells for 3 days 0.1–100 µM sunitinib was applied for 72 h. Therapy-sensitive (parental) RCC subcell lines served as controls. RCC cells were designated as sunitinib-resistant when the IC50 under 72 h sunitinib application was approximately doubled.

Artesunate (ART) (Sigma-Aldrich, Darmstadt, Germany) was applied at a concentration of 1–100 µM. Controls (parental and sunitinib-resistant) remained ART-untreated. The IC50 of ART in parental and sunitinib-resistant RCC cells was evaluated analog to sunitinib using the 72 h growth data at a concentration of 1–100 µM ART. To evaluate possible toxic effects of sunitinib and/or ART, cell viability was determined in parallel to experimentation by testing aliquoted cells with trypan blue (Sigma-Aldrich, Darmstadt, Germany). Only viable cells were employed.

4.3. Tumor Cell Growth

Cell growth was assessed using 3-(4,5-dimethylthiazol- 2-yl)-2,5-diphenyltetrazolium bromide (MTT) dye. RCC cells (50 µL, 1×10^5 cells/mL) were seeded onto 96-well-plates. After 24, 48, and 72 h, 10 µL MTT (0.5 mg/mL) (Sigma-Aldrich, Darmstadt, Germany) was added for 4 h. Cells were then lysed in 100 µL solubilization buffer containing 10% SDS in 0.01 M HCl. The 96-well-plates were subsequently incubated overnight at 37 °C, 5% CO_2. Absorbance at 570 nm was determined for each well using a multi-mode microplate-reader (Tecan, Spark 10 M, Crailsheim, Germany). After subtracting background absorbance and offsetting with a standard curve, results were expressed as mean cell number. To illustrate dose-response kinetics, mean cell number after 24 h incubation was set to 100%. Each experiment was done in triplicate.

4.4. Proliferation

Cell proliferation was measured using a BrdU (Bromodeoxyuridine / 5-bromo-2′-deoxyuridine) cell proliferation enzyme-linked immunosorbent assay (ELISA) kit (Calbiochem/Merck Biosciences, Darmstadt, Germany). Tumor cells (50 μL, 1×10^5 cells/mL), seeded onto 96-well-plates, were incubated with 20 μL BrdU-labeling solution per well for 24 h, fixed and stained using anti-BrdU mAb according to the manufacturer's protocol. Absorbance was measured at 450 nm using a multi-mode microplate-reader (Tecan, Spark 10 M, Crailsheim, Germany). Values were presented as percentage compared to untreated controls set to 100%.

4.5. Clonogenic Assay

The clonogenic recovery potential gives insight into the capability of the cells to form a new tumor (metastasis). Therefore, 500 cells/well were seeded on a 6-well-plate and treated for 10 days with ART. Untreated cells served as controls. RCC cells were subsequently fixed with 85% MeOH/15% AcOH and stained with Coomassie (0.5 g Coomassie Blue G250 (Sigma-Aldrich, Darmstadt, Germany), 75 mL AcOH, 200 mL MeOH, 725 mL distilled water). Amount and size of cell clone colonies were measured with a biomolecular imager (Sapphire, Azure Biosystems, Biozym, Hess. Oldendorf, Germany). Colony forming efficiency was evaluated by ImageJ analysis. A colony was defined as consisting of at least 50 cells with an area of 50.8 μm^2. Untreated controls were set to 100%.

4.6. Cell Cycle Phase Distribution

For cell cycle analysis cell cultures were grown to sub-confluency. A total of 1×10^6 cells was stained with propidium iodide (50 μg/mL) (Invitrogen, Thermo Fisher Scientific, Darmstadt, Germany) and then subjected to flow cytometry (Fortessa X20, BD Biosciences, Heidelberg, Germany). Ten thousand events were collected from each sample. Data acquisition was carried out using DIVA software (BD Biosciences, Heidelberg, Germany), and cell cycle distribution was analyzed by ModFit LT 5.0 software (Verity Software House, Topsham, ME, USA). The number of cells in the G0/G1, S, or G2/M phases was expressed as a percentage.

4.7. Western Blot Analysis of Cell Cycle Regulating Proteins, GPX4 and p53

To explore the expression and activity of cell cycle and cell death regulating proteins, western blot analysis was performed. Tumor cell lysates (50 μg) were applied to 10% or 12% polyacrylamide gel and separated for 10 min at 80 V and 1 h at 120 V. The protein was then transferred to nitrocellulose membranes (1 h, 100 V). After blocking with 10% non-fat dry milk for 1 h, the membranes were incubated overnight with the following primary antibodies directed against cell cycle proteins: p21 (Rabbit IgG, clone 12D1, Cell Signaling, Frankfurt am Main, Germany), p27 (Mouse IgG_1, clone 57/Kip1, BD Biosciences, Heidelberg, Germany), Cyclin A (Mouse IgG_1, clone 25, BD Biosciences, Heidelberg, Germany), Cyclin B (Mouse IgG_1, clone 18, BD Biosciences, Heidelberg, Germany), CDK1 (Mouse IgG_1, clone 2, BD Biosciences, Heidelberg, Germany), pCDK1 (Rabbit, clone 10A11, Cell Signaling, Frankfurt am Main, Germany), CDK2 (Mouse IgG_{2a}, clone 55, BD Biosciences, Heidelberg, Germany).

To indicate lipid peroxidation and ferroptosis related proteins the following primary antibodies were used: GPX4 (Rabbit IgG, ab41787, Abcam, Berlin, Germany), p53 (Rabbit, clone 7F5, Cell Signaling, Frankfurt am Main, Germany). HRP-conjugated rabbit-anti-mouse IgG or goat-anti-rabbit IgG served as secondary antibodies (IgG, both: dilution 1:1000, Dako, Glostrup, Denmark). The membranes were incubated with ECL detection reagent (AC2204, Azure Biosystems, Munich, Germany) to visualize proteins with a Sapphire Imager (Azure Biosystems, Munich, Germany). β-actin (clone AC-1; Sigma Aldrich, Taufenkirchen, Germany) served as the internal control, except for p53, which was normalized to total protein. To quantify total protein all membranes were stained by Coomassie brilliant blue and measured by Sapphire Imager. AlphaView software (ProteinSimple, San Jose, CA, USA) was used for pixel density analysis of the protein bands. The ratio of protein intensity/β-actin intensity or whole protein intensity was calculated and expressed in percentage, related to the untreated controls, set to 100%.

4.8. Apoptosis and Ferroptosis

To investigate apoptotic and necrotic events, the FITC-Annexin V Apoptosis Detection kit (BD Biosciences, Heidelberg, Germany) was used to quantify binding of Annexin V/propidium iodide (PI). After washing tumor cells twice with PBS, 1×10^5 cells were suspended in 500 μL of 1 × binding buffer and incubated with 5 μL Annexin V-FITC and (or) 5 μL PI in the dark for 15 min. Staining was measured by flow cytometer (Fortessa X20, BD Biosciences, Heidelberg, Germany). Ten thousand events were collected from each sample. The percentage of apoptotic and necrotic cells in each quadrant was calculated using DIVA software (BD Biosciences, Heidelberg, Germany). Further analysis was done by FlowJo software (BD Biosciences, Heidelberg, Germany).

A BrdU cell proliferation enzyme-linked immunosorbent assay (ELISA) kit (Calbiochem/Merck Biosciences, Darmstadt, Germany) was used to evaluate ferroptosis and ROS generation. To evaluate ferroptosis, tumor cells were treated for 48 h with 20, 50, and 100 μM ART or ART combined with 20 μM ferrostatin-1 (Sigma-Aldrich, Darmstadt, Germany), a ferroptosis inhibitor. ROS generation during ferroptosis was verified by treating the RCC cells for 48 h with 20, 50, and 100 μM ART in combination with 0.5 mM Trolox (Sigma-Aldrich, Taufkirchen, Germany), an antioxidant. For more details see "Proliferation" (4.4), as described above.

4.9. GSH-Assay

The GSH level was evaluated with the GSH-Glo™ Glutathione Assay (Promega Corporation, Madison, Wisconsin, USA). Five thousand cells/well were seeded onto a 96-well-plate and incubated for 24 h with 50 μM ART or ART combined with 20 μg/mL holo-Transferrin (Fe; Sigma-Aldrich, Taufkirchen, Germany). Experiments were performed according to the manufacturer's protocol. Luminescence was measured using a multi-mode microplate-reader (Tecan, Spark 10 M, Tecan, Grödig, Austria).

4.10. Evaluation of Mitochondrial Respiration and Anaerobic Glycolytic Activity

Mitochondrial respiration (OCR = oxygen consumption rate) and anaerobic glycolytic activity (EACR = extracellular acidification rate) were assessed in real time by the Seahorse XFp Extracellular Flux Analyzer using the Seahorse XF Cell Mito Stress Test Kit (both: Agilent Technologies, Waldbronn, Germany). The EACR indicating anaerobic glycolytic activity was used to determine compensatory glycolysis. OCR was obtained by multiple parameters, including basal respiration, ATP production-coupled respiration, maximal and reserve capacities, and non-mitochondrial respiration. Cells stained with CellTracker Green CMFDA (Thermo Fisher Scientific, Darmstadt, Germany) were plated at a density of 2×10^4 cells/well and media was replaced with XF Assay media the following day 1h prior to the assay and incubated without CO_2. Five measurements of OCR and ECAR were taken at baseline and after each injection of the following mitochondrial modulators: Oligomycin (1.5 μM, Inhibitor of ATP synthase), carbonylcyanide 4-(trifluoromethoxy)phenylhydrazone (FCCP) (1 μM, proton gradient uncoupler), and rotenone/actinomycin A (0.5 μM, inhibitors of complex I/Complex III). Data were normalized by using Wave 2.6.1 (Agilent Technologies, Waldbronn, Germany) desktop software to the mean fluorescent intensity of cells in the area of measurement in each well. Data pertaining to the OCR were normalized to total basal respiration (set to 100%) consisting of mitochondrial and non-mitochondrial respiration. Basal and maximal respiration were calculated by subtracting non-mitochondrial OCR. Respiratory reserve capacity was calculated as the difference between maximal and basal OCR. ATP-linked OCR was estimated as the difference between basal and rotenone/actinomycin A inhibited OCR.

4.11. Statistical Analysis

All experiments were performed at least three times. The evaluation and generation of mean values, the associated standard deviation, and normalization in percent were done by Microsoft Excel. Statistical significance was calculated with GraphPad Prism 7.0 (GraphPad Software Inc., San Diego, CA, USA): Two-sided T-test (Western blot, apoptosis, cell cycle), one-way ANOVA test (BrdU), and two-way ANOVA test (MTT). Correction for multiple comparisons was done using the conservative Bonferroni method. Differences were considered statistically significant at a p-value ≤ 0.05.

5. Conclusions

ART induced cell-type specific anti-tumor effects in both parental and sunitinib-resistant RCC cells. In three of the four tested cell lines, Caki-1, 786-O, and A-498, ART induced a strong G0/G1 phase arrest. In the KTCTL-26 cell line, the phase arrest was not as pronounced, but ART exposure additionally induced ferroptosis. In this cell line, the anti-tumor activity of ART was much stronger than in the other three cell lines where ferroptosis was not induced by ART. p53 was only detectable in the KTCTL-26 cells, possibly making it a predictive marker for ferroptosis and a better response to ART. Since RCC exhibits intra-tumor heterogeneity, this might be a clinically relevant aspect. The results presented here suggest that ART may hold promise as a new additive therapy option for selected patients with advanced and even sunitinib-resistant RCC.

Author Contributions: Conceptualization, E.J.; methodology, S.D.M., J.L., P.S. and K.S.S.; software, S.D.M. and O.V.; validation, O.V., R.M. and T.E.; formal analysis, S.D.M. and O.V.; investigation, S.D.M., O.V., E.J. and T.E.; resources, E.J. and A.H.; data curation, R.M.; writing—original draft preparation, S.D.M.; writing—review and editing, E.J., A.H. and T.E.; visualization, S.D.M.; supervision, E.J.; project administration, E.J.; funding acquisition, E.J. All authors have read and agree to the published version of the manuscript.

Acknowledgments: The main portion of the results presented here stem from work connected with the PhD thesis of S.D.M. Some elements stem from the bachelor thesis of J.L.

References

1. Fornara, P.; Hoda, M.R. Renal cell carcinoma. *Urol. A* **2011**, *50* (Suppl. S1), 219–222. [CrossRef]
2. Janzen, N.K.; Kim, H.L.; Figlin, R.A.; Belldegrun, A.S. Surveillance after radical or partial nephrectomy for localized renal cell carcinoma and management of recurrent disease. *Urol. Clin. N. Am.* **2003**, *30*, 843–852. [CrossRef]
3. Deng, H.; Liu, W.; He, T.; Hong, Z.; Yi, F.; Wei, Y.; Zhang, W. Comparative Efficacy, Safety, and Costs of Sorafenib vs. Sunitinib as First-Line Therapy for Metastatic Renal Cell Carcinoma: A Systematic Review and Meta-Analysis. *Front. Oncol.* **2019**, *9*, 479. [CrossRef] [PubMed]
4. Busch, J.; Seidel, C.; Weikert, S.; Wolff, I.; Kempkensteffen, C.; Weinkauf, L.; Hinz, S.; Magheli, A.; Miller, K.; Grunwald, V. Intrinsic resistance to tyrosine kinase inhibitors is associated with poor clinical outcome in metastatic renal cell carcinoma. *BMC Cancer* **2011**, *11*, 295. [CrossRef] [PubMed]
5. Zhou, X.; Hou, W.; Gao, L.; Shui, L.; Yi, C.; Zhu, H. Synergies of Antiangiogenic Therapy and Immune Checkpoint Blockade in Renal Cell Carcinoma: From Theoretical Background to Clinical Reality. *Front. Oncol.* **2020**, *10*, 1321. [CrossRef] [PubMed]
6. Ahrens, M.; Hartmann, A.; Bergmann, L. What is new in the diagnosis and therapy of renal cell carcinoma? *Dtsch. Med. Wochenschr.* **2020**, *145*, 734–739. [CrossRef] [PubMed]
7. Rini, B.I.; Battle, D.; Figlin, R.A.; George, D.J.; Hammers, H.; Hutson, T.; Jonasch, E.; Joseph, R.W.; McDermott, D.F.; Motzer, R.J.; et al. The Society for Immunotherapy of Cancer consensus statement on immunotherapy for the treatment of advanced renal cell carcinoma (RCC). *J. Immunother. Cancer* **2019**, *7*, 354. [CrossRef] [PubMed]
8. Massari, F.; Mollica, V.; Rizzo, A.; Cosmai, L.; Rizzo, M.; Porta, C. Safety evaluation of immune-based combinations in patients with advanced renal cell carcinoma: A systematic review and meta-analysis. *Expert Opin. Drug Saf.* **2020**, 1–10. [CrossRef]

9. Chau, V.; Bilusic, M. Pembrolizumab in Combination with Axitinib as First-Line Treatment for Patients with Renal Cell Carcinoma (RCC): Evidence to Date. *Cancer Manag. Res.* **2020**, *12*, 7321–7330. [CrossRef]
10. Poonthananiwatkul, B.; Howard, R.L.; Williamson, E.M.; Lim, R.H. Cancer patients taking herbal medicines: A review of clinical purposes, associated factors, and perceptions of benefit or harm. *J. Ethnopharmacol.* **2015**, *175*, 58–66. [CrossRef]
11. Saghatchian, M.; Bihan, C.; Chenailler, C.; Mazouni, C.; Dauchy, S.; Delaloge, S. Exploring frontiers: Use of complementary and alternative medicine among patients with early-stage breast cancer. *Breast* **2014**, *23*, 279–285. [CrossRef]
12. Christensen, C.M.; Morris, R.S.; Kapsandoy, S.C.; Archer, M.; Kuang, J.; Shane-McWhorter, L.; Bray, B.E.; Zeng-Treitler, Q. Patient needs and preferences for herb-drug-disease interaction alerts: A structured interview study. *BMC Complement. Altern. Med.* **2017**, *17*, 272. [CrossRef]
13. Mani, J.; Juengel, E.; Arslan, I.; Bartsch, G.; Filmann, N.; Ackermann, H.; Nelson, K.; Haferkamp, A.; Engl, T.; Blaheta, R.A. Use of complementary and alternative medicine before and after organ removal due to urologic cancer. *Patient Prefer Adherence* **2015**, *9*, 1407–1412. [CrossRef]
14. Ebel, M.-D.; Rudolph, I.; Keinki, C.; Hoppe, A.; Muecke, R.; Micke, O.; Muenstedt, K.; Huebner, J. Perception of cancer patients of their disease, self-efficacy and locus of control and usage of complementary and alternative medicine. *J. Cancer Res. Clin. Oncol.* **2015**, *141*, 1449–1455. [CrossRef] [PubMed]
15. Horneber, M.; Bueschel, G.; Dennert, G.; Less, D.; Ritter, E.; Zwahlen, M. How Many Cancer Patients Use Complementary and Alternative Medicine: A Systematic Review and Metaanalysis. *Integr. Cancer Ther.* **2011**, *11*, 187–203. [CrossRef] [PubMed]
16. Huebner, J.; Micke, O.; Muecke, R.; Buentzel, J.; Prott, F.J.; Kleeberg, U.; Senf, B.; Muenstedt, K. User rate of complementary and alternative medicine (CAM) of patients visiting a counseling facility for CAM of a German comprehensive cancer center. *Anticancer Res.* **2014**, *34*, 943–948.
17. Kessel, K.A.; Lettner, S.; Kessel, C.; Bier, H.; Biedermann, T.; Friess, H.; Herrschbach, P.; Gschwend, J.E.; Meyer, B.; Peschel, C.; et al. Use of Complementary and Alternative Medicine (CAM) as Part of the Oncological Treatment: Survey about Patients' Attitude towards CAM in a University-Based Oncology Center in Germany. *PLoS ONE* **2016**, *11*, e0165801. [CrossRef]
18. Juengel, E.; Thomas, A.; Rutz, J.; Makarevic, J.; Tsaur, I.; Nelson, K.; Haferkamp, A.; Blaheta, R.A. Amygdalin inhibits the growth of renal cell carcinoma cells in vitro. *Int. J. Mol. Med.* **2016**, *37*, 526–532. [CrossRef]
19. Rutz, J.; Maxeiner, S.; Juengel, E.; Bernd, A.; Kippenberger, S.; Zoller, N.; Chun, F.K.; Blaheta, R.A. Growth and Proliferation of Renal Cell Carcinoma Cells Is Blocked by Low Curcumin Concentrations Combined with Visible Light Irradiation. *Int. J. Mol. Sci.* **2019**, *20*, 1464. [CrossRef] [PubMed]
20. Lee, H.M.; Moon, A. Amygdalin Regulates Apoptosis and Adhesion in Hs578T Triple-Negative Breast Cancer Cells. *Biomol. Ther.* **2016**, *24*, 62–66. [CrossRef]
21. Wang, F.; Wang, W.; Li, J.; Zhang, J.; Wang, X.; Wang, M. Sulforaphane reverses gefitinib tolerance in human lung cancer cells via modulation of sonic hedgehog signaling. *Oncol. Lett.* **2018**, *15*, 109–114. [CrossRef] [PubMed]
22. Hsu, E. The history of qing hao in the Chinese materia medica. *Trans. R Soc. Trop. Med. Hyg.* **2006**, *100*, 505–508. [CrossRef]
23. Efferth, T.; Dunstan, H.; Sauerbrey, A.; Miyachi, H.; Chitambar, C.R. The anti-malarial artesunate is also active against cancer. *Int. J. Oncol.* **2001**, *18*, 767–773. [CrossRef] [PubMed]
24. Konstat-Korzenny, E.; Ascencio Aragon, J.; Niezen, S.; Vazquez, R. Artemisinin and Its Synthetic Derivatives as a Possible Therapy for Cancer. *Med. Sci.* **2018**, *6*, 19. [CrossRef] [PubMed]
25. Roh, J.-L.; Kim, E.H.; Jang, H.; Shin, D. Nrf2 inhibition reverses the resistance of cisplatin-resistant head and neck cancer cells to artesunate-induced ferroptosis. *Redox Biol.* **2017**, *11*, 254–262. [CrossRef] [PubMed]
26. Nunes, J.J.; Pandey, S.K.; Yadav, A.; Goel, S.; Ateeq, B. Targeting NF-kappa B Signaling by Artesunate Restores Sensitivity of Castrate-Resistant Prostate Cancer Cells to Antiandrogens. *Neoplasia* **2017**, *19*, 333–345. [CrossRef] [PubMed]
27. Slezakova, S.; Ruda-Kucerova, J. Anticancer Activity of Artemisinin and its Derivatives. *Anticancer Res.* **2017**, *37*, 5995–6003. [CrossRef]

28. Newton, P.; Suputtamongkol, Y.; Teja-Isavadharm, P.; Pukrittayakamee, S.; Navaratnam, V.; Bates, I.; White, N. Antimalarial Bioavailability and Disposition of Artesunate in Acute Falciparum Malaria. *Antimicrob. Agents Chemother.* **2000**, *44*, 972–977. [CrossRef]
29. Lai, H.C.; Singh, N.P.; Sasaki, T. Development of artemisinin compounds for cancer treatment. *Investig. New Drugs* **2013**, *31*, 230–246. [CrossRef]
30. Efferth, T.; Giaisi, M.; Merling, A.; Krammer, P.H.; Li-Weber, M. Artesunate induces ROS-mediated apoptosis in doxorubicin-resistant T leukemia cells. *PLoS ONE* **2007**, *2*, e693. [CrossRef]
31. Krishna, S.; Ganapathi, S.; Ster, I.C.; Saeed, M.E.; Cowan, M.; Finlayson, C.; Kovacsevics, H.; Jansen, H.; Kremsner, P.G.; Efferth, T.; et al. A Randomised, Double Blind, Placebo-Controlled Pilot Study of Oral Artesunate Therapy for Colorectal Cancer. *EBioMedicine* **2015**, *2*, 82–90. [CrossRef] [PubMed]
32. Hamacher-Brady, A.; Stein, H.A.; Turschner, S.; Toegel, I.; Mora, R.; Jennewein, N.; Efferth, T.; Eils, R.; Brady, N.R. Artesunate activates mitochondrial apoptosis in breast cancer cells via iron-catalyzed lysosomal reactive oxygen species production. *J. Biol. Chem.* **2011**, *286*, 6587–6601. [CrossRef]
33. Efferth, T.; Volm, M. Glutathione-related enzymes contribute to resistance of tumor cells and low toxicity in normal organs to artesunate. *In Vivo* **2005**, *19*, 225–232. [PubMed]
34. Efferth, T.; Benakis, A.; Romero, M.R.; Tomicic, M.; Rauh, R.; Steinbach, D.; Hafer, R.; Stamminger, T.; Oesch, F.; Kaina, B.; et al. Enhancement of cytotoxicity of artemisinins toward cancer cells by ferrous iron. *Free Radic. Biol. Med.* **2004**, *37*, 998–1009. [CrossRef] [PubMed]
35. Kong, Z.; Liu, R.; Cheng, Y. Artesunate alleviates liver fibrosis by regulating ferroptosis signaling pathway. *Biomed. Pharmacother.* **2019**, *109*, 2043–2053. [CrossRef]
36. Eling, N.; Reuter, L.; Hazin, J.; Hamacher-Brady, A.; Brady, N.R. Identification of artesunate as a specific activator of ferroptosis in pancreatic cancer cells. *Oncoscience* **2015**, *2*, 517–532. [CrossRef]
37. Gopalakrishnan, A.M.; Kumar, N. Antimalarial action of artesunate involves DNA damage mediated by reactive oxygen species. *Antimicrob. Agents Chemother.* **2015**, *59*, 317–325. [CrossRef]
38. Ooko, E.; Saeed, M.E.; Kadioglu, O.; Sarvi, S.; Colak, M.; Elmasaoudi, K.; Janah, R.; Greten, H.J.; Efferth, T. Artemisinin derivatives induce iron-dependent cell death (ferroptosis) in tumor cells. *Phytomedicine* **2015**, *22*, 1045–1054. [CrossRef]
39. Jung, M.; Mertens, C.; Tomat, E.; Brune, B. Iron as a Central Player and Promising Target in Cancer Progression. *Int. J. Mol. Sci.* **2019**, *20*, 273. [CrossRef] [PubMed]
40. Schnetz, M.; Meier, J.K.; Rehwald, C.; Mertens, C.; Urbschat, A.; Tomat, E.; Akam, E.A.; Baer, P.; Roos, F.C.; Brune, B.; et al. The Disturbed Iron Phenotype of Tumor Cells and Macrophages in Renal Cell Carcinoma Influences Tumor Growth. *Cancers* **2020**, *12*, 530. [CrossRef] [PubMed]
41. Greene, C.J.; Attwood, K.; Sharma, N.J.; Gross, K.W.; Smith, G.J.; Xu, B.; Kauffman, E.C. Transferrin receptor 1 upregulation in primary tumor and downregulation in benign kidney is associated with progression and mortality in renal cell carcinoma patients. *Oncotarget* **2017**, *8*, 107052–107075. [CrossRef]
42. Chen, H.H.; Zhou, H.J.; Wu, G.D.; Lou, X.E. Inhibitory effects of artesunate on angiogenesis and on expressions of vascular endothelial growth factor and VEGF receptor KDR/flk-1. *Pharmacology* **2004**, *71*, 1–9. [CrossRef] [PubMed]
43. Dell'Eva, R.; Pfeffer, U.; Vene, R.; Anfosso, L.; Forlani, A.; Albini, A.; Efferth, T. Inhibition of angiogenesis in vivo and growth of Kaposi's sarcoma xenograft tumors by the anti-malarial artesunate. *Biochem. Pharm.* **2004**, *68*, 2359–2366. [CrossRef] [PubMed]
44. Anfosso, L.; Efferth, T.; Albini, A.; Pfeffer, U. Microarray expression profiles of angiogenesis-related genes predict tumor cell response to artemisinins. *Pharmacol. J.* **2006**, *6*, 269–278. [CrossRef] [PubMed]
45. Soomro, S.; Langenberg, T.; Mahringer, A.; Konkimalla, V.B.; Horwedel, C.; Holenya, P.; Brand, A.; Cetin, C.; Fricker, G.; Dewerchin, M.; et al. Design of novel artemisinin-like derivatives with cytotoxic and anti-angiogenic properties. *J. Cell. Mol. Med.* **2011**, *15*, 1122–1135. [CrossRef]
46. Wang, N.; Chen, H.; Teng, Y.; Ding, X.; Wu, H.; Jin, X. Artesunate inhibits proliferation and invasion of mouse hemangioendothelioma cells in vitro and of tumor growth in vivo. *Oncol. Lett.* **2017**, *14*, 6170–6176. [CrossRef]

47. Jeong, D.E.; Song, H.J.; Lim, S.; Lee, S.J.; Lim, J.E.; Nam, D.H.; Joo, K.M.; Jeong, B.C.; Jeon, S.S.; Choi, H.Y.; et al. Repurposing the anti-malarial drug artesunate as a novel therapeutic agent for metastatic renal cell carcinoma due to its attenuation of tumor growth, metastasis, and angiogenesis. *Oncotarget* **2015**, *6*, 33046–33064. [CrossRef]
48. Li, J.; Cao, F.; Yin, H.-L.; Huang, Z.-J.; Lin, Z.-T.; Mao, N.; Sun, B.; Wang, G. Ferroptosis: Past, present and future. *Cell Death Dis.* **2020**, *11*, 88. [CrossRef]
49. Kang, R.; Kroemer, G.; Tang, D. The tumor suppressor protein p53 and the ferroptosis network. *Free Radic. Biol. Med.* **2019**, *133*, 162–168. [CrossRef]
50. Gnanapradeepan, K.; Basu, S.; Barnoud, T.; Budina-Kolomets, A.; Kung, C.-P.; Murphy, M.E. The p53 Tumor Suppressor in the Control of Metabolism and Ferroptosis. *Front. Endocrinol.* **2018**, *9*, 124. [CrossRef]
51. Zhang, P.; Luo, H.-S.; Li, M.; Tan, S.-Y. Artesunate inhibits the growth and induces apoptosis of human gastric cancer cells by downregulating COX-2. *Oncotargets Ther.* **2015**, *8*, 845–854. [CrossRef]
52. Xu, Q.; Li, Z.-X.; Peng, H.-Q.; Sun, Z.-W.; Cheng, R.-L.; Ye, Z.-M.; Li, W.-X. Artesunate inhibits growth and induces apoptosis in human osteosarcoma HOS cell line in vitro and in vivo. *J. Zhejiang Univ. Sci. B* **2011**, *12*, 247–255. [CrossRef] [PubMed]
53. Greenshields, A.L.; Shepherd, T.G.; Hoskin, D.W. Contribution of reactive oxygen species to ovarian cancer cell growth arrest and killing by the anti-malarial drug artesunate. *Mol. Carcinog.* **2017**, *56*, 75–93. [CrossRef] [PubMed]
54. Ma, L.; Fei, H. Antimalarial drug artesunate is effective against chemoresistant anaplastic thyroid carcinoma via targeting mitochondrial metabolism. *J. Bioenerg. Biomembr.* **2020**, *52*, 123–130. [CrossRef]
55. Zhang, H.-T.; Wang, Y.-L.; Zhang, J.; Zhang, Q.-X. Artemisinin inhibits gastric cancer cell proliferation through upregulation of p53. *Tumor Biol.* **2014**, *35*, 1403–1409. [CrossRef] [PubMed]
56. Efferth, T.; Sauerbrey, A.; Olbrich, A.; Gebhart, E.; Rauch, P.; Weber, H.O.; Hengstler, J.G.; Halatsch, M.E.; Volm, M.; Tew, K.D.; et al. Molecular modes of action of artesunate in tumor cell lines. *Mol. Pharmacol.* **2003**, *64*, 382–394. [CrossRef]
57. Disbrow, G.L.; Baege, A.C.; Kierpiec, K.A.; Yuan, H.; Centeno, J.A.; Thibodeaux, C.A.; Hartmann, D.; Schlegel, R. Dihydroartemisinin is cytotoxic to papillomavirus-expressing epithelial cells in vitro and in vivo. *Cancer Res.* **2005**, *65*, 10854–10861. [CrossRef]
58. Yu, C.; Sun, P.; Zhou, Y.; Shen, B.; Zhou, M.; Wu, L.; Kong, M. Inhibition of AKT enhances the anti-cancer effects of Artemisinin in clear cell renal cell carcinoma. *Biomed. Pharmacother.* **2019**, *118*, 109383. [CrossRef]
59. Zhang, X.; Yang, M.; Shi, H.; Hu, J.; Wang, Y.; Sun, Z.; Xu, S. Reduced E-cadherin facilitates renal cell carcinoma progression by WNT/β-catenin signaling activation. *Oncotarget* **2017**, *8*, 19566–19576. [CrossRef]
60. Juengel, E.; Maxeiner, S.; Rutz, J.; Justin, S.; Roos, F.; Khoder, W.; Tsaur, I.; Nelson, K.; Bechstein, W.O.; Haferkamp, A.; et al. Sulforaphane inhibits proliferation and invasive activity of everolimus-resistant kidney cancer cells in vitro. *Oncotarget* **2016**, *7*, 85208. [CrossRef]
61. Juengel, E.; Kim, D.; Makarevic, J.; Reiter, M.; Tsaur, I.; Bartsch, G.; Haferkamp, A.; Blaheta, R.A. Molecular analysis of sunitinib resistant renal cell carcinoma cells after sequential treatment with RAD001 (everolimus) or sorafenib. *J. Cell. Mol. Med.* **2015**, *19*, 430–441. [CrossRef] [PubMed]
62. Juengel, E.; Nowaz, S.; Makarevi, J.; Natsheh, I.; Werner, I.; Nelson, K.; Reiter, M.; Tsaur, I.; Mani, J.; Harder, S.; et al. HDAC-inhibition counteracts everolimus resistance in renal cell carcinoma in vitro by diminishing cdk2 and cyclin A. *Mol. Cancer* **2014**, *13*, 152. [CrossRef]
63. Juengel, E.; Dauselt, A.; Makarević, J.; Wiesner, C.; Tsaur, I.; Bartsch, G.; Haferkamp, A.; Blaheta, R.A. Acetylation of histone H3 prevents resistance development caused by chronic mTOR inhibition in renal cell carcinoma cells. *Cancer Lett.* **2012**, *324*, 83–90. [CrossRef] [PubMed]
64. Juengel, E.; Makarević, J.; Tsaur, I.; Bartsch, G.; Nelson, K.; Haferkamp, A.; Blaheta, R.A. Resistance after Chronic Application of the HDAC-Inhibitor Valproic Acid Is Associated with Elevated Akt Activation in Renal Cell Carcinoma In Vivo. *PLoS ONE* **2013**, *8*, e53100. [CrossRef]

65. Jiang, Z.; Chai, J.; Chuang, H.H.F.; Li, S.; Wang, T.; Cheng, Y.; Chen, W.; Zhou, D. Artesunate induces G0/G1 cell cycle arrest and iron-mediated mitochondrial apoptosis in A431 human epidermoid carcinoma cells. *Anticancer Drugs* **2012**, *23*, 606–613. [CrossRef] [PubMed]
66. Tran, K.Q.; Tin, A.S.; Firestone, G.L. Artemisinin triggers a G1 cell cycle arrest of human Ishikawa endometrial cancer cells and inhibits cyclin-dependent kinase-4 promoter activity and expression by disrupting nuclear factor-κB transcriptional signaling. *Anticancer Drugs* **2014**, *25*, 270–281. [CrossRef] [PubMed]
67. Greenshields, A.L.; Fernando, W.; Hoskin, D.W. The anti-malarial drug artesunate causes cell cycle arrest and apoptosis of triple-negative MDA-MB-468 and HER2-enriched SK-BR-3 breast cancer cells. *Exp. Mol. Pathol.* **2019**, *107*, 10–22. [CrossRef]
68. Zhang, H.; Kobayashi, R.; Galaktionov, K.; Beach, D. pl9skp1 and p45skp2 are essential elements of the cyclin A-CDK2 S phase kinase. *Cell* **1995**, *82*, 915–925. [CrossRef]
69. Gavet, O.; Pines, J. Progressive activation of CyclinB1-Cdk1 coordinates entry to mitosis. *Dev. Cell* **2010**, *18*, 533–543. [CrossRef]
70. Bates, S.; Ryan, K.M.; Phillips, A.C.; Vousden, K.H. Cell cycle arrest and DNA endoreduplication following p21Waf1/Cip1 expression. *Oncogene* **1998**, *17*, 1691–1703. [CrossRef]
71. Wang, S.-T.; Ho, H.J.; Lin, J.-T.; Shieh, J.-J.; Wu, C.-Y. Simvastatin-induced cell cycle arrest through inhibition of STAT3/SKP2 axis and activation of AMPK to promote p27 and p21 accumulation in hepatocellular carcinoma cells. *Cell Death Dis.* **2017**, *8*, e2626. [CrossRef] [PubMed]
72. Currier, A.W.; Kolb, E.A.; Gorlick, R.G.; Roth, M.E.; Gopalakrishnan, V.; Sampson, V.B. p27/Kip1 functions as a tumor suppressor and oncoprotein in osteosarcoma. *Sci. Rep.* **2019**, *9*, 6161. [CrossRef] [PubMed]
73. Hedberg, Y.; Ljungberg, B.; Roos, G.; Landberg, G. Expression of cyclin D1, D3, E, and p27 in human renal cell carcinoma analysed by tissue microarray. *Br. J. Cancer* **2003**, *88*, 1417–1423. [CrossRef] [PubMed]
74. Gerlinger, M.; Horswell, S.; Larkin, J.; Rowan, A.J.; Salm, M.P.; Varela, I.; Fisher, R.; McGranahan, N.; Matthews, N.; Santos, C.R.; et al. Genomic architecture and evolution of clear cell renal cell carcinomas defined by multiregion sequencing. *Nat. Genet.* **2014**, *46*, 225–233. [CrossRef] [PubMed]
75. Dagogo-Jack, I.; Shaw, A.T. Tumour heterogeneity and resistance to cancer therapies. *Nat. Rev. Clin. Oncol.* **2018**, *15*, 81–94. [CrossRef]
76. Li, Z.-J.; Dai, H.-Q.; Huang, X.-W.; Feng, J.; Deng, J.-H.; Wang, Z.-X.; Yang, X.-M.; Liu, Y.-J.; Wu, Y.; Chen, P.-H.; et al. Artesunate synergizes with sorafenib to induce ferroptosis in hepatocellular carcinoma. *Acta Pharmacol. Sin.* **2020**. [CrossRef]
77. Xiao, Y.; Meierhofer, D. Glutathione Metabolism in Renal Cell Carcinoma Progression and Implications for Therapies. *Int. J. Mol. Sci.* **2019**, *20*, 3672. [CrossRef]
78. Hatakeyama, H.; Fujiwara, T.; Sato, H.; Terui, A.; Hisaka, A. Investigation of Metabolomic Changes in Sunitinib-Resistant Human Renal Carcinoma 786-O Cells by Capillary Electrophoresis-Time of Flight Mass Spectrometry. *Biol. Pharm. Bull.* **2018**, *41*, 619–627. [CrossRef]
79. Mou, Y.; Zhang, Y.; Wu, J.; Hu, B.; Zhang, C.; Duan, C.; Li, B. The Landscape of Iron Metabolism-Related and Methylated Genes in the Prognosis Prediction of Clear Cell Renal Cell Carcinoma. *Front. Oncol.* **2020**, *10*, 788. [CrossRef]
80. Yang, W.S.; SriRamaratnam, R.; Welsch, M.E.; Shimada, K.; Skouta, R.; Viswanathan, V.S.; Cheah, J.H.; Clemons, P.A.; Shamji, A.F.; Clish, C.B.; et al. Regulation of ferroptotic cancer cell death by GPX4. *Cell* **2014**, *156*, 317–331. [CrossRef]
81. Gaschler, M.M.; Andia, A.A.; Liu, H.; Csuka, J.M.; Hurlocker, B.; Vaiana, C.A.; Heindel, D.W.; Zuckerman, D.S.; Bos, P.H.; Reznik, E.; et al. FINO(2) initiates ferroptosis through GPX4 inactivation and iron oxidation. *Nat. Chem. Biol.* **2018**, *14*, 507–515. [CrossRef]
82. Sui, X.; Zhang, R.; Liu, S.; Duan, T.; Zhai, L.; Zhang, M.; Han, X.; Xiang, Y.; Huang, X.; Lin, H.; et al. RSL3 Drives Ferroptosis through GPX4 Inactivation and ROS Production in Colorectal Cancer. *Front. Pharmacol.* **2018**, *9*, 1371. [CrossRef] [PubMed]

83. Jiang, L.; Kon, N.; Li, T.; Wang, S.J.; Su, T.; Hibshoosh, H.; Baer, R.; Gu, W. Ferroptosis as a p53-mediated activity during tumour suppression. *Nature* **2015**, *520*, 57–62. [CrossRef] [PubMed]
84. Våtsveen, T.K.; Myhre, M.R.; Steen, C.B.; Wälchli, S.; Lingjærde, O.C.; Bai, B.; Dillard, P.; Theodossiou, T.A.; Holien, T.; Sundan, A.; et al. Artesunate shows potent anti-tumor activity in B-cell lymphoma. *J. Hematol. Oncol.* **2018**, *11*, 23. [CrossRef] [PubMed]
85. Zhang, W.; Du, Q.; Bian, P.; Xiao, Z.; Wang, X.; Feng, Y.; Feng, H.; Zhu, Z.; Gao, N.; Zhu, D.; et al. Artesunate exerts anti-prolactinoma activity by inhibiting mitochondrial metabolism and inducing apoptosis. *Ann. Transl. Med.* **2020**, *8*, 858. [CrossRef] [PubMed]

12

Therapeutic Targeting of Autophagy for Renal Cell Carcinoma Therapy

Trace M. Jones, Jennifer S. Carew and Steffan T. Nawrocki *

Division of Translational and Regenerative Medicine, Department of Medicine and The University of Arizona Cancer Center, Tucson, AZ 85724, USA; tracejones@email.arizona.edu (T.M.J.); jcarew@email.arizona.edu (J.S.C.)
* Correspondence: snawrocki@email.arizona.edu

Abstract: Kidney cancer is the 7th most prevalent form of cancer in the United States with the vast majority of cases being classified as renal cell carcinoma (RCC). Multiple targeted therapies have been developed to treat RCC, but efficacy and resistance remain a challenge. In recent years, the modulation of autophagy has been shown to augment the cytotoxicity of approved RCC therapeutics and overcome drug resistance. Inhibition of autophagy blocks a key nutrient recycling process that cancer cells utilize for cell survival following periods of stress including chemotherapeutic treatment. Classic autophagy inhibitors such as chloroquine and hydroxychloroquine have been introduced into phase I/II clinical trials, while more experimental compounds are moving forward in preclinical development. Here we examine the current state and future directions of targeting autophagy to improve the efficacy of RCC therapeutics.

Keywords: renal cell carcinoma; autophagy; hydroxychloroquine; chloroquine; ROC-325

---

1. Introduction

It is estimated that over 73,000 new cases of renal cancer will be diagnosed in the United States this year, with upwards of 14,000 individuals succumbing to their disease [1]. The most common malignancy of the kidney is renal cell carcinoma (RCC), which accounts for 85% of cases [2]. RCC can be divided into three distinct histological subtypes. Clear cell RCC (ccRCC) is the predominant subtype (~75%), with papillary RCC (PRCC) and chromophobe RCC (ChRCC) accounting for ~20% and ~5% of cases, respectively [3]. Disease stage at the time of diagnosis is the most important factor when considering the best course of treatment. Localized disease, generally TNM stage I or II, has a positive prognosis with a 5-year relative survival rate of 92.6% [4]. Localized neoplasms can be effectively treated with either a partial or radical nephrectomy, depending on the location of the primary mass [5]. After successful surgery, patients are often simply surveyed for signs of recurrence. It is estimated that 20–30% of patients who have undergone a successful nephrectomy will experience a recurrence, often presenting between one to three years following surgery [6]. Following a relapse, patients often undergo treatment with chemotherapy or immunotherapy depending on their histologic subtype. Patients presenting with regionally or distantly invasive tumors have a less favorable prognosis. A nephrectomy is still the primary first line treatment. However, patients are often administered chemotherapy, immunotherapy, or enrolled in a clinical trial in order to manage metastases and tumors that are surgically unresectable [5].

Given that metastatic, relapsed, and surgically unresectable tumors must be treated by systemic chemotherapy or immunotherapy, great interest has been shown in the past decade in developing targeted therapeutics for RCC. The most commonly mutated gene in RCC is the *von Hippel-Lindau (VHL)* tumor suppressor gene. Approximately 50% of RCC cases contain a mutation in this gene, with an additional 20% of cases presenting with a hypermethylated gene [7]. The VHL protein is an E3 ubiquitin ligase that controls the conjugation of ubiquitin molecules onto hypoxia-inducible factors (HIFs), proteins that are vital to the cellular hypoxia response pathway. Upon ubiquitylation, HIFs are processed and degraded through the ubiquitin proteasome pathway. Without a functional copy of *VHL*, HIFs are free to translocate to the nucleus and activate transcription of HIF responsive genes. A few of these HIF responsive genes code for vascular endothelial growth factor (VEGF), platelet-derived growth factor B (PDGF-B), transforming growth factor alpha (TGFα), and glucose transporter 1 (GLUT1) [7]. The overexpression of these factors is often a driving force in RCC tumorigenesis. In addition to *VHL*, genes involved in the mammalian target of rapamycin (mTOR) pathway are mutated in 28% of RCC cases [8,9]. These include genes encoding for phosphatidylinositol-3-kinase (PI3K), phosphatase and tensin homolog (PTEN), protein kinase B (AKT), and mTOR itself. These frequent mutation profiles provide the rationale for therapeutically targeting various receptor tyrosine kinases (RTKs) and downstream effector proteins currently being developed and used in the clinic (Figure 1).

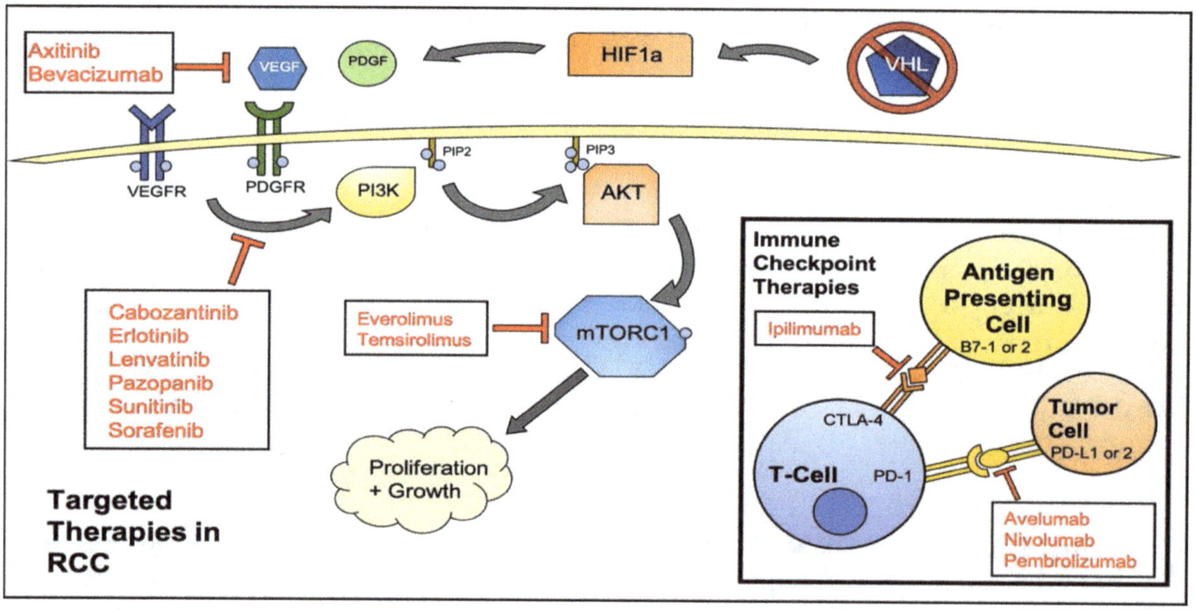

Figure 1. Federal Drug Administration (FDA) approved agents to treat renal cell carcinoma (RCC). Various kinase and mammalian target of rapamycin (mTOR) inhibitors are amongst the most common drugs used, however, immune checkpoint inhibitors are becoming a mainstay of RCC treatment.

Although targeted tyrosine kinase and mTOR inhibitors are effective first-line treatment options, many, if not all, cases of RCC will eventually become resistant to these drugs. The median time to a resistant tumor phenotype is 6–15 months depending on the therapeutic regimen [10]. A better understanding of the mechanistic drivers of drug resistance in RCC will facilitate the development of new and more effective treatment options for the relapsed/refractory patient population.

A hallmark of cancer is evasion of the immune response [11]. Cancer cells are capable of evading immune surveillance by expressing various signals that act as "off" switches to T-cells and natural killer (NK) cells. The most well-characterized of these signals are cytotoxic T-lymphocyte associated protein 4 (CTLA-4) and programmed cell death ligand 1 (PD-L1). When these surface proteins come in contact with the appropriate receptor on T-cells, they effectively trick the lymphocyte into recognizing the cancer cell as normal self-cells. Given this, an immense amount of energy has been dedicated to developing monoclonal antibody therapies to block the binding of cancer cell expressed PD-L1 and CTLA-4 allowing the immune cells to recognize the tumor cells as a foreign entity. These immune checkpoint inhibitor therapies enable the immune system to both eliminate tumor cells and also develop a lasting immune response. A persistent remission state is observed in two thirds of patients who experience an initial response to these therapies [12]. Importantly, immune checkpoint inhibitors have demonstrated significant efficacy in patients with RCC.

2. Targeted Therapeutics for RCC

For multiple decades, the standard therapy for RCC patients was a regimen of cytokines. While more effective than traditional chemotherapy options, interferon-alpha, and interleukin-2 as single agents or in combination yielded low response rates in patients with the combination generating an 18.6% response rate [13]. In addition, cytokine therapy was often associated with severe adverse effects and the incidence of comorbidities was high. With the advent of targeted therapies for cancer patients came an influx of approved therapeutics for RCC patients. There are now a multitude of Federal Drug Administration (FDA)-approved targeted treatments for RCC. The target-specific therapies can roughly be broken down into three distinct categories: small molecule kinase inhibitors, mTOR inhibitors, and monoclonal antibodies. The monoclonal antibodies frequently used to treat advanced RCC can be further classified as immune checkpoint inhibitors and non-immunomodulatory antibodies. A listing of targeted therapies approved for use in RCC can be found in Table 1.

Table 1. FDA-approved treatments for RCC.

Category	Therapeutic Name	Target(s)	Comparator	PFS (in Months) vs. Comparator
Small Molecule Kinase Inhibitors	Axitinib [14]	VEGF, PDGF	Sorafenib	6–7 vs. 4–7
	Cabozantinib [15]	VEGFR-1,2,3, MET, FLT3, TIE-2, AXL, TRKB	Everolimus	7.4–9.1 vs. 3.7–5.1
	Erlotinib [16]	EGFR	Bevacizumab	9.9 vs. 8.5
	Lenvatinib [17]	VEGFR2	Everolimus	7.4 vs. 5.5
	Pazopanib [18]	VEGFR-1,2,3, PDGFR, c-kit	Placebo	9.2 vs. 4.2
	Sorafenib [19]	RAF, VEGFR, PDGFR	Placebo	5.5 vs. 2.8
	Sunitinib [20]	VEGFR2, PDGFRb, c-kit, FLT3	Interferon-alpha	11 vs. 5
mTOR Inhibitors	Everolimus [21]	FKBP-12	Placebo	4 vs. 1.9
	Temsirolimus [22]	mTOR	Interferon-alpha	5.5 vs. 3.1
Monoclonal Antibodies	Avelumab [23]	PD-L1	Sunitinib	13.8 vs. 8.4
	Bevacizumab [24]	VEGF	Interferon-alpha	10.2 vs. 5.4
	Ipilimumab [25]	CTLA4	Sunitinib	11.6 vs. 8.4
	Nivolumab [26]	PD-1	Everolimus	4.6 vs. 4.4
	Pembrolizumab [27]	PD-1	Sunitinib	15.1 vs. 11.1
Cytokine Therapy	Interferon alfa-2a [28]	Immunostimulatory	N/A	10% Response Rate
	Interleukin-2 [29]	Immunostimulatory	N/A	14% Response Rate

Abbreviations: VEGF—vascular endothelial growth factor; PDGF—platelet-derived growth factor; VEGFR—vascular endothelial growth factor receptor; MET—tyrosine-protein kinase Met; FLT3—fms like tyrosine kinase 3; TIE-2—angiopoietin-1 receptor; AXL—AXL receptor tyrosine kinase; TRKB—tropomyosin receptor kinase B; EGFR—epidermal growth factor receptor; RAF—rapidly accelerated fibrosarcoma; FKBP-12—FK506 binding protein 12; mTOR—mammalian target of rapamycin; PD-L1—programmed death ligand 1; CTLA4—cytotoxic t-lymphocyte associated protein 4; PD-1—programmed cell death protein 1; PFS—progression free survival.

Due to the frequent inactivation of VHL and subsequent overexpression of HIF1a, RCC often presents as a highly vascularized tumor type. Hence, many of the small molecule therapeutics approved for use in RCC target various effectors in the angiogenesis pathway (VEGF, VEGFR). The goal of these drugs is to abrogate the formation of new blood vessels in the tumor microenvironment via growth factor withdrawal, which deprives the cancer cells of oxygen and nutrients that are needed to fuel their growth and survival. Many of these therapies provide an initial response. However, oxygen deprivation and nutrient withdrawal activates various stress response pathways in the cancer cell. Autophagy is one such stress response, and allows for survival during periods of therapeutic insult.

3. Autophagy

3.1. Molecular Mechanisms of Autophagy

Autophagy is a catabolic process by which cells internally break down and recycle cellular components through non-specific, lysosome-mediated degradation. Autophagy is highly conserved in eukaryotes and is a vital mechanism to mediate cellular stress and damage that results from hypoxia and starvation, as well as therapeutic intervention. Mammalian target of rapamycin complex 1 (mTORC1) is often regarded as the master regulatory kinase of cellular metabolism. Activation of mTORC1 is generally thought of as a pro-proliferation signal. mTORC1 activity can be stimulated from activated upstream tyrosine kinases such as PDGFR and VEGFR, often through the phosphoinositide 3 kinase (PI3K)/ protein kinase B (AKT) pathway. This mechanism of mTORC1 activation is especially important in RCC, given the genes encoding the proteins involved are frequently mutated. Importantly, activated mTORC1 is responsible for adding an inhibitory phosphate at Serine 757 to the Unc-51-like kinase (ULK1) complex, which prevents the initiation of autophagy [30]. Both direct and indirect inhibition of mTORC1 leads to potent activation of the autophagy inducer ULK1, which in turn promotes activity of the Beclin1-Vacuolar protein sorting 34 (VPS34) complex. The Beclin1-VPS34 complex is vital to the nucleation of the premature phagophore.

Maturation of the phagophore into a complete autophagosome involves elongation of the vesicle's lipid membrane. This process is regulated by a complex containing autophagy-related 12, autophagy-related 5 and autophagy-related 16L (ATG12-ATG5-ATG16L). Another crucial protein involved in the elongation of the autophagosome membrane is microtubule-associated protein 1A/1B light chain 3 (LC3). Cytosolic LC3 is referred to as LC3-I. LC3-I is conjugated in a ubiquitin-like fashion to phosphatidylethanolamines (PE) on the autophagosome membrane by the autophagy protein, autophagy-related 7 (ATG7). It must be mentioned that autophagy related 4B (ATG4B), a widely conserved cysteine protease, must first make a specific cleavage to allow conjugation of LC3 [31]. PE-associated LC3 protein is referred to as LC3-II, and is often considered a reliable marker of autophagosome formation and autophagy. LC3-II is vital for cargo recruitment as it binds Sequestosome-1 (p62) to the autophagosome membrane. p62 is responsible for binding misfolded proteins or dysfunctional organelles and subsequently delivering them to the autophagosome for degradation [32]. Finally, the mature autophagosome, with its contents localized and completely enclosed will fuse with the lysosome. The fusion of membranes will release the cargo of the autophagosome into the lysosome where the acidic pH, as well as various enzymes will facilitate their degradation. After degradation has occurred, the remaining molecules are released back into the cytoplasm where they can be used as building blocks for new proteins, organelles, or energy sources. We will specifically focus on the role of autophagy in RCC pathogenesis and its involvement related to emerging targeted therapies in RCC. For a more extensive review of the molecular machinery and regulation of autophagy, refer to the following articles [33–35].

3.2. Targeting Autophagy to Improve RCC Therapeutic Outcome

Autophagy is an essential lysosomal degradation process that can be used by cancer cells to generate alternative sources of energy via nutrient recycling under stress conditions [36,37]. Although many studies have demonstrated that autophagy may function as a mechanism of tumor suppression through the degradation of defective pre-malignant cells, significant data indicates a key role for autophagic degradation in the maintenance of energy balance under stress conditions including nutrient deprivation and hypoxia [38]. Futhermore, autophagy has emerged as an important mechanism of resistance to radiation, conventional chemotherapy, and targeted anticancer agents due to its ability to enhance the stress tolerance of malignant cells [39–43]. Collectively, these data support a role for autophagy as a promoter of drug resistance and cancer progression as well as a target for therapeutic inhibition. Importantly, several new studies demonstrate that alterations in the autophagy pathway may be particularly relevant for patients with RCC and impact overall survival [44,45].

RCC cell lines inherently exhibit an elevated basal level of autophagy. One study found that across many RCC cell lines, 30–60% of growing cells display prominent LC3-II puncta [46]. This compares to just 1–5% of cells in normal primary kidney cell cultures. Autophagy has been shown to counteract growth factor and nutrient withdrawal and maintain cell viability under stress conditions [47]. Importantly, inhibiting autophagy in RCC increases the efficacy of many therapeutic strategies. Sorafenib, a general RTK inhibitor, shows a significant increase in activity when combined with autophagy inhibitors [48]. The efficacy of AKT/mTOR inhibition is also significantly augmented through the use of a variety of autophagy inhibitors [49]. It has been demonstrated that RCC cells that have adopted an aggressive metastatic phenotype also rely on an increase in cellular autophagic flux. These highly aggressive cells can be rendered sensitive to the mTOR inhibitor temsirolimus by chloroquine, an anti-malarial drug that inhibits autophagy [50]. Successful enhancement of therapeutic efficacy via in vitro autophagy inhibition has provided a solid foundation for the development and clinical testing of autophagy inhibitors in RCC.

4. Inhibition of Autophagy for Therapy of RCC

4.1. Chloroquine and Hydroxychloroquine

Chloroquine (CQ) and hydroxychloroquine (HCQ) are quinone-containing compounds that have been used to combat malaria for decades. These compounds work via their accumulation in and subsequent deacidification of lysosomes [51]. This deacidification disrupts autophagy as the low pH of lysosomes is a necessity in degrading the cargo of the autophagosome. CQ and HCQ have been repurposed to pharmacologically target autophagy in a broad range of cancer types for over a decade [52]. To date, CQ and HCQ are the only autophagy inhibitors to be evaluated in clinical trials. A number of clinical trials involving the use of CQ or HCQ alone or in combination with standard of care agents for the treatment of many different malignancies are ongoing and completed. However, limited clinical studies have evaluated HCQ in patients with RCC (Table 2).

Table 2. Clinical trials with hydroxychloroquine (HCQ) in patients with RCC.

Clinical Trial Identifier	Autophagy-Modulating Compound	Interventions	Phase	Neoplasm	DLTs	Response Rate
NCT01510119 [53]	HCQ	Everolimus	I/II	Previously Treated RCC	None in Phase I; Grades 3–4 AE's <10%	SD or PR: 67%; Median PFS 6.3 Months
NCT01144169	HCQ	Surgery	I	Primary RCC	N/A	N/A
NCT01480154	HCQ	MK2206	I	Advanced Solid Tumors	N/A	N/A
NCT01550367	HCQ	IL-2	I/II	Metastatic RCC	Grades 3–5 AE's 96.6%	SD/PR/CR: 69%; Median PFS 5.5 Months
NCT01023737 [54]	HCQ	Vorinostat	I	Advanced Solid Tumors	Grades 3–4 AE's 18.5%	RCC Patient: PR for >50 cycles

A recent study in RCC combined the mTOR inhibitor, everolimus, with twice daily doses of HCQ in a metastatic patient population refractory to at least one prior treatment [53]. No dose-limiting toxicities (DLTs) were attributed to the HCQ in the phase I portion of the trial. The median progression-free survival (PFS) for the patient population was 6.3 months, an improvement over the median PFS of 4 months, which was observed in the clinical testing of everolimus alone [21]. A separate phase I trial sought to elucidate the toxicity and efficacy of combining HCQ with an AKT inhibitor, MK-2206, in a multitude of advanced solid tumors [55]. Patients were administered 135–200 mg of MK-2206 weekly in combination with 200–600 mg HCQ twice a day. 31 of the 35 patients enrolled were taken off treatment due to relapsed or progressive disease. In addition, 94% of participants experienced an adverse event (AE) attributed to treatment with MK-2206, while only 13% experienced an AE from the HCQ. Due to high toxicity and the low enrollment on the study, no anti-tumor activity data could be interpreted. One phase I trial has provided an exciting preliminary example of the power of HCQ in combination with vorinostat, an FDA approved histone deacetylase (HDAC) inhibitor [54]. This trial included patients with a variety of advanced solid tumors who had failed conventional therapy. Of these patients, a single person presented with advanced RCC. This particular patient had failed seven previous lines of therapy. A durable, partial response was obtained with a regimen of 400 mg vorinostat and 400 mg HCQ, administered daily. This response was maintained for more than 50 three-week cycles of the drug combination. This remarkable result in an RCC patient has sparked follow-up studies to evaluate tumor characteristics that may be indicative of a positive response to concurrent HDAC and autophagy inhibition.

4.2. *Lucanthone*

In addition to HCQ and CQ, several other agents used for non-cancer indications that disrupt lysosomal function have been repurposed as autophagy inhibitors for cancer therapy [41]. Lucanthone has been used as an anti-schistosome agent for many years and is also being developed as an anticancer agent due to its inhibitory effects on topoisomerase II and AP endonuclease (APE1). In cell culture experiments, lucanthone demonstrated lysosomal disruption and inhibition of autophagy [56]. In addition, strong pro-apoptotic effects were evident in various breast cancer cell lines and the lysosomal protease, cathepsin D, was shown to be an important mediator for the apoptotic effects of lucanthone. The chemical structure of lucanthone has provided clues to the construction of novel, lysosome-targeting agents.

4.3. *ROC-325*

While the clinical benefits of adjuvant CQ and HCQ treatment have not been fully elucidated, a substantial amount of funding and effort has been put forth to develop more efficient autophagy inhibitors. Initial results stemming from the use of CQ or HCQ have indicated that while these drugs partially block the degradation of cellular components in the lysosome, the compounds may not be potent enough to completely shut off the autophagy degradation. Thus, it is essential to generate new and more potent autophagy inhibitors that may improve clinical efficacy. A complete listing of next generation autophagy inhibitors discussed in this review, as well as the cancer types they have been explored in, can be found in Table 3.

ROC-325 is a water-soluble, small molecule developed by our group that shows significantly higher efficacy than HCQ [57–60]. ROC-325 is a dimeric compound that was designed to contain core motifs of HCQ as well as lucanthone. Much like HCQ, ROC-325 targets the late stages of autophagy. We have shown that ROC-325 does not affect the formation of autophagosomes but rather accumulates in and deacidifies the lysosome. In vitro treatment with ROC-325 shows stabilization of LC3-II and p62, indicators that are consistent with autophagy inhibition. In addition, treatment with ROC-325 results in near-complete loss of acridine orange fluorescence, a strong marker for lysosome membrane permeability and lysosome deacidification. ROC-325 reduced cell viability in RCC cell lines at much lower concentrations than HCQ, with half maximal inhibitory concentration (IC50) values of 2–10 μM vs. 50–100 μM, respectively.

Table 3. Selected agents that inhibit autophagy.

Inhibitor	Autophagy Target	Cancer Type	References
Hydroxychloroquine	Lysosome	RCC, etc.	[21,53–55]
Chloroquine	Lysosome	RCC, etc.	[51,52]
ROC-325	Lysosome	RCC, AML	[57–60]
Lucanthone	Lysosome	Breast	[41,56]
STF-62247	Lysosome	RCC, Glioblastoma, T-cell Leukemia	[45,61–63]
Lys05, DQ661, DC661	Lysosome, PPT1	Melanoma, Colon, Glioma	[64–67]
SAR405, SB02024	VPS34	RCC, Cervical	[68–70]
SBI-0206965, ULK-100, ULK-101	ULK1	Lung	[71,72]
S130, FMK-9a, NSC185058	ATG4B	Cervical, Colon, Osteosarcoma, GBM	[73–76]

Abbreviations: PPT1—palmitoyl-protein thioesterase 1; VPS34—vacuolar protein sorting 34; ULK1—unc51-like-kinase 1; ATG4B—autophagy related 4B; AML—acute myeloid leukemia; RCC—renal cell carcinoma; GBM—glioblastoma.

In vivo experiments also demonstrated the improved anticancer activity of ROC-325 over HCQ. Mice treated with orally-administered ROC-325 displayed significantly decreased 786-O RCC xenograft burden when compared to both control and HCQ-treated mice. Importantly, no significant toxicities were observed in mice treated with ROC-325. Tumors taken from each group were analyzed using immunohistochemistry (IHC). Tumors treated with ROC-325 showed elevated levels of LC3-II, p62, and cleaved caspase-3, thereby confirming in vitro findings. Further study of ROC-325 especially in combination with conventional and targeted therapy is warranted.

4.4. STF-62247

STF-62247 is an experimental agent that was first discovered over a decade ago. This particular compound was identified to have potent cytotoxic effects in VHL-deficient cancer cells, but very little efficacy in wild-type (WT) VHL cells [45]. Due to this selective anti-tumor activity, this compound is a potentially exciting therapeutic option for RCC. The exact mechanism by which STF-62247 acts is not fully understood. STF-62247 is believed to induce autophagy in cancer cells, as treatment produces large, cytoplasmic vacuoles in both WT-VHL and VHL-deficient cells. However, VHL-deficient cells contain much larger vacuoles and show significantly brighter acridine orange staining [45]. This indicates that VHL-deficient cells form large, highly acidic vesicles in response to STF-62247. Upon further investigation, it was shown that Golgi vesicle trafficking proteins played a pivotal role in sensitizing cells to the compound. However, the mechanistic links between VHL and autophagy were not fully elucidated.

Bouhamdani et al. recently confirmed these findings in RCC and also noted that while VHL-proficient cells also form large vacuoles, they are capable of resolving them within 48 hours of treatment [44]. Interestingly, in this study, STF-62247 was not shown to induce autophagy, but rather blocked the late stages of autophagy. No known upstream markers of increased autophagy were shown to be affected by the drug and inhibiting the vacuolar H^+ ATPase pump with bafilomycin A1 (BAF) showed very little, if any, additive stabilization of LC3-II or p62 when combined with STF-62247. These results cast doubt on the idea that STF-62247 is inducing autophagy. This also suggests that STF-62247 is potentially obstructing a similar stage of autophagy as BAF, indicating that it is a late-stage autophagy inhibitor, much like HCQ, CQ and ROC-325. However, much of this work is still controversial as STF-62247 has been shown to induce an autophagy-dependent cell death response in multiple malignancy types regardless of VHL status [61–63]. More data is needed in order for STF-62247 to be effectively transitioned into the clinical setting.

4.5. Lys05, DQ661, and DC661

Lys05 is a lysosome-disrupting, water-soluble salt of the compound Lys01. Lys01 consists of a pair of aminoquinolines, the major motif of CQ, connected by a methylamine-containing spacer [64,65]. Much like the previously discussed compounds, Lys01 produces an accumulation of LC3-II at a much lower dosage than CQ or HCQ. LN229 cells containing a green fluorescent protein tagged LC3 protein (GFP-LC3) treated with Lys01 display localization of LC3 to autophagic vesicles with 10x greater potency than HCQ, and electron microscopy confirms the presence of large autophagic vesicles in cells treated with Lys01. The anticancer profile of Lys01 is greater than that of HCQ when tested across colon cancer, glioma, and melanoma cell lines, with IC50 values ranging from 4–8 μM compared to 15–42 μM with HCQ. In vivo studies exhibited moderate, single agent, antitumor activity against orthotopically injected 1205Lu melanoma xenografts. Using HPLC tandem mass spectrometry, Lys05 was shown to accumulate in tumors in vivo at a much greater concentration than HCQ.

In addition to Lys05, two second-generation compounds have been developed—DQ661 and DC661 [66,67]. Interestingly, all these compounds were recently reported to block the lysosomal enzyme palmitoyl-protein thioesterase 1 (PPT1), which plays a key role in palmitoylation-mediated intracellular protein trafficking. These preclinical results imply that Lys05, DQ661, and DC661 have the potential to combat many different types of tumors. However, investigation of these compounds for RCC therapy has not been tested. It is worth noting that each of these lysosome-disrupting compounds has a similar mechanism of action, but contain unique chemical motifs. These novel structures will most likely lead to toxicity differences when clinical testing is initiated. This, in turn, could prove to be fundamental to approval and widespread therapeutic use.

4.6. VPS34 Inhibitors

The compounds discussed thus far act on the most distal component of the autophagy pathway, the lysosome. The lysosome acts as the common end point to this cellular process. The upstream, initiating machineries of autophagy show a great amount of complexity and have proven quite difficult to target. Nonetheless, multiple research groups are developing molecules to inhibit these proteins.

VPS34 is a PI3K lipid kinase family member, responsible for the addition of a phosphate group at the 3 position of the inositol ring of phosphatidylinositol (PI) on cellular membranes. This lipid phosphorylation is a vital step in the initiation and elongation of autophagosome membranes. While many pan-PI3K inhibitors currently exist, a few compounds have been developed to specifically target VPS34, including SAR405 and SB02024. SAR405 is a small molecule that targets the ATP binding pocket of VPS34 with high affinity [68,69]. In vitro work with this compound shows a reduction in autophagosome formation in GFP-LC3 tagged HeLa cells. In addition, concomitant treatment with everolimus in RCC cell lines eliminates the enhanced autophagic flux seen with mTOR inhibition. SAR405 also significantly enhanced the anticancer activity of everolimus in these same RCC cells. These preliminary findings have opened the door for combining VPS34 inhibitors with current standard-of-care therapeutics in RCC. SB02024, another recently discovered VPS34 inhibitor, shows significant anticancer activity when combined with standard RTK inhibitors, sunitinib and erlotinib, in breast cancer cell lines [70]. While this particular compound has not been tested in RCC, these findings highlight the potential of SB02024 to be paired with standard of care RCC agents.

4.7. ULK1 Inhibitors

UNC-51-like kinase 1 (ULK1) is a proximal serine/threonine kinase that is responsible for autophagy initiation. ULK1 acts as one of the key signaling regulators linking mTORC1, 5′ adenosine monophosphate-activated protein kinase (AMPK), starvation, and autophagy. Due to its vital role in integrating cellular stress signals, successful inhibition of ULK1 is an attractive therapeutic strategy. SBI-0206965 was developed in 2015 as a selective ULK1 inhibitor [71]. This compound displayed potent inhibition of ULK1 activity with an in vitro IC50 of 108 nM. Treatment of A549 human lung cancer cells in vitro with a combination of SBI-0206965 and the mTOR inhibitor AZD8055 led to a significantly enhanced apoptotic response. This result further supports the rationale of inhibiting autophagy to augment the activity of other target-specific molecules. More recently, two closely related compounds, ULK-100 and ULK-101, have also been developed as more potent inhibitors of ULK1 [72]. Martin et al. demonstrated that these two small molecules show increased antitumor activity when combined with nutrient starvation in non-small-cell lung cancer cell lines. All three of these novel compounds have the potential for therapeutic impact in RCC. However, their specific efficacy in RCC models has not yet been evaluated.

4.8. ATG4B Inhibitors

ATG4B is a cysteine protease that activates LC3 for lipidation and recent studies suggest that it may be another promising target to inhibit autophagy upstream of the lysosome. Consistent with this idea, several ATG4B inhibitors have been developed including FMK-9a, NSC185058, and S130 [73–76]. NSC185058 and S130 have demonstrated significant in vivo activity against osteosarcoma and colon tumors, respectively [74,75]. Additionally, NSC185058 treatment decreased glioma xenograft growth in mice and augmented the antitumor efficacy of radiation therapy [76]. Collectively, these studies demonstrate that inhibiting ATG4B may be a suitable anti-autophagy target for the treatment of various cancers. However, these compounds remain in the earliest stages of preclinical development (Figure 2).

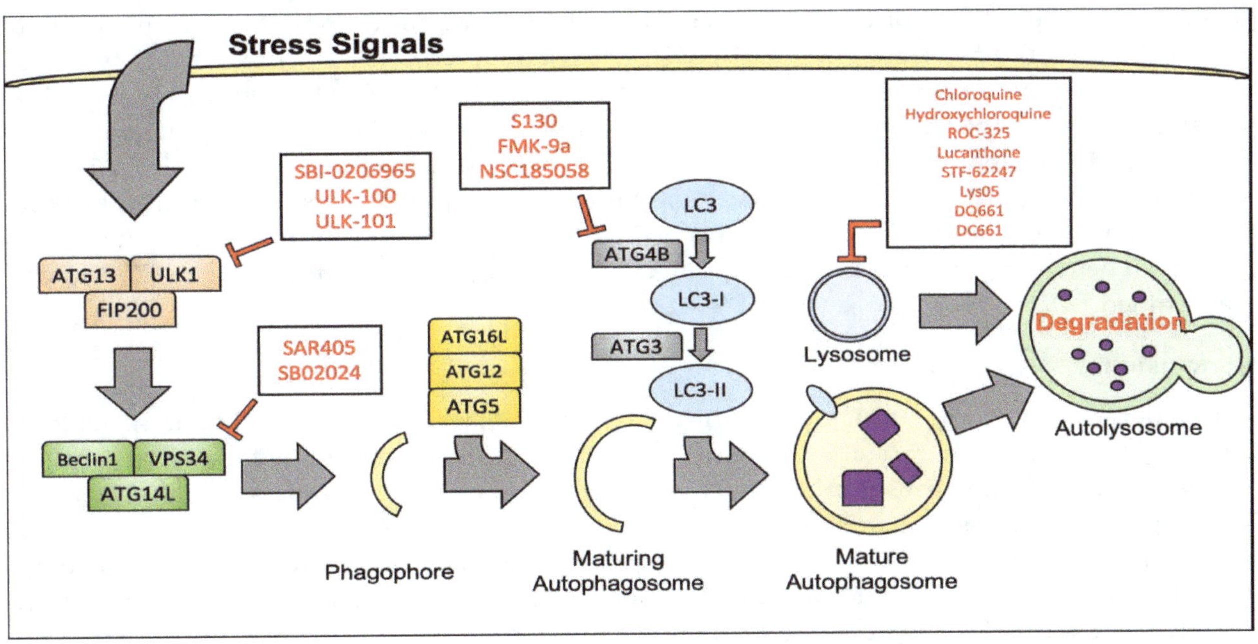

Figure 2. Selected agents that target autophagy at different points in the pathway. Hydroxychloroquine, chloroquine, and ROC-325 are amongst the compounds that target the lysosome. Compounds such as SBI-0206965 and SAR405 are being developed to inhibit autophagy factors near the proximal end of the cascade.

5. Immune Checkpoint Inhibitor Therapy and Autophagy

The clinical efficacy of novel immune checkpoint inhibitors has been variable. Through further research and testing, cancer types are now generally thought of as "immune hot" and "immune cold". Tumors that have significant infiltration of immune cells are considered "hot" and are generally responsive to immune checkpoint inhibitor therapy. The greatest immune checkpoint inhibitor therapy success to date has been the treatment of metastatic melanoma with a monoclonal antibody-targeting CTLA-4, Ipilimumab [77]. The FDA has now approved six different immune checkpoint inhibitors in a variety of cancer types. This number only stands to grow with over 200 active clinical trials involving immune checkpoint inhibitor therapies.

RCC is characterized as being responsive to immune checkpoint inhibitor therapy. As previously mentioned, cytokine therapy, a precursor to modern day immunotherapy, was long used as the primary treatment for advanced RCC. Nivolumab, a monoclonal antibody-targeting PD-1, was approved for use in RCC in 2015 after demonstrating improved progression-free survival (4.6 months vs. 4.4 months) over everolimus in a phase III clinical trial [26]. While more traditional small molecule therapy options, such as kinase inhibitors will remain a mainstay in RCC treatment, immunomodulatory therapies are becoming increasingly common as frontline and adjuvant therapies [78,79].

The connection between autophagy and immune cell activation is not well established, particularly in RCC. However, preliminary findings in different cancer models have provided conflicting findings. Early work has suggested that autophagy inhibition can interfere with hematopoiesis and systemic immunity indicating that combination autophagy and immune checkpoint inhibitor therapy may not be beneficial [80–82]. However, recent studies demonstrate that autophagy inhibition does not block T-cell activity [83–86]. Treatment of subcutaneous B16 melanoma xenografts with CQ in immunocompetent mice has provided evidence that autophagy inhibition promotes macrophage phenotype switching from an alternatively activated (M2) to a classically activated (M1) state [87]. This switch in macrophage phenotype gave rise to an increase in CD3+/CD8+ tumor-infiltrating lymphocytes as well as increased interferon gamma (IFNγ) expression, a key marker of cytotoxic T-lymphocyte (CTL) activation. Importantly, the antitumor effects of CQ in vivo were completely reversed in T-cell deficient mice, confirming that the activity of CQ was indeed a product of immunomodulation in this particular model. Recent work has also shown that HCQ, when delivered to E.G7-OVA murine lymphoma xenografts via nanoparticle vaccination, is capable of enhancing tumor cell major histocompatibility complex (MHC)-I antigen presentation, a key event in CTL activation [88]. A significant increase in the production of IFNγ was also observed in this model. Both of these recent studies highlight a potential relationship between autophagy inhibition and responsiveness to immune checkpoint inhibitor therapy, but additional studies are needed to better understand this interaction. Furthermore, the potential benefit of dual immune checkpoint and autophagy inhibitor therapy to RCC remains to be determined.

6. Conclusions

Two decades ago, patients diagnosed with advanced, metastatic, or surgically unresectable RCC had very few approved therapeutic options. However, significant research efforts have resulted in the development of numerous targeted agents and immune-related therapies for the treatment of RCC. Despite this success, patients that are refractory to these treatments or develop drug resistance continues to be a major clinical issue. Autophagy has now been established as a key mechanism by which cancer cells are capable of surviving periods of therapy-induced stress leading to drug resistance. This provides the rationale for the development and testing of autophagy-modulating compounds to use in conjunction with the ever-expanding list of approved RCC treatments. While HCQ has demonstrated some promising activity in combination with standard agents in clinical trials, its effectiveness appears to be limited by a variety of factors. Considering this, there is a need for new and more potent autophagy inhibitors that can be tested in clinical trials. Additional information is also required to determine the differences between upstream and lysosomal autophagy targeting in regards to therapeutic efficacy. The development and classification of compounds targeting autophagy is an ongoing process, but one can hope that a breakthrough is on the horizon.

Author Contributions: Conceptualization, writing—original draft preparation, writing—review and editing; T.M.J., J.S.C., S.T.N. All authors have read and agreed to the published version of the manuscript.

Abbreviations

The following abbreviations are used in this manuscript:

RCC	renal cell carcinoma
VHL	Von-Hippel Lindau tumor suppressor
VEGF	vascular endothelial growth factor
PDGF	platelet-derived growth factor
ATG	autophagy-related gene
PFS	progression-free survival
PR	partial response
DLT	dose-limiting toxicity
SD	stable disease
CR	complete response
HDAC	histone deacetylase
AE	adverse event
HCQ	hydroxychloroquine
CQ	chloroquine
IHC	immunohistochemistry
ULK	UNC-51 like kinase
CTLA-4	cytotoxic t-lymphocyte associated protein 4
PD-L1	Programmed cell death ligand 1

References

1. Siegel, R.L.; Miller, K.D.; Jemal, A. Cancer statistics, 2019. *CA A Cancer J. Clin.* **2019**, *69*, 7–34. [CrossRef] [PubMed]
2. Barata, P.C.; Rini, B.I. Treatment of renal cell carcinoma: Current status and future directions. *CA A Cancer J. Clin.* **2017**, *67*, 507–524. [CrossRef] [PubMed]
3. Ricketts, C.J.; De Cubas, A.A.; Fan, H.; Smith, C.C.; Lang, M.; Reznik, E.; Bowlby, R.; Gibb, E.A.; Akbani, R.; Beroukhim, R.; et al. The Cancer Genome Atlas Comprehensive Molecular Characterization of Renal Cell Carcinoma. *Cell Rep.* **2018**, *23*, 313–326. [CrossRef] [PubMed]
4. Noone, A.; Howlander, N.; Krapcho, M.; Miller, D.; Brest, A.; Yu, M.; Ruhl, J.; Tatalovich, Z.; Mariotto, A.; Lewis, D.; et al. *Cancer Statistics Review*; SEER: Bethesda, MD, USA, 2018.
5. National Comprehensive Cancer Network. NCCN Clinical Practice Guidelines in Oncology: Kidney Cancer; Version 2.2020. Available online: https://www.nccn.org/professionals/physician_gls/pdf/kidney.pdf (accessed on 1 November 2019).
6. Eggener, S.E.; Yossepowitch, O.; Pettus, J.A.; Snyder, M.E.; Motzer, R.J.; Russo, P. Renal cell carcinoma recurrence after nephrectomy for localized disease: Predicting survival from time of recurrence. *J. Clin. Oncol.* **2006**, *24*, 3101–3106. [CrossRef]
7. Kim, W.Y.; Kaelin, W.G. Role of VHL gene mutation in human cancer. *J. Clin. Oncol.* **2004**, *22*, 4991–5004. [CrossRef]
8. Creighton, C.J.; Morgan, M.; Gunaratne, P.H.; Wheeler, D.A.; Gibbs, R.A.; Robertson, G.; Chu, A.; Beroukhim, R.; Cibulskis, K.; Signoretti, S.; et al. Comprehensivemolecular characterization of clear cell renal cell carcinoma. *Nature* **2013**, *499*, 43–49. [CrossRef]
9. Duran, I.; Lambea, J.; Maroto, P.; González-Larriba, J.L.; Flores, L.; Granados-Principal, S.; Graupera, M.; Sáez, B.; Vivancos, A.; Casanovas, O. Resistance to Targeted Therapies in Renal Cancer: The Importance of Changing the Mechanism of Action. *Target. Oncol.* **2017**, *12*, 19–35. [CrossRef]

10. Rini, B.I.; Atkins, M.B. Resistance to targeted therapy in renal-cell carcinoma. *Lancet Oncol.* **2009**, *10*, 992–1000. [CrossRef]
11. Hanahan, D.; Weinberg, R.A. Hallmarks of cancer: The next generation. *Cell* **2011**, *144*, 646–674. [CrossRef]
12. Ribas, A.; Wolchok, J.D. Cancer immunotherapy using checkpoint blockade. *Science* **2018**, *359*, 1350–1355. [CrossRef]
13. Negrier, S.; Escudier, B.; Lasset, C.; Douillard, J.-Y.; Savary, J.; Chevreau, C.; Ravaud, A.; Mercatello, A.; Peny, J.; Mousseau, M.; et al. Recombinant Human Interleukin-2, Recombinant Human Interferon Alfa-2a, or Both in Metastatic Renal-Cell Carcinoma. *N. Engl. J. Med.* **2002**, *338*, 1272–1278. [CrossRef] [PubMed]
14. Rini, B.I.; Escudier, B.; Tomczak, P.; Kaprin, A.; Szczylik, C.; Hutson, T.E.; Michaelson, M.D.; Gorbunova, V.A.; Gore, M.E.; Rusakov, I.G.; et al. Comparative effectiveness of axitinib versus sorafenib in advanced renal cell carcinoma (AXIS): A randomised phase 3 trial. *Lancet* **2011**, *378*, 1931–1939. [CrossRef]
15. Powles, T.; Motzer, R.J.; Escudier, B.; Pal, S.; Kollmannsberger, C.; Pikiel, J.; Gurney, H.; Rha, S.Y.; Park, S.H.; Geertsen, P.F.; et al. Outcomes based on prior therapy in the phase 3 METEOR trial of cabozantinib versus everolimus in advanced renal cell carcinoma. *Br. J. Cancer* **2018**, *119*, 663–669. [CrossRef] [PubMed]
16. Bukowski, R.M.; Kabbinavar, F.F.; Figlin, R.A.; Flaherty, K.; Srinivas, S.; Vaishampayan, U.; Drabkin, H.A.; Dutcher, J.; Ryba, S.; Xia, Q.; et al. Randomized phase II study of erlotinib combined with bevacizumab compared with bevacizumab alone in metastatic renal cell cancer. *J. Clin. Oncol.* **2007**, *25*, 4536–4541. [CrossRef]
17. Motzer, R.J.; Hutson, T.E.; Glen, H.; Michaelson, M.D.; Molina, A.; Eisen, T.; Jassem, J.; Zolnierek, J.; Maroto, J.P.; Mellado, B.; et al. Lenvatinib, everolimus, and the combination in patients with metastatic renal cell carcinoma: A randomised, phase 2, open-label, multicentre trial. *Lancet Oncol.* **2015**, *16*, 1473–1482. [CrossRef]
18. Sternberg, C.N.; Davis, I.D.; Mardiak, J.; Szczylik, C.; Lee, E.; Wagstaff, J.; Barrios, C.H.; Salman, P.; Gladkov, O.A.; Kavina, A.; et al. Pazopanib in locally advanced or metastatic renal cell carcinoma: Results of a randomized phase III trial. *J. Clin. Oncol.* **2010**, *28*, 1061–1068. [CrossRef]
19. Escudier, B.; Eisen, T.; Stadler, W.M.; Szczylik, C.; Oudard, S.; Siebels, M.; Negrier, S.; Chevreau, C.; Solska, E.; Desai, A.A.; et al. Sorafenib in advanced clear-cell renal-cell carcinoma. *N. Engl. J. Med.* **2007**, *356*, 125–134. [CrossRef]
20. Motzer, R.J.; Hutson, T.E.; Tomczak, P.; Michaelson, M.D.; Bukowski, R.M.; Rixe, O.; Oudard, S.; Negrier, S.; Szczylik, C.; Kim, S.T.; et al. Sunitinib versus interferon alfa in metastatic renal-cell carcinoma. *N. Engl. J. Med.* **2007**, *356*, 115–124. [CrossRef]
21. Motzer, R.J.; Escudier, B.; Oudard, S.; Hutson, T.E.; Porta, C.; Bracarda, S.; Grünwald, V.; Thompson, J.A.; Figlin, R.A.; Hollaender, N.; et al. Efficacy of everolimus in advanced renal cell carcinoma: A double-blind, randomised, placebo-controlled phase III trial. *Lancet* **2008**, *372*, 449–456. [CrossRef]
22. Hudes, G.; O'Toole, T.; Tomczak, P.; Bodrogi, I.; Sosman, J.; Kapoor, A.; Staroslawska, E.; Kovacevic, Z.; McDermott, D.; Dutcher, J.; et al. Temsirolimus, Interferon Alfa, or Both for Advanced Renal-Cell Carcinoma. *N. Engl. J. Med.* **2007**, *356*, 2271–2281. [CrossRef]
23. Motzer, R.J.; Penkov, K.; Haanen, J.; Rini, B.; Albiges, L.; Campbell, M.T.; Venugopal, B.; Kollmannsberger, C.; Negrier, S.; Uemura, M.; et al. Avelumab plus axitinib versus sunitinib for advanced renal-cell carcinoma. *N. Engl. J. Med.* **2019**, *380*, 1103–1115. [CrossRef] [PubMed]
24. Escudier, B.; Bellmunt, J.; Négrier, S.; Bajetta, E.; Melichar, B.; Bracarda, S.; Ravaud, A.; Golding, S.; Jethwa, S.; Sneller, V. Bevacizumab plus interferon alfa-2a for treatment of metastatic renal cell carcinoma: A randomised, double-blind phase III trial. *Lancet* **2007**, *370*, 2103–2111. [CrossRef]
25. Motzer, R.J.; Tannir, N.M.; McDermott, D.F.; Arén Frontera, O.; Melichar, B.; Choueiri, T.K.; Plimack, E.R.; Barthélémy, P.; Porta, C.; George, S.; et al. Nivolumab plus Ipilimumab versus Sunitinib in advanced renal-cell carcinoma. *N. Engl. J. Med.* **2018**, *378*, 1277–1290. [CrossRef] [PubMed]
26. Motzer, R.J.; Escudier, B.; McDermott, D.F.; George, S.; Hammers, H.J.; Srinivas, S.; Tykodi, S.S.; Sosman, J.A.; Procopio, G.; Plimack, E.R.; et al. Nivolumab versus everolimus in advanced renal-cell carcinoma. *N. Engl. J. Med.* **2015**, *373*, 1803–1813. [CrossRef] [PubMed]
27. Rini, B.I.; Plimack, E.R.; Stus, V.; Gafanov, R.; Hawkins, R.; Nosov, D.; Pouliot, F.; Alekseev, B.; Soulières, D.; Melichar, B.; et al. Pembrolizumab plus axitinib versus sunitinib for advanced renal-cell carcinoma. *N. Engl. J. Med.* **2019**, *380*, 1116–1127. [CrossRef]

28. Minasian, L.M.; Motzer, R.J.; Gluck, L.; Mazumdar, M.; Vlamis, V.; Krown, S.E. Interferon alfa-2a in advanced renal cell carcinoma: Treatment results and survival in 159 patients with long-term follow-up. *J. Clin. Oncol.* **1993**, *11*, 1368–1375. [CrossRef]
29. Fyfe, G.; Fisher, R.I.; Rosenberg, S.A.; Sznol, M.; Parkinson, D.R.; Louie, A.C. Results of treatment of 255 patients with metastatic renal cell carcinoma who received high-dose recombinant interleukin-2 therapy. *J. Clin. Oncol.* **1995**, *13*, 688–696. [CrossRef]
30. Kim, J.; Kundu, M.; Viollet, B.; Guan, K.L. AMPK and mTOR regulate autophagy through direct phosphorylation of Ulk1. *Nat. Cell Biol.* **2011**, *13*, 132–141. [CrossRef]
31. Satoo, K.; Noda, N.N.; Kumeta, H.; Fujioka, Y.; Mizushima, N.; Ohsumi, Y.; Inagaki, F. The structure of Atg4B-LC3 complex reveals the mechanism of LC3 processing and delipidation during autophagy. *EMBO J.* **2009**, *28*, 1341–1350. [CrossRef]
32. Pankiv, S.; Clausen, T.H.; Lamark, T.; Brech, A.; Bruun, J.A.; Outzen, H.; Øvervatn, A.; Bjørkøy, G.; Johansen, T. p62/SQSTM1 binds directly to Atg8/LC3 to facilitate degradation of ubiquitinated protein aggregates by autophagy*[S]. *J. Biol. Chem.* **2007**, *282*, 24131–24145. [CrossRef]
33. He, C.; Klionsky, D.J. Regulation Mechanisms and Signaling Pathways of Autophagy. *Ann. Rev. Genet.* **2009**, *43*, 67–93. [CrossRef] [PubMed]
34. Barth, S.; Glick, D.; Macleod, K.F. Autophagy: Assays and artifacts. *J. Pathol.* **2010**, *221*, 117–124. [CrossRef] [PubMed]
35. Meijer, A.J.; Codogno, P. Regulation and role of autophagy in mammalian cells. *Int. J. Biochem. Cell Biol.* **2004**, *36*, 2445–2462. [CrossRef]
36. Rubinsztein, D.C.; Codogno, P.; Levine, B. Autophagy modulation as a potential therapeutic target for diverse diseases. *Nat. Rev. Drug Discov.* **2012**, *11*, 709–730. [CrossRef] [PubMed]
37. Yang, Z.; Klionsky, D.J. Mammalian autophagy: Core molecular machinery and signaling regulation. *Curr. Opin. Cell Biol.* **2010**, *22*, 124–131. [CrossRef]
38. White, E. Deconvoluting the context-dependent role for autophagy in cancer. *Nat. Rev. Cancer* **2012**, *12*, 401. [CrossRef]
39. Janku, F.; McConkey, D.J.; Hong, D.S.; Kurzrock, R. Autophagy as a target for anticancer therapy. *Nat. Rev. Clin. Oncol.* **2011**, *8*, 528–539. [CrossRef]
40. Amaravadi, R.K.; Lippincott-Schwartz, J.; Yin, X.M.; Weiss, W.A.; Takebe, N.; Timmer, W.; DiPaola, R.S.; Lotze, M.T.; White, E. Principles and current strategies for targeting autophagy for cancer treatment. *Clin. Cancer Res.* **2011**, *17*, 654–666. [CrossRef]
41. Carew, J.S.; Kelly, K.R.; Nawrocki, S.T. Autophagy as a target for cancer therapy: New developments. *Cancer Manag. Res.* **2012**, *4*, 357–365. [CrossRef]
42. Carew, J.S.; Nawrocki, S.T.; Cleveland, J.L. Modulating autophagy for therapeutic benefit. *Autophagy* **2007**, *3*, 464–467. [CrossRef]
43. Chen, S.; Zhou, L.; Zhang, Y.; Leng, Y.; Pei, X.Y.; Lin, H.; Jones, R.; Orlowski, R.Z.; Dai, Y.; Grant, S. Targeting SQSTM1/p62 induces cargo loading failure and converts autophagy to apoptosis via NBK/Bik. *Mol. Cell Biol.* **2014**, *34*, 3435–3449. [CrossRef]
44. Bouhamdani, N.; Comeau, D.; Cormier, K.; Turcotte, S. STF-62247 accumulates in lysosomes and blocks late stages of autophagy to selectively target von Hippel-Lindau-inactivated cells. *Am. J. Physiol. Cell Physiol.* **2019**, *316*, C605–C620. [CrossRef]
45. Turcotte, S.; Chan, D.A.; Sutphin, P.D.; Hay, M.P.; Denny, W.A.; Giaccia, A.J. A Molecule Targeting VHL-Deficient Renal Cell Carcinoma that Induces Autophagy. *Cancer Cell* **2008**, *14*, 90–102. [CrossRef]
46. Bray, K.; Mathew, R.; Lau, A.; Kamphorst, J.J.; Fan, J.; Chen, J.; Chen, H.Y.; Ghavami, A.; Stein, M.; DiPaola, R.S.; et al. Autophagy suppresses RIP kinase-dependent necrosis enabling survival to mTOR inhibition. *PLoS ONE* **2012**, *7*. [CrossRef]
47. Lum, J.J.; Bauer, D.E.; Kong, M.; Harris, M.H.; Li, C.; Lindsten, T.; Thompson, C.B. Growth factor regulation of autophagy and cell survival in the absence of apoptosis. *Cell* **2005**, *120*, 237–248. [CrossRef]
48. Zheng, B.; Zhu, H.; Gu, D.; Pan, X.; Qian, L.; Xue, B.; Yang, D.; Zhou, J.; Shan, Y. MiRNA-30a-mediated autophagy inhibition sensitizes renal cell carcinoma cells to sorafenib. *Biochem. Biophys. Res. Comun.* **2015**, *459*, 234–239. [CrossRef]

49. Li, H.; Jin, X.; Zhang, Z.; Xing, Y.; Kong, X. Inhibition of autophagy enhances apoptosis induced by the PI3K/AKT/mTor inhibitor NVP-BEZ235 in renal cell carcinoma cells. *Cell Biochem. Funct.* **2013**, *31*, 427–433. [CrossRef]
50. Singla, M.; Bhattacharyya, S. Autophagy as a potential therapeutic target during epithelial to mesenchymal transition in renal cell carcinoma: An in vitro study. *Biomed. Pharmacother.* **2017**, *94*, 332–340. [CrossRef]
51. Homewood, C.A.; Warhurst, D.C.; Peters, W.; Baggaley, V.C. Lysosomes, pH and the anti-malarial action of chloroquine. *Nature* **1972**, *235*, 50–52. [CrossRef]
52. Amaravadi, R.K.; Yu, D.; Lum, J.J.; Bui, T.; Christophorou, M.A.; Evan, G.I.; Thomas-Tikhonenko, A.; Thompson, C.B. Autophagy inhibition enhances therapy-induced apoptosis in a Myc-induced model of lymphoma. *J. Clin. Investig.* **2007**, *117*, 326–336. [CrossRef]
53. Haas, N.B.; Appleman, L.J.; Stein, M.; Redlinger, M.; Wilks, M.; Xu, X.; Onorati, A.; Kalavacharla, A.; Kim, T.; Zhen, C.J.; et al. Autophagy inhibition to augment mTOR inhibition: A phase I/II trial of everolimus and hydroxychloroquine in patients with previously treated renal cell carcinoma. *Clin. Cancer Res.* **2019**, *25*, 2080–2087. [CrossRef] [PubMed]
54. Mahalingam, D.; Mita, M.; Sarantopoulos, J.; Wood, L.; Amaravadi, R.K.; Davis, L.E.; Mita, A.C.; Curiel, T.J.; Espitia, C.M.; Nawrocki, S.T.; et al. Combined autophagy and HDAC inhibition: A phase I safety, tolerability, pharmacokinetic, and pharmacodynamic analysis of hydroxychloroquine in combination with the HDAC inhibitor vorinostat in patients with advanced solid tumors. *Autophagy* **2014**, *10*, 1403–1414. [CrossRef] [PubMed]
55. Mehnert, J.M.; Kaveney, A.D.; Malhotra, J.; Spencer, K.; Portal, D.; Goodin, S.; Tan, A.R.; Aisner, J.; Moss, R.A.; Lin, H.; et al. A phase I trial of MK-2206 and hydroxychloroquine in patients with advanced solid tumors. *Cancer Chemother. Pharmacol.* **2019**. [CrossRef]
56. Carew, J.S.; Espitia, C.M.; Esquivel, J.A., 2nd; Mahalingam, D.; Kelly, K.R.; Reddy, G.; Giles, F.J.; Nawrocki, S.T. Lucanthone is a novel inhibitor of autophagy that induces cathepsin D-mediated apoptosis. *J. Biol. Chem.* **2011**, *286*, 6602–6613. [CrossRef]
57. Carew, J.S.; Nawrocki, S.T. Drain the lysosome: Development of the novel orally available autophagy inhibitor ROC-325. *Autophagy* **2017**, *13*, 765–766. [CrossRef]
58. Carew, J.S.; Espitia, C.M.; Zhao, W.; Han, Y.; Visconte, V.; Phillips, J.; Nawrocki, S.T. Disruption of autophagic degradation with ROC-325 antagonizes renal cell carcinoma pathogenesis. *Clin. Cancer Res.* **2017**, *23*, 2869–2879. [CrossRef]
59. Jones, T.M.; Espitia, C.; Wang, W.; Nawrocki, S.T.; Carew, J.S. Moving beyond hydroxychloroquine: The novel lysosomal autophagy inhibitor ROC-325 shows significant potential in preclinical studies. *Cancer Commun.* **2019**, *39*, 72. [CrossRef]
60. Nawrocki, S.T.; Han, Y.; Visconte, V.; Przychodzen, B.; Espitia, C.M.; Phillips, J.; Anwer, F.; Advani, A.; Carraway, H.E.; Kelly, K.R.; et al. The novel autophagy inhibitor ROC-325 augments the antileukemic activity of azacitidine. *Leukemia* **2019**, *33*, 2971–2974. [CrossRef]
61. Zielke, S.; Meyer, N.; Mari, M.; Abou-El-Ardat, K.; Reggiori, F.; van Wijk, S.J.L.; Kögel, D.; Fulda, S. Loperamide, pimozide, and STF-62247 trigger autophagy-dependent cell death in glioblastoma cells. *Cell Death Dis.* **2018**, *9*, 1–16. [CrossRef]
62. Anbalagan, S.; Pires, I.M.; Blick, C.; Hill, M.A.; Ferguson, D.J.P.; Chan, D.A.; Hammond, E.M. Radiosensitization of renal cell carcinoma in vitro through the induction of autophagy. *Radiother. Oncol.* **2012**, *103*, 388–393. [CrossRef]
63. Kozako, T.; Sato, K.; Uchida, Y.; Kato, N.; Aikawa, A.; Ogata, K.; Kamimura, H.; Uemura, H.; Yoshimitsu, M.; Ishitsuka, K.; et al. The small molecule STF-62247 induces apoptotic and autophagic cell death in leukemic cells. *Oncotarget* **2018**, *9*, 27645–27655. [CrossRef]
64. Amaravadi, R.K.; Winkler, J.D. Lys05: A new lysosomal autophagy inhibitor. *Autophagy* **2012**, *8*, 1383–1384. [CrossRef]
65. McAfee, Q.; Zhang, Z.; Samanta, A.; Levi, S.M.; Ma, X.H.; Piao, S.; Lynch, J.P.; Uehara, T.; Sepulveda, A.R.; Davis, L.E.; et al. Autophagy inhibitor Lys05 has single-agent antitumor activity and reproduces the phenotype of a genetic autophagy deficiency. *Proc. Natl. Acad. Sci. USA* **2012**, *109*, 8253–8258. [CrossRef]
66. Rebecca, V.W.; Nicastri, M.C.; McLaughlin, N.; Fennelly, C.; McAfee, Q.; Ronghe, A.; Nofal, M.; Lim, C.Y.; Witze, E.; Chude, C.I.; et al. A Unified Approach to Targeting the Lysosome's Degradative and Growth Signaling Roles. *Cancer Discov.* **2017**, *7*, 1266–1283. [CrossRef]

67. Rebecca, V.W.; Nicastri, M.C.; Fennelly, C.; Chude, C.I.; Barber-Rotenberg, J.S.; Ronghe, A.; McAfee, Q.; McLaughlin, N.P.; Zhang, G.; Goldman, A.R.; et al. PPT1 Promotes Tumor Growth and Is the Molecular Target of Chloroquine Derivatives in Cancer. *Cancer Discov.* **2019**, *9*, 220–229. [CrossRef]
68. Pasquier, B. SAR405, a PIK3C3/VPS34 inhibitor that prevents autophagy and synergizes with MTOR inhibition in tumor cells. *Autophagy* **2015**, *11*, 725–726. [CrossRef]
69. Ronan, B.; Flamand, O.; Vescovi, L.; Dureuil, C.; Durand, L.; Fassy, F.; Bachelot, M.F.; Lamberton, A.; Mathieu, M.; Bertrand, T.; et al. A highly potent and selective Vps34 inhibitor alters vesicle trafficking and autophagy. *Nat. Chem. Biol.* **2014**, *10*, 1013–1019. [CrossRef]
70. Dyczynski, M.; Yu, Y.; Otrocka, M.; Parpal, S.; Braga, T.; Henley, A.B.; Zazzi, H.; Lerner, M.; Wennerberg, K.; Viklund, J.; et al. Targeting autophagy by small molecule inhibitors of vacuolar protein sorting 34 (Vps34) improves the sensitivity of breast cancer cells to Sunitinib. *Cancer Lett.* **2018**, *435*, 32–43. [CrossRef]
71. Egan, D.F.; Chun, M.G.H.; Vamos, M.; Zou, H.; Rong, J.; Miller, C.J.; Lou, H.J.; Raveendra-Panickar, D.; Yang, C.C.; Sheffler, D.J.; et al. Small Molecule Inhibition of the Autophagy Kinase ULK1 and Identification of ULK1 Substrates. *Mol. Cell* **2015**, *59*, 285–297. [CrossRef]
72. Martin, K.R.; Celano, S.L.; Solitro, A.R.; Gunaydin, H.; Scott, M.; O'Hagan, R.C.; Shumway, S.D.; Fuller, P.; MacKeigan, J.P. A Potent and Selective ULK1 Inhibitor Suppresses Autophagy and Sensitizes Cancer Cells to Nutrient Stress. *Iscience* **2018**, *8*, 74–84. [CrossRef]
73. Chu, J.; Fu, Y.; Xu, J.; Zheng, X.; Gu, Q.; Luo, X.; Dai, Q.; Zhang, S.; Liu, P.; Hong, L.; et al. ATG4B inhibitor FMK-9a induces autophagy independent on its enzyme inhibition. *Arch. Biochem. Biophys.* **2018**, *644*, 29–36. [CrossRef]
74. Fu, Y.; Hong, L.; Xu, J.; Zhong, G.; Gu, Q.; Gu, Q.; Guan, Y.; Zheng, X.; Dai, Q.; Luo, X.; et al. Discovery of a small molecule targeting autophagy via ATG4B inhibition and cell death of colorectal cancer cells in vitro and in vivo. *Autophagy* **2019**, *15*, 295–311. [CrossRef] [PubMed]
75. Akin, D.; Wang, S.K.; Habibzadegah-Tari, P.; Law, B.; Ostrov, D.; Li, M.; Yin, X.M.; Kim, J.S.; Horenstein, N.; Dunn, W.A., Jr. A novel ATG4B antagonist inhibits autophagy and has a negative impact on osteosarcoma tumors. *Autophagy* **2014**, *10*, 2021–2035. [CrossRef] [PubMed]
76. Huang, T.; Kim, C.K.; Alvarez, A.A.; Pangeni, R.P.; Wan, X.; Song, X.; Shi, T.; Yang, Y.; Sastry, N.; Horbinski, C.M.; et al. MST4 Phosphorylation of ATG4B Regulates Autophagic Activity, Tumorigenicity, and Radioresistance in Glioblastoma. *Cancer Cell* **2017**, *32*, 840–855. [CrossRef] [PubMed]
77. Hodi, F.S.; O'Day, S.J.; McDermott, D.F.; Weber, R.W.; Sosman, J.A.; Haanen, J.B.; Gonzalez, R.; Robert, C.; Schadendorf, D.; Hassel, J.C.; et al. Improved survival with ipilimumab in patients with metastatic melanoma. *N. Engl. J. Med.* **2010**, *363*, 711–723. [CrossRef] [PubMed]
78. Choueiri, T.K.; Larkin, J.; Oya, M.; Thistlethwaite, F.; Martignoni, M.; Nathan, P.; Powles, T.; McDermott, D.; Robbins, P.B.; Chism, D.D.; et al. Preliminary results for avelumab plus axitinib as first-line therapy in patients with advanced clear-cell renal-cell carcinoma (JAVELIN Renal 100): An open-label, dose-finding and dose-expansion, phase 1b trial. *Lancet Oncol.* **2018**, *19*, 451–460. [CrossRef]
79. Mitchell, T.C.; Hamid, O.; Smith, D.C.; Bauer, T.M.; Wasser, J.S.; Olszanski, A.J.; Luke, J.J.; Balmanoukian, A.S.; Schmidt, E.V.; Zhao, Y.; et al. Epacadostat plus pembrolizumab in patients with advanced solid tumors: Phase I results from a multicenter, open-label phase I/II trial (ECHO-202/KEYNOTE-037). *J. Clin. Oncol.* **2018**, *36*, 3223–3230. [CrossRef]
80. Phadwal, K.; Alegre-Abarrategui, J.; Watson, A.S.; Pike, L.; Anbalagan, S.; Hammond, E.M.; Wade-Martins, R.; McMichael, A.; Klenerman, P.; Simon, A.K. A novel method for autophagy detection in primary cells: Impaired levels of macroautophagy in immunosenescent T cells. *Autophagy* **2012**, *8*, 677–689. [CrossRef]
81. Clarke, A.J.; Riffelmacher, T.; Braas, D.; Cornall, R.J.; Simon, A.K. B1a B cells require autophagy for metabolic homeostasis and self-renewal. *J. Exp. Med.* **2018**, *215*, 399–413. [CrossRef]
82. Xu, X.; Araki, K.; Li, S.; Han, J.H.; Ye, L.; Tan, W.G.; Konieczny, B.T.; Bruinsma, M.W.; Martinez, J.; Pearce, E.L.; et al. Autophagy is essential for effector CD8(+) T cell survival and memory formation. *Nat. Immunol.* **2014**, *15*, 1152–1161. [CrossRef]
83. Starobinets, H.; Ye, J.; Broz, M.; Barry, K.; Goldsmith, J.; Marsh, T.; Rostker, F.; Krummel, M.; Debnath, J. Antitumor adaptive immunity remains intact following inhibition of autophagy and antimalarial treatment. *J. Clin. Investig.* **2016**, *126*, 4417–4429. [CrossRef]

84. Baginska, J.; Viry, E.; Berchem, G.; Poli, A.; Noman, M.Z.; van Moer, K.; Medves, S.; Zimmer, J.; Oudin, A.; Niclou, S.P.; et al. Granzyme B degradation by autophagy decreases tumor cell susceptibility to natural killer-mediated lysis under hypoxia. *Proc. Natl. Acad. Sci. USA* **2013**, *110*, 17450–17455. [CrossRef] [PubMed]
85. Noman, M.Z.; Janji, B.; Kaminska, B.; Van Moer, K.; Pierson, S.; Przanowski, P.; Buart, S.; Berchem, G.; Romero, P.; Mami-Chouaib, F.; et al. Blocking hypoxia-induced autophagy in tumors restores cytotoxic T-cell activity and promotes regression. *Cancer Res.* **2011**, *71*, 5976–5986. [CrossRef] [PubMed]
86. Khazen, R.; Muller, S.; Gaudenzio, N.; Espinosa, E.; Puissegur, M.P.; Valitutti, S. Melanoma cell lysosome secretory burst neutralizes the CTL-mediated cytotoxicity at the lytic synapse. *Nat. Commun.* **2016**, *7*, 10823. [CrossRef] [PubMed]
87. Chen, D.; Xie, J.; Fiskesund, R.; Dong, W.; Liang, X.; Lv, J.; Jin, X.; Liu, J.; Mo, S.; Zhang, T.; et al. Chloroquine modulates antitumor immune response by resetting tumor-associated macrophages toward M1 phenotype. *Nat. Commun.* **2018**, *9*, 1–15. [CrossRef]
88. Liu, J.; Liu, X.; Han, Y.; Zhang, J.; Liu, D.; Ma, G.; Li, C.; Liu, L.; Kong, D. Nanovaccine Incorporated with Hydroxychloroquine Enhances Antigen Cross-Presentation and Promotes Antitumor Immune Responses. *ACS Appl. Mater. Interfaces* **2018**, *10*, 30983–30993. [CrossRef]

13

The Value of PD-L1 Expression as Predictive Biomarker in Metastatic Renal Cell Carcinoma Patients

Alberto Carretero-González [1], David Lora [2], Isabel Martín Sobrino [3], Irene Sáez Sanz [3], María T. Bourlon [4], Urbano Anido Herranz [5], Nieves Martínez Chanzá [6], Daniel Castellano [1] and Guillermo de Velasco [1,*]

1 Medical Oncology Department, University Hospital 12 de Octubre, 28041 Madrid, Spain; carretero_88@hotmail.com (A.C.-G.); cdanicas@hotmail.com (D.C.)
2 Clinical Research Unit, IMAS12-CIBERESP, University Hospital 12 de Octubre, 28041 Madrid, Spain; david@h12o.es
3 School of Medicine, Universidad Complutense de Madrid, University Hospital 12 de Octubre, 28040 Madrid, Spain; isabelms95@hotmail.com (I.M.S.); irenesaezsanz@gmail.com (I.S.S.)
4 Hemato-Oncology Department, Instituto Nacional de Ciencias Médicas y Nutrición Salvador Zubirán, 14080 Mexico City, Mexico; maitebourlon@gmail.com
5 Medical Oncology Department, University Clinical Hospital of Santiago de Compostela, 15076 Santiago de Compostela, Spain; urbanoanido@gmail.com
6 Medical Oncology Department, Jules Bordet Institute, Université Libre de Bruxelles, 1000 Brussels, Belgium; n.martinezchanza@gmail.com
* Correspondence: gdvelasco.gdv@gmail.com

Abstract: Immune checkpoint inhibitors (ICIs) are soluble antibodies that have dramatically changed the outcomes including overall survival in a subset of kidney tumors, specifically in renal cell carcinoma (RCC). To date, there is no a single predictive biomarker approved to be used to select the patients that achieve benefit from ICIs targeting. It seems reasonable to analyze whether the programmed death-ligand 1 (PD-L1) expression could be useful. To assess the role of PD-L1 expression as a potential predictive biomarker for benefit of ICIs in RCC patients, we performed a search of randomized clinical trials (RCTs) comparing ICIs (monotherapy or in combination with other therapies) to standard of care in metastatic RCC patients according to PRISMA guidelines. Trials must have included subgroup analyses evaluating the selected outcomes (progression-free survival (PFS) and overall survival (OS)) in different subsets of patients according to PD-L1 expression on tumor samples. Hazard ratios with confidence intervals were used as the measure of efficacy between groups. A total of 4635 patients (six studies) were included (ICIs arm: 2367 patients; standard of care arm: 2268 patients). Globally, PFS and OS results favored ICIs. Differential expression of PD-L1 on tumor samples could select a subset of patients who could benefit more in terms of PFS (those with higher levels; *p*-value for difference between subgroups: <0.0001) but it did not seem to impact in OS results (*p*-value for difference: 0.63). As different methods to assess PD-L1 positivity were used among trials, this heterogeneity could have an influence on the results. PD-L1 could represent a biomarker to test PFS in clinical trials but its value for OS is less clear. In this meta-analysis, the usefulness of PD-L1 expression as a predictive biomarker to select treatment in metastatic RCC patients was not clearly shown.

Keywords: renal cell carcinoma; PD-L1; predictive; biomarker; treatment

1. Introduction

Kidney cancer represents about 5% and 3% of all solid tumors in adults in men and women, respectively [1]. Renal cell carcinomas (RCC), considering only parenchymal tumors and excluding urothelial tumors, involve 80% of all renal malignancies. Metastatic disease is found in 20% of patients at diagnosis. In addition, 25% of those with localized disease will relapse after radical treatment. The expected 5-year overall survival (OS) rate for advanced disease is estimated to be around 20% [2].

Antiangiogenic drugs and immunotherapy shape the landscape of treatment for metastatic RCC. Recently, immune checkpoint inhibitors (ICIs) have transformed the management of metastatic clear-cell RCC (ccRCC) [3–8]. Specially, monoclonal antibodies directed against programmed cell death 1 (PD-1) or programmed death-ligand 1 (PD-L1) combined with either cytotoxic T-lymphocyte associated protein 4 (CTLA-4) or with tyrosine kinase inhibitors (TKIs) have shown significant survival improvement in the first-line setting [4–8].

Despite the numerous efforts to identify predictive markers, none were robust enough to be implemented in clinical practice for RCC patients. The International Metastatic Renal Cell Carcinoma Database Consortium (IMDC) [9] is one of the most validated scores to characterize the prognosis of metastatic RCC patients [10].

The IMDC criteria have been recognized as an aid to select the most appropriate treatment for patients, specifically in the case of nivolumab (anti-PD-1) and ipilimumab (anti-CTLA-4) combination in the first-line setting [4]. Recently, the score has been included in the guidelines as a treatment selection strategy [11,12]. Nevertheless, it remains unknown which patient subgroups will benefit the most within the IMDC categories with the different combinations.

2. PD-L1 Expression: Immunohistochemistry Antibody and Cutoff

PD-L1 expression on tumor tissue has been determined to be present in 25–60% of the patients depending upon the employed assay. Largely, PD-L1 expression has been identified as a negative prognostic factor in metastatic RCC [3]. In addition, high PD-L1 levels are associated with unfavorable outcomes of TKI therapy [13].

First data on expression of PD-L1 in RCC come from early trials. The first anti-PD-1 drugs tested were MDX-1106 (ClinicalTrials.gov Identifier: NCT00441337) in a phase 1 trial that included five metastatic RCC patients and nivolumab, in a phase 1 trial that included 34 metastatic RCC patients. PD-L1 expression was studied on the surface of tumor cells. None of the patients with PD-L1–negative tumors had an objective response [14,15]. In this study PD-L1 expression was studied by the murine antihuman PD-L1 monoclonal antibody 5H1. Tumors were considered PD-L1-positive if ≥5% of tumor cells showed membranous staining with 5H1.

Studies with atezolizumab (anti-PD-L1) have used an anti-human PD-L1 monoclonal antibody (Clone SP142) but instead of analyzing tumor cell, immune cell (IC) were studied (all types of ICs, including macrophages, dendritic cells, and lymphocytes, were counted together). The number of patients IC0 (low to no PD-L1 expression) was about 75% if the cutoff is >5% and around 50% if the cutoff is >1% [8,16].

Most recent trials have used alternative antibodies and different locations within the tumor sample in order to improve the accuracy of the technique. Two main strategies assessing PD-L1 expression include those focusing only on tumor cell expression (e.g., Tumor Proportion Score (TPS)), and those incorporating also immune cells (e.g., Combined Positive Score (CPS)). A rabbit anti-human PD-L1 antibody (clone 28-8) has been used in several studies testing the anti-PD-1 drug nivolumab. Distinctive limits for PD-L1 positivity were also investigated containing cutoffs of 1% and more or equal than 5% [17,18].

3. PD-L1 Antibodies: Pharmacokinetics and Pharmacodynamics

After the intravenous administration of anti-PD-1/PD-L1 antibodies, the highest concentration is reached between 1 and 4 h. The pharmacokinetics of these soluble antibodies has been described as linear. The increase of concentration during the peak is dose-proportional [14,15].

Early studies showed that the levels of anti-PD-L1 antibodies in the blood are amplified as well in a dose-dependent manner. The half-life of anti-PD-L1 antibody has been calculated over 2 weeks. Importantly, median PD-L1 receptor use on $CD3^+$ peripheral-blood mononuclear cells after anti-PD-1 therapy has been shown to exceed 65%.

4. Data on PD-L1 Expression and Anti-PD-1/PD-L1 Treatment

The predictive value of PD-L1 expression as a biomarker in metastatic RCC patients treated with anti-PD-1/PD-L1 therapy remains indeterminate [3–8]. Selected studies have shown that either tumor cell or tumor-infiltrating immune cell PD-L1 overexpression is associated with deeper response rates with ICIs across different solid tumors, not only metastatic RCC [19]. Indeed, PD-L1 expression has already been used for treatment selection in solid tumors such as lung cancer [20,21]. Nevertheless, tumors that do not express PD-L1 may benefit from ICI. One theory is that the expression of PD-L2 modifies the response; current available tests do not assess this protein [22].

Trials have explored different efficacy parameters according to PD-L1-expression status at a 5% cutoff. In a randomized trial with nivolumab, the group of patients (27%) with tumors PD-L1 expression ≥5% had a median progression-free survival (PFS) of 4.9 months versus 2.9 months in the PD-L1 < 5% subgroup; overall response rate (ORR) was 31% in the PD-L1 ≥ 5% subgroup and 18% in the PD-L1 < 5% subgroup; median OS was not reached in the PD-L1 ≥ 5% subgroup and 18.2 months in the PD-L1 < 5% subgroup. The authors did not find differences with the cutoff ≥1% for PD-L1 expression [17].

In a phase 1 trial testing atezolizumab, there was no correlation between tumor cell score of PD-L1 and outcomes. However, the subgroup of patients with low-to-no PD-L1 expression (IC0) tended to have worse survival [16]. In the phase 3 JAVELIN Renal 101 trial, the combination of avelumab plus axitinib showed an improvement on median PFS in those patients with at least 1% of immune cells staining positive within the tested tumor area (primary endpoint) [6]. On the other side, in the phase 3 KEYNOTE-426 trial, treatment with pembrolizumab plus axitinib resulted in longer OS and PFS compared to sunitinib and regardless of PD-L1 expression measured by CPS (tumor and immune cells); however there was a trend of a greater benefit in patients with higher PD-L1 expression [5].

5. PD-L1 Expression and Duration of Response

There is lack of data showing whether the duration of response is associated with PD-L1 expression [16]. PD-L1 expression is associated with high expression of the T-effector (Teff) gene signature and $CD8^+$ T cell infiltration. The predictive relevance of PD-L1 expression on IC is further supported by the strong correlation of PD-L1 IC as determined by immunohistochemistry with the Teff immune gene signature.

6. PD-L1 Expression: Differences in Primary Tumor Versus Metastases

PD-L1 expression has been associated with poor pathologic features and high nuclear grade areas. Discrepancies in tumor cell PD-L1 expression by immunohistochemistry between primary tumors and metastases counterparts have been described in around 20% of metastatic RCC patients. Based on published data, the PD-L1 expression in the primary tumor seems more common than in the metastases. Largely, PD-L1 expression in multiple metastases from the same primary tumor is consistent [23]. These fluctuations could be predisposed by the particular tumor microenvironment and hypoxia status in each individual tumor location [24,25].

7. PD-L1 Expression: Differences Localized Versus Metastatic Tumors

In RCC, increased PD-L1 expression has been found to be considerably associated with large tumor size and TNM stage [26]. In a series of 194 nephrectomies from the Mayo Clinic, 33% of RCC patients were PD-L1 negative [27]. Slightly higher data are presented in a recent pivotal trial ranging from 25% to 40% of PD-L1 negative patients.

8. PD-L1 Expression: Evolution with Treatment

In a phase 2 trial with nivolumab, PD-L1 expression on tumor cells was assessed by immunohistochemistry in fresh biopsies obtained at baseline and at the second cycle. There was no consistent change in tumor PD-L1 expression following nivolumab treatment relative to baseline [18]. While baseline PD-L1 expression by immunohistochemistry did not correlate with response to atezolizumab in combination with bevacizumab, upregulation of PD-L1 was only detected in one patient, who demonstrated a partial response on a phase 1 trial [28].

9. Gene Expression Profiles

Different studies have shown that tumors with an angiogenic signature present an enhanced response to tyrosine kinase inhibitors such as sunitinib, whereas tumors with a Teff gene signature had better correlation with higher PD-L1 expression, $CD8^+$ T cell infiltration, and better response to anti-PD-L1 treatment. Interestingly, a subanalysis of a randomized clinical trial showed that a myeloid inflammatory signature (a subgroup with Teff gene signature) benefited from receiving the combination treatment with an anti-Vascular Endothelial Growth Factor (VEGF) antibody (bevacizumab) and an anti-PD-L1 antibody (atezolizumab) while presenting a poor response to atezolizumab in monotherapy [8].

In the Javelin 101 trial, an association between a signature with 26 gene (including several genes implicated in T cell signaling, proliferation, chemokine expression, and other immune response genes) and improved PFS was observed with the combination of axitinib (TKI) and avelumab (anti-PD-L1). However, this association was not observed with sunitinib monotherapy [6].

10. Other Potential Biomarkers

Tumor mutational or tumor neoantigen burden have arisen as promising biomarkers for response to ICIs. The evidence seems to be solid in lung cancer although the biomarker is not flawless [29]. RCC has been shown to express a high frequency of clonal indel mutations, potentially related to neoantigen abundance and $CD8^+$ T cell activation [30]; however the association between these features and response to ICIs in RCC has yet to be confirmed [8].

Although further studies are necessary to confirm the findings, loss-of-function mutations in specific genes such as *PBRM1* might predict clinical response to anti-PD-1 antibodies in metastatic RCC according to whole-exome sequencing studies in patients treated with nivolumab [31,32].

$CD8^+$ T cell infiltration has been shown to be an adverse prognostic factor for RCC [33]. Contrary, increased amounts of tumor $CD8^+$ T cells have been associated with an improved PFS in those patients treated with axitinib plus avelumab but not in patients treated with sunitnib [6]. $CD8^+$ infiltration has been shown to be associated with PD-L1 expression. Further data are needed to determine the value of $CD8^+$ T cell density and its relationship with PD-L1 as a biomarker for ICI in RCC.

From a different angle, the microbiome (the genetic material within the microbiota) and its variations could be associated with the benefit of ICIs. The microbiome influences the processes of antitumor immunity, and the variations of some bacterial species have been associated with an increased likelihood of response [34,35]. In fact, studies in RCC have shown that antibiotic use could decrease the response to ICI in RCC [36]. Whether the microbiome may alter PD-L1 expression has not been really studied. Further studies focusing on microbiome manipulation in RCC are ongoing [37].

Finally, liquid biopsy is another promising source of information currently under investigation in RCC. Soluble immune checkpoint-related proteins (including PD-1, PD-L1, and CTLA-4 among others) have been shown to be associated with advanced disease, recurrence, and survival in a study with RCC patients, highlighting the potential prognostic value of these biomarkers [38]. In lung cancer, the molecular characterization of PD-L1 expression in circulating tumor cells (CTC) might be supportive to identify a subgroup of patients that will most likely benefit from ICI therapies [39].

11. PD-L1 by Immunohistochemistry as a Biomarker in RCC

Currently, the most valuable biomarker due to availability and worldwide access is the determination of PD-L1 by immunohistochemistry. Due to the current uncertain value for metastatic RCC, we performed a meta-analysis of published randomized clinical trials (RCTs) in order to analyze the predictive role of PD-L1 expression and its potential usefulness in treatment decisions in metastatic RCC patients.

12. Material and Methods

12.1. Literature Search and Inclusion Criteria

The literature search was accomplished by May 1 2019. Two different databases were reviewed: MEDLINE and EMBASE. Only agents targeting PD-1/PD-L1 approved or extensively studied in RCC were included in the search: (a) anti-PD-1 antibodies: nivolumab (Opdivo®), pembrolizumab (Keytruda®), (b) anti-PD-L1 antibodies: atezolizumab (Tecentric®) and avelumab (Bavencio®). The specific words used during the search were ("nivolumab" OR "pembrolizumab" OR "atezolizumab" OR "avelumab" OR "PD-1" OR "PD-L1") AND ("renal cell carcinoma" OR "RCC" OR "kidney cancer"). Additionally, the manufacturers' package inserts for drugs included in the meta-analysis were also analyzed to spot original or different data not reported in published trials.

All RCTs that compared ICIs based therapy (either in monotherapy or in combination with another ICI or VEGF-targeted therapy) versus the previous standard of care (TKIs or mammalian Target of Rapamycin (mTOR) inhibitors in monotherapy) in any line of treatment in adults (≥18 years-old) with metastatic ccRCC were included. The review was restricted to RCTs in humans and published in English. Non clear-cell RCC studies were excluded. Every publication was reviewed, but only the most complete report of the RCTs was included when duplicate publications were identified. We tried to decrease the heterogeneity among the results gathering only comparisons of ICIs based therapy (defined previously) with TKIs or mTOR inhibitors in monotherapy; other combinations were excluded. We selected the most validated endpoints for efficacy: PFS and OS. Trials that met the following criteria were included in the meta-analysis: randomized phase II or III trials, prospective clinical studies in patients with metastatic ccRCC, and trials with at least one of the previous efficacy endpoints mentioned above available. Two reviewers (A.C-G. and G.d.V.) independently evaluated studies for eligibility.

12.2. Data Extraction and Clinical Endpoints

Two investigators (A.C-G. and G.d.V.) extracted the data individually, discordances were resolved by consensus. Data was reported agreeing to Preferred Reporting Items for Systematic reviews and Meta-Analyses (PRISMA) guidelines [40]. Collected variables included the first author's surname, year of publication, National Clinical Trials (NCT) registry number, study phase, number of previous treatment lines received, selection of population by PD-L1 expression on tumor samples (yes/no), method employed to assess PD-L1 expression, percentage of PD-L1 considered as a positive result, number of enrolled subjects, number of enrolled patients according to PD-L1 expression status, criteria used for assessing efficacy (Response Evaluation Criteria In Solid Tumors (RECIST) or others), blinding (yes/no), treatment arms, number of patients per treatment arm in the total population, and according to PD-L1 expression subgroups, and median age. The efficacy endpoints selected for the analysis (hazard ratios (HR) with confidence intervals (CI) for PFS and OS between treatment arms) were obtained in the total population and according to PD-L1 expression subgroups when available.

12.3. Statistical Analysis

Stata version 16 (https://www.stata.com) was the software used for the main statistical analysis. HRs with CIs were the parameters considered to assess the impact on OS and PFS of treatment based on ICIs as compared to standard of care. I2 statistics were used to assess the study heterogeneity among the included trials; these evaluations estimate the significance of heterogeneity compared to chance in relation to the variation observed across the studies [41]. Random and fixed-effects models were used to pool studies depending on the heterogeneity of the studies included. PD-L1 expression on tumor samples (positive or negative depending on the techniques used in each trial) was the clinical feature employed to perform subgroup analyses. Egger's test, the test for asymmetry of the funnel plot, was performed to reject publication bias [42]. In addition, as other causes of asymmetry could exist, contour-enhanced meta-analysis and trim-and-fill method were used to distinguish publication bias from these other possibilities [43].

13. Results

13.1. Study Selection

Studies that met criteria for the final analysis are shown in the flow chart (Figure 1). A total of 265 studies were reviewed through our screening process for RCTs. We did not include (i) duplicate studies and/or no-clinical trial type studies (n = 250) and (ii) no-only renal cell carcinoma studies and/or early phase I/II or non-RCTs (n = 9). Six RCTs met the standards for inclusion in the meta-analysis.

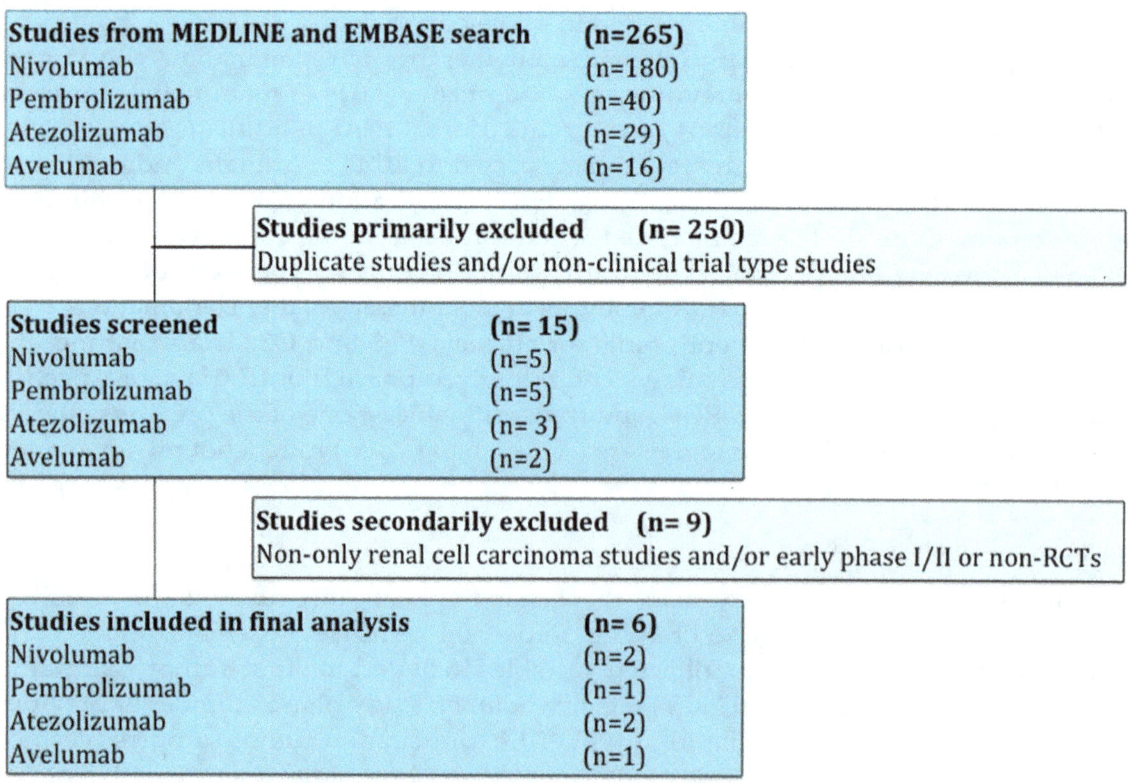

Figure 1. Flow diagram for identification and selection of studies.

The baseline characteristics of each trial are displayed in Table 1. All trials but one [3] were performed in the first-line setting for metastatic RCC (treatment naïve). One trial reported the results only in the intermediate and poor risk-groups according to the IMDC score (https://www.imdconline.com) [4]. All studies had two treatment arms except one, which had three arms [8]. In one study, everolimus (mTOR inhibitor) was the control arm (in the second- and third-line setting) [3]; the remaining studies used sunitinib in monotherapy as the control arm. There were no placebo-controlled trials that met the criteria of the study. None of the studies restricted eligible populations according to PD-L1 expression; different assays and thresholds were used among trials to measure PD-L1 expression by immunochemistry. Only three studies included primary endpoints involving exclusively PD-L1 positive patients [6–8] but the rest of them only performed primary endpoints in the intent-to-treat (ITT) population [3–5]. A total of 4635 patients were available for the meta-analysis: 2367 patients were assigned to the therapy based on ICIs arm (432 to pembrolizumab plus axitinib, 555 to atezolizumab plus bevacizumab, 103 to atezolizumab in monotherapy, 425 to nivolumab plus ipilimumab, 442 to avelumab plus axitinib, and 410 to nivolumab in monotherapy), and 2268 were assigned to the control arm (1857 received sunitinib and 411 received everolimus). PFS was assessed in all trials according to the RECIST v1.1. All RCTs were sponsored by pharmaceutical companies.

Table 1. Summary of randomized clinical trials included in the meta-analysis.

Author/Year	Phase	Number of Patients (N)	Line of Treatment	PD-L1 Assay	Experimental Arm	Control Arm	Primary Endpoint
B.I. Rini/2019 [5]	3	861	1	PD-L1 IHC 22C3 pharmDx assay (combined score: <1; ≥1)	Pembrolizumab + Axitinib (*n* = 432; PD-L1 positive: 243)	Sunitinib (*n* = 429; PD-L1 positive: 254)	OS and PFS in the intent-to-treat population
D.F. McDermott/2018 [8]	2	305	1	PD-L1 on IC by SP142 IHC assay (<1; ≥1)	Atezolizumab (*n* = 103; PD-L1 positive: 54)	Sunitinib (*n* = 101; PD-L1 positive: 60)	PFS in the intent-to-treat and PD-L1 positive populations
					Atezolizumab + Bevacizumab (*n* = 101; PD-L1 positive: 50)	Sunitinib (*n* = 101; PD-L1 positive: 60)	
R.J. Motzer/2018 [4]	3	847	1 (intermediate risk- and poor risk-groups)	Dako PD-L1 IHC 28-8 pharmDx test (<1; ≥1)	Nivolumab + Ipilimumab (*n* = 425; PD-L1 positive: 100)	Sunitinib (*n* = 422; PD-L1 positive: 114)	OS, objective response rate and PFS in the intermediate risk- and poor risk-patients
R.J. Motzer/2019 [6]	3	886	1	Ventana PD-L1 (SP263) assay (<1; ≥1)	Avelumab + Axitinib (*n* = 442; PD-L1 positive: 270)	Sunitinib (*n* = 444; PD-L1 positive: 290)	PFS and OS in the PD-L1 positive population
R.J. Motzer/2015 [3]	3	821	2 and 3	Dako PD-L1 IHC (<1; ≥1)	Nivolumab (*n* = 410; PD-L1 positive: 94)	Everolimus (*n* = 411; PD-L1 positive: 87)	OS in the intent-to-treat population
B.I. Rini/2019 [7]	3	915	1	VENTANA PD-L1 SP142 assay (<1; ≥1)	Atezolizumab + Bevacizumab (*n* = 454; PD-L1 positive: 178)	Sunitinib (*n* = 461; PD-L1 positive: 184)	PFS in the PD-L1 positive population and OS in the intent-to-treat population

13.2. Global PFS and OS Results

Globally, both PFS and OS results favored therapy based on ICIs. The HR for PFS was improved in those patients treated with ICIs compared to standard of care (HR 0.82; 95% CI 0.73–0.92, $p = 0.0006$), as well as the HR for OS (HR 0.73; 95% CI 0.60–0.88, $p = 0.0012$).

Evidence of asymmetry in the studies addressing OS was observed ($p = 0.0192$); by using contour-enhanced meta-analysis funnel plots we can conclude that small studies with negative results have not been published. Evidence of asymmetry in the results of those studies addressing PFS was not verified ($p = 0.110$).

13.3. PFS Results According to PD-L1 Expression

In PD-L1 negative patients (only three studies with available information) receiving therapy based on anti-PD-1/PD-L1 antibodies, PFS was not improved compared to those patients receiving standard of care (HR 0.95; 95% CI 0.82–1.09). The PD-L1 positive patients receiving therapy based on anti-PD-1/PD-L1 antibodies had better PFS compared to those patients receiving standard of care (HR 0.65; 95% CI 0.56–0.76). The difference in terms of PFS between these two groups (PD-L1 negative versus PD-L1 positive populations) was statistically significant ($p < 0.0001$; Figure 2).

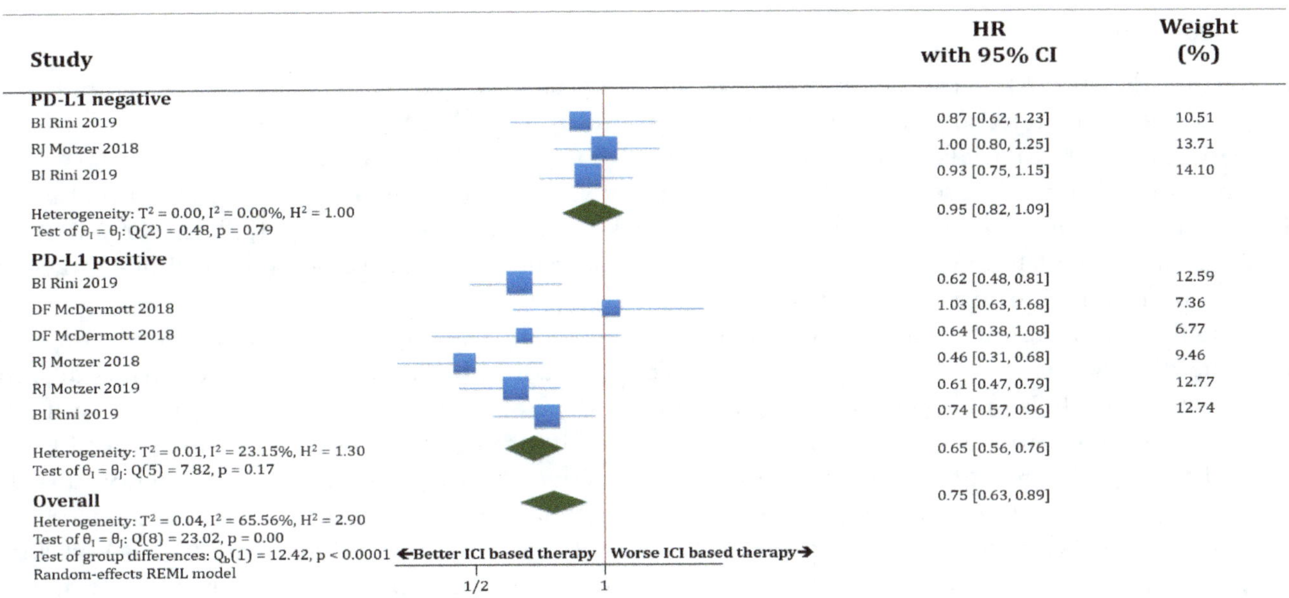

Figure 2. Forest plot diagram: hazard ratio (HR) with 95% confidence interval of progression-free survival (PFS) between arms according to programmed death-ligand 1 (PD-L1) expression subgroups.

13.4. OS Results According to PD-L1 Expression

In terms of OS, both populations, PD-L1 negative (only three trials with available data) and PD-L1 positive patients, benefited from receiving therapy based on anti-PD-1/PD-L1 antibodies compared to standard of care. HR for OS was improved in PD-L1 negative patients treated with ICIs compared to standard of care (HR 0.73; 95% CI 0.62–0.87) as well as in PD-L1 positive patients (HR 0.68; 95% CI 0.54–0.87). There was no statistically significant difference in OS between the populations PD-L1 negative versus PD-L1 positive patients ($p = 0.63$; Figure 3).

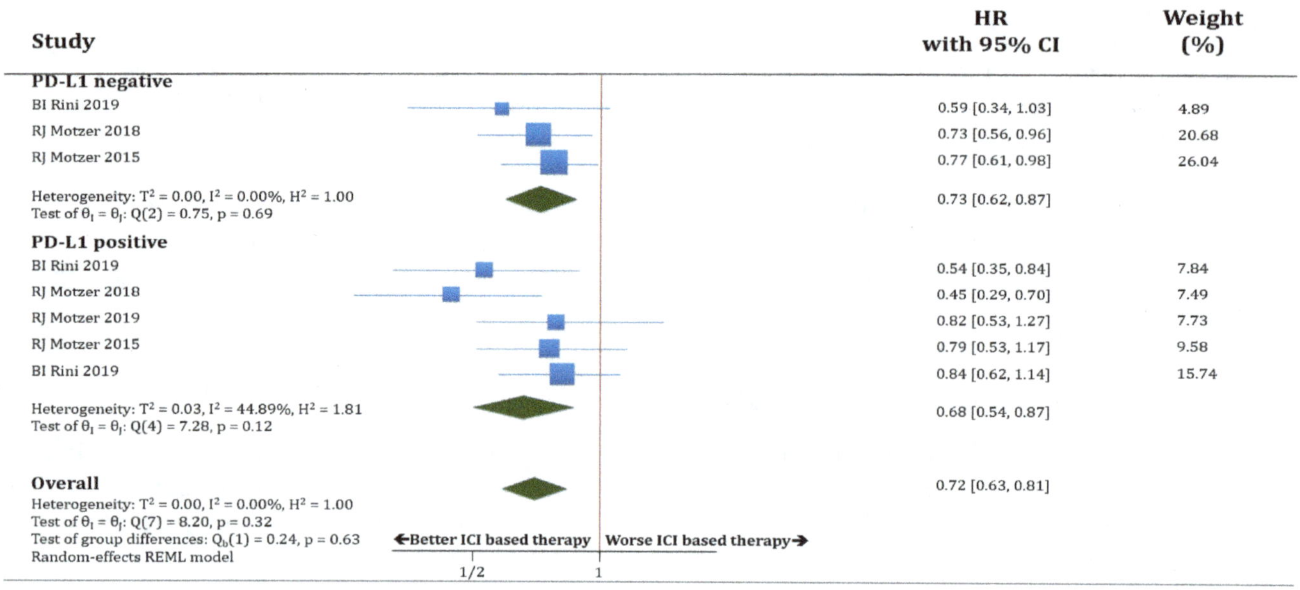

Figure 3. Forest plot diagram: hazard ratio (HR) with 95% confidence interval of overall survival (OS) between arms according to PD-L1 expression subgroups.

14. Discussion

In recent years, the therapeutic landscape of metastatic ccRCC has been broadening as a consequence of the incorporation of different ICIs to the antiangiogenic agents.

Most of the clinical trials were not developed based on predictive biomarkers. Currently, the IMDC score remains as the only useful strategy for treatment selection (restricting the use of the nivolumab plus ipilimumab combination for the intermediate risk- and poor risk-patients) [4]. There are no other validated biomarkers to inform patients about their best treatment choice available in clinical practice. This fact highlights the current lack of personalized therapy in RCC.

The results of this meta-analysis, focused on metastatic RCC, support that PD-L1 expression may be a reliable biomarker for PFS but not for OS. This fact could be relevant for clinical trials design. Therapy based on ICIs improved PFS compared to standard of care in PD-L1 positive patients but not in PD-L1 negative patients. However, OS was improved with immunotherapy regardless of PD-L1 status. Therefore, the role of PD-L1 expression as a predictive biomarker is not flawless and not suitable for selecting the therapeutic strategy. Despite the fact that PFS is considered a validated surrogate endpoint for OS [44] in RCC patients treated with TKIs, its value in those treated with ICIs is less clear, as it has been shown in different trials [3,20]. A long-term "delayed" positive effect has been pointed as a typical characteristic of ICI treatment. This phenomenon, partially reflected by lasting durations of response to ICI therapy, explains the existence of long-term survivor groups with these drugs in different solid tumors even in the absence of benefit in terms of PFS. This fact might help to explain the results obtained in the PD-L1 negative population (benefit in OS but not in PFS). On the other hand, as a consequence of their worse prognosis, PD-L1 positive patients could present shorter median PFS with TKIs compared to PD-L1 negative patients and this feature could explain the difference observed between these groups in terms of PFS but not OS; in this case the positive effect of immunotherapy would manifest earlier in the PD-L1 positive population.

The results obtained in OS should overrule those in PFS, reaching the conclusion that PD-L1 expression has not been shown to be useful for treatment selection in metastatic RCC so far. However, for testing new drugs or combinations targeting PD-1 or PD-L1 it may be useful to consider that PD-L1 expression may predict PFS benefit.

In addition to seeking to optimize and homogenize the assessment of PD-L1 expression among trials, other factors beyond this biomarker that may improve its value are also being studied. Tumor mutational burden, $CD8^+$ T lymphocytes infiltration or gene expression profiles could represent alternative biomarkers of response for a better selection of individuals for specific therapies and to optimize the outcomes of this disease [8]. In this sense, gene expression profiles that focus on angiogenic or immunological pathways have shown promising results in patients treated with the combination of atezolizumab plus bevacizumab [8]. In addition, blood constitutes a source for obtaining oncological material and is the basis for the development of liquid biopsy [45]. Due to the improvement of molecular characterization in last years, different nucleic acids as well as exosomes (nanovesicles arisen from endocytosis processes) found in blood may inform about the efficacy of treatments and disease status in a dynamic way [46,47]. As PD-L1 expression is a dynamic biomarker, real time assessment could provide a more accurate evaluation of current status improving the predictive value. As example, in metastatic melanoma patients, it has been shown that expression levels of PD-L1 on circulating exosomes can be modified during treatment with ICIs and those changes might be related to the development of therapy resistance and the type of responses obtained [48].

The future of PD-L1 could be less relevant in the future. This fact will depend on the success of different ICIs being tested or how drugs may change the expression of PD-L1. Bempegaldesleukin (NKTR-214) combined with nivolumab has been shown to change PD-L1 negative tumors (PD-L1 $< 1\%$) to PD-L1 positive tumors (PD-L1 $\geq 1\%$) [49]. Indeed, several immune checkpoints, such as T cell immunoglobulin 3 (TIM3), lymphocyte activation gene 3 (LAG3), or T cell immunoglobulin and ITIM domain (TIGIT), are potential regulators contributing to the immunosuppressive tumor microenvironment in RCC [50].

A new generation of ICIs, targeting LAG3, VISTA, TIM3, or TIGIT are currently under evaluation. The combination of nivolumab with relatlimab (BMS-986016), an antibody directed against LAG3, has been shown to achieve an ORR of 16% in patients with advanced melanoma progressing after PD-1 or PD-L1 blockade [51]; relatlimab is being tested in a phase III trial (ClinicalTrials.gov Identifier: NCT03470922) [52]. Eftilagimod alpha (IMP321) is a soluble version of LAG3 that preferentially binds to a subset of major histocompatibility complex (MHC) class II molecules and activates antigen-presenting cells. A phase I trial (NCT00351949) tested this drug as monotherapy in 21 metastatic RCC showing both sustained $CD8^+$ T cell activation and an increase in the percentage of long-lived effector-memory $CD8^+$ T cell in all patients at doses above 6 mg; seven of eight evaluable patients dosed at 6 mg experienced stable disease at 3 months compared with only three of 11 in the lower dose group ($p = 0.015$) [53]. As a consequence of its good safety profile and demonstration of efficacy, the drug is currently being tested in different solid tumors [54]. INCAGN02385 (monoclonal antibody anti-LAG3) and XmAb®22841 (bispecific antibody anti-LAG3 and anti-CTLA-4) are also drugs being tested as monotherapy or in combination with anti-PD-1 drugs in a variety of solid tumors including RCC [55,56]. Early-phase trials of anti-TIM3 and anti-TIGIT antibodies are also ongoing in multiple tumor types [57–59]. INCAGN02390 (as monotherapy) and MBG453 (as monotherapy or in combination with anti-PD-1) are, both of them, examples of anti-TIM3 antibodies currently being tested in RCC among other tumors [60,61].

OX40 (also known as CD134) is a secondary co-stimulatory molecule whose expression is dependent on full activation of the T cell. OX40 agonists, such as PF-04518600 (in combination with axitinib or avelumab) are other types of molecules undergoing clinical development in RCC [62,63].

Finally, high-dose IL-2 has long been used in RCC as a promoter of T cell proliferation and activation and it is known that a subgroup of patients may achieve complete responses with this therapy [64]. Newer formulations of IL-2 are being developed, such as bempegaldesleukin that is currently being evaluated in combination with nivolumab in RCC in a phase III trial (NCT03729245) [65].

Combination of ICI with cancer cell vaccines, oncolytic viruses, or chimeric antigen receptor CAR T cells is also biologically plausible.

The study has numerous limitations. Primarily, there is not a unique standardized method to assess PD-L1 regardless of the tumor type and potential equivalence among the different techniques is unknown at this moment. Different antibodies, thresholds, and evaluated cells are used to consider the positivity for this marker on the tumor samples with very heterogeneous results. For all these reasons, conclusions obtained from different clinical trials in relation to the role of PD-L1 as a predictive biomarker in ccRCC have to be confirmed.

Patient-level data was not accessible, but trial-level and patient-level meta-analyses may eventually reach comparable conclusions [66]. Finally, response rates (due to lack of data) were not studied. This could be relevant because it is possible that higher PD-L1 expression could be associated with higher probability of response; as this parameter is related to OS, it would be interesting to study it thoroughly and assess its relevance as an endpoint for clinical trials.

15. Conclusions

In conclusion, in this meta-analysis, PD-L1 expression did not show to be an accurate and solid biomarker to select treatment for ccRCC patients as both groups (PD-L1 negative and PD-L1 positive) benefited from immunotherapy. The improvement of the assessment of PD-L1 expression status and the introduction of new biomarkers are ongoing; hopefully personalization of systemic therapy in RCC will become a reality in the near future.

References

1. Siegel, R.L.; Miller, K.D.; Jemal, A. Cancer statistics, 2019. *Cancer J. Clin.* **2019**, *69*, 7–34. [CrossRef] [PubMed]
2. Cancer of the Kidney: Section 3. In *Cancer: Principles & Practice of Oncology*, 8th ed.; DeVita, V.T., Jr.; Hellman, S.; Rosenberg, S.A. (Eds.) Lipincott-Raven: Philadelphia, PA, USA, 2001.
3. Motzer, R.J.; Escudier, B.; McDermott, D.F.; George, S.; Hammers, H.J.; Srinivas, S.; Tykodi, S.S.; Sosman, J.A.; Procopio, G.; Plimack, E.R.; et al. Nivolumab versus Everolimus in Advanced Renal-Cell Carcinoma. *N. Engl. J. Med.* **2015**, *373*, 1803–1813. [CrossRef]
4. Motzer, R.J.; Tannir, N.M.; McDermott, D.F.; Frontera, O.A.; Melichar, B.; Choueiri, T.K.; Plimack, E.R.; Barthelemy, P.; Porta, C.; George, S.; et al. Nivolumab plus Ipilimumab versus Sunitinib in Advanced Renal-Cell Carcinoma. *N. Engl. J. Med.* **2018**, *378*, 1277–1290. [CrossRef] [PubMed]
5. Rini, B.I.; Plimack, E.R.; Stus, V.; Gafanov, R.; Hawkins, R.; Nosov, D.; Pouliot, F.; Alekseev, B.; Soulières, D.; Melichar, B.; et al. Pembrolizumab plus Axitinib versus Sunitinib for Advanced Renal-Cell Carcinoma. *N. Engl. J. Med.* **2019**, *380*, 1116–1127. [CrossRef]
6. Motzer, R.J.; Penkov, K.; Haanen, J.; Rini, B.; Albiges, L.; Campbell, M.T.; Venugopal, B.; Kollmannsberger, C.; Negrier, S.; Uemura, M.; et al. Avelumab plus Axitinib versus Sunitinib for Advanced Renal-Cell Carcinoma. *N. Engl. J. Med.* **2019**, *380*, 1103–1115. [CrossRef] [PubMed]
7. Rini, B.; Powles, T.; Atkins, M.B.; Escudier, B.; McDermott, D.F.; Suarez, C.; Bracarda, S.; Stadler, W.M.; Donskov, F.; Lee, J.L.; et al. Atezolizumab plus bevacizumab versus sunitinib in patients with previously untreated metastatic renal cell carcinoma (IMmotion151): A multicentre, open-label, phase 3, randomised controlled trial. *Lancet* **2019**, *393*, 2404–2415. [CrossRef]
8. McDermott, D.F.; Huseni, M.A.; Atkins, M.B.; Motzer, R.J.; Rini, B.I.; Escudier, B.; Fong, L.; Joseph, R.W.; Pal, S.K.; Reeves, J.A.; et al. Clinical activity and molecular correlates of response to atezolizumab alone or in combination with bevacizumab versus sunitinib in renal cell carcinoma. *Nat. Med.* **2018**, *24*, 749–757. [CrossRef]
9. Heng, D.Y.; Xie, W.; Regan, M.M.; Warren, M.A.; Golshayan, A.R.; Sahi, C.; Eigl, B.J.; Ruether, J.D.; Cheng, T.; North, S.; et al. Prognostic Factors for Overall Survival in Patients With Metastatic Renal Cell Carcinoma Treated With Vascular Endothelial Growth Factor–Targeted Agents: Results From a Large, Multicenter Study. *J. Clin. Oncol.* **2009**, *27*, 5794–5799. [CrossRef]
10. Heng, D.Y.; Xie, W.; Regan, M.M.; Harshman, L.C.; Bjarnason, G.A.; Vaishampayan, U.N.; MacKenzie, M.; Wood, L.; Donskov, F.; Tan, M.-H.; et al. External validation and comparison with other models of the International Metastatic Renal-Cell Carcinoma Database Consortium prognostic model: A population-based study. *Lancet Oncol.* **2013**, *14*, 141–148. [CrossRef]
11. Escudier, B.; Porta, C.; Schmidinger, M.; Rioux-Leclercq, N.; Bex, A.; Khoo, V.; Grünwald, V.; Gillessen, S.; Horwich, A. ESMO Guidelines Committee Renal cell carcinoma: ESMO Clinical Practice Guidelines for diagnosis, treatment and follow-up. *Ann. Oncol.* **2019**, *30*, 706–720. [CrossRef]
12. Jonasch, E. NCCN Guidelines Updates: Management of Metastatic Kidney Cancer. *J. Natl. Compr. Cancer Netw.* **2019**, *17*, 587–589.

13. Choueiri, T.K.; Figueroa, D.J.; Fay, A.P.; Signoretti, S.; Liu, Y.; Gagnon, R.; Deen, K.; Carpenter, C.; Benson, P.; Ho, T.H.; et al. Correlation of PD-L1 Tumor Expression and Treatment Outcomes in Patients with Renal Cell Carcinoma Receiving Sunitinib or Pazopanib: Results from COMPARZ, a Randomized Controlled Trial. *Clin. Cancer Res.* **2014**, *21*, 1071–1077. [CrossRef] [PubMed]
14. Topalian, S.L.; Hodi, F.S.; Brahmer, J.R.; Gettinger, S.N.; Smith, D.C.; McDermott, D.F.; Powderly, J.D.; Carvajal, R.D.; Sosman, J.A.; Atkins, M.B.; et al. Safety, Activity, and Immune Correlates of Anti–PD-1 Antibody in Cancer. *N. Engl. J. Med.* **2012**, *366*, 2443–2454. [CrossRef] [PubMed]
15. Brahmer, J.R.; Drake, C.G.; Wollner, I.; Powderly, J.D.; Picus, J.; Sharfman, W.H.; Stankevich, E.; Pons, A.; Salay, T.M.; McMiller, T.L.; et al. Phase I Study of Single-Agent Anti–Programmed Death-1 (MDX-1106) in Refractory Solid Tumors: Safety, Clinical Activity, Pharmacodynamics, and Immunologic Correlates. *J. Clin. Oncol.* **2010**, *28*, 3167–3175. [CrossRef]
16. McDermott, D.F.; Sosman, J.A.; Sznol, M.; Massard, C.; Gordon, M.S.; Hamid, O.; Powderly, J.D.; Infante, J.R.; Fassò, M.; Wang, Y.V.; et al. Atezolizumab, an Anti–Programmed Death-Ligand 1 Antibody, in Metastatic Renal Cell Carcinoma: Long-Term Safety, Clinical Activity, and Immune Correlates From a Phase Ia Study. *J. Clin. Oncol.* **2016**, *34*, 833–842. [CrossRef]
17. Motzer, R.J.; Rini, B.I.; McDermott, D.F.; Redman, B.G.; Kuzel, T.M.; Harrison, M.R.; Vaishampayan, U.N.; Drabkin, H.A.; George, S.; Logan, T.F.; et al. Nivolumab for Metastatic Renal Cell Carcinoma: Results of a Randomized Phase II Trial. *J. Clin. Oncol.* **2015**, *33*, 1430–1437. [CrossRef]
18. Choueiri, T.K.; Fishman, M.N.; Escudier, B.; Kim, J.J.; Kluger, H.M.; Stadler, W.M.; Perez-Gracia, J.L.; McNeel, D.G.; Curti, B.D.; Harrison, M.R.; et al. Immunomodulatory activity of nivolumab in previously treated and untreated metastatic renal cell carcinoma (mRCC): Biomarker-based results from a randomized clinical trial. *J. Clin. Oncol.* **2014**, *32*, 5012. [CrossRef]
19. Khunger, M.; Hernandez, A.V.; Pasupuleti, V.; Rakshit, S.; Pennell, N.A.; Stevenson, J.; Mukhopadhyay, S.; Schalper, K.; Velcheti, V. Programmed Cell Death 1 (PD-1) Ligand (PD-L1) Expression in Solid Tumors As a Predictive Biomarker of Benefit From PD-1/PD-L1 Axis Inhibitors: A Systematic Review and Meta-Analysis. *JCO Precis. Oncol.* **2017**, *1*, 1–15. [CrossRef]
20. Borghaei, H.; Paz-Ares, L.; Horn, L.A.; Spigel, D.R.; Steins, M.; Ready, N.E.; Chow, L.Q.; Vokes, E.E.; Felip, E.; Holgado, E.; et al. Nivolumab versus Docetaxel in Advanced Nonsquamous Non-Small-Cell Lung Cancer. *N. Engl. J. Med.* **2015**, *373*, 1627–1639. [CrossRef]
21. Reck, M.; Rodríguez-Abreu, D.; Robinson, A.G.; Hui, R.; Csőszi, T.; Fülöp, A.; Gottfried, M.; Peled, N.; Tafreshi, A.; Cuffe, S.; et al. Pembrolizumab versus Chemotherapy for PD-L1–Positive Non–Small-Cell Lung Cancer. *N. Engl. J. Med.* **2016**, *375*, 1823–1833. [CrossRef]
22. Yearley, J.H.; Gibson, C.; Yu, N.; Moon, C.; Murphy, E.; Juco, J.; Lunceford, J.; Cheng, J.; Chow, L.Q.; Seiwert, T.Y.; et al. PD-L2 Expression in Human Tumors: Relevance to Anti-PD-1 Therapy in Cancer. *Clin. Cancer Res.* **2017**, *23*, 3158–3167. [CrossRef] [PubMed]
23. Callea, M.; Albiges, L.; Gupta, M.; Cheng, S.-C.; Genega, E.M.; Fay, A.P.; Song, J.; Carvo, I.; Bhatt, R.S.; Atkins, M.B.; et al. Differential Expression of PD-L1 between Primary and Metastatic Sites in Clear-Cell Renal Cell Carcinoma. *Cancer Immunol. Res.* **2015**, *3*, 1158–1164. [CrossRef]
24. Barsoum, I.B.; Smallwood, C.A.; Siemens, D.R.; Graham, C.H. A Mechanism of Hypoxia-Mediated Escape from Adaptive Immunity in Cancer Cells. *Cancer Res.* **2013**, *74*, 665–674. [CrossRef] [PubMed]
25. Chen, S.; Crabill, G.A.; Pritchard, T.S.; McMiller, T.L.; Wei, P.; Pardoll, D.M.; Pan, F.; Topalian, S.L. Mechanisms regulating PD-L1 expression on tumor and immune cells. *J. Immunother. Cancer* **2019**, *7*, 305–312. [CrossRef] [PubMed]
26. Xu, F.; Xu, L.; Wang, Q.; An, G.; Feng, G.; Liu, F. Clinicopathological and prognostic value of programmed death ligand-1 (PD-L1) in renal cell carcinoma: A meta-analysis. *Int. J. Clin. Exp. Med.* **2015**, *8*, 14595–14603. [PubMed]
27. Thompson, R.H.; Gillett, M.D.; Cheville, J.C.; Lohse, C.M.; Dong, H.; Webster, W.S.; Krejci, K.G.; Lobo, J.R.; Sengupta, S.; Chen, L.; et al. Costimulatory B7-H1 in renal cell carcinoma patients: Indicator of tumor aggressiveness and potential therapeutic target. *Proc. Natl. Acad. Sci. USA* **2004**, *101*, 17174–17179. [CrossRef]
28. Wallin, J.J.; Bendell, J.C.; Funke, R.; Sznol, M.; Korski, K.; Jones, S.; Hernandez, G.; Mier, J.; He, X.; Hodi, F.S.; et al. Atezolizumab in combination with bevacizumab enhances antigen-specific T-cell migration in metastatic renal cell carcinoma. *Nat. Commun.* **2016**, *7*, 12624. [CrossRef]

29. Hellmann, M.D.; Ciuleanu, T.-E.; Pluzanski, A.; Lee, J.S.; Otterson, G.A.; Audigier-Valette, C.; Minenza, E.; Linardou, H.; Burgers, S.; Salman, P.; et al. Nivolumab plus Ipilimumab in Lung Cancer with a High Tumor Mutational Burden. *N. Engl. J. Med.* **2018**, *378*, 2093–2104. [CrossRef]
30. Turajlic, S.; Litchfield, K.; Xu, H.; Rosenthal, R.; McGranahan, N.; Reading, J.L.; Wong, Y.N.S.; Rowan, A.; Kanu, N.; Al Bakir, M.; et al. Insertion-and-deletion-derived tumour-specific neoantigens and the immunogenic phenotype: A pan-cancer analysis. *Lancet Oncol.* **2017**, *18*, 1009–1021. [CrossRef]
31. Miao, D.; Margolis, C.A.; Gao, W.; Voss, M.H.; Li, W.; Martini, D.J.; Norton, C.; Bosse, D.; Wankowicz, S.M.; Cullen, D.; et al. Genomic correlates of response to immune checkpoint therapies in clear cell renal cell carcinoma. *Science* **2018**, *359*, 801–806. [CrossRef]
32. Carril-Ajuria, L.; Santos, M.; Roldán-Romero, J.M.; Rodríguez-Antona, C.; De Velasco, G. Prognostic and Predictive Value of PBRM1 in Clear Cell Renal Cell Carcinoma. *Cancers* **2019**, *12*, 16. [CrossRef] [PubMed]
33. Giraldo, N.; Becht, E.; Pagès, F.; Skliris, G.P.; Verkarre, V.; Vano, Y.; Mejean, A.; Saint-Aubert, N.; Lacroix, L.; Natario, I.; et al. Orchestration and Prognostic Significance of Immune Checkpoints in the Microenvironment of Primary and Metastatic Renal Cell Cancer. *Clin. Cancer Res.* **2015**, *21*, 3031–3040. [CrossRef] [PubMed]
34. Sivan, A.; Corrales, L.; Hubert, N.; Williams, J.B.; Aquino-Michaels, K.; Earley, Z.M.; Benyamin, F.W.; Lei, Y.M.; Jabri, B.; Alegre, M.-L.; et al. Commensal Bifidobacterium promotes antitumor immunity and facilitates anti-PD-L1 efficacy. *Science* **2015**, *350*, 1084–1089. [CrossRef] [PubMed]
35. Vétizou, M.; Pitt, J.M.; Daillère, R.; Lepage, P.; Waldschmitt, N.; Flament, C.; Rusakiewicz, S.; Routy, B.; Roberti, M.P.; Duong, C.P.M.; et al. Anticancer immunotherapy by CTLA-4 blockade relies on the gut microbiota. *Science* **2015**, *350*, 1079–1084. [CrossRef] [PubMed]
36. DeRosa, L.; Routy, B.; Enot, D.; Bacciarelo, G.; Massard, C.; Loriot, Y.; Fizazi, K.; Escudier, B.; Zitvogel, L.; Albiges, L. Impact of antibiotics on outcome in patients with metastatic renal cell carcinoma treated with immune checkpoint inhibitors. *J. Clin. Oncol.* **2017**, *35*, 462. [CrossRef]
37. Routy, B.; Le Chatelier, E.; DeRosa, L.; Duong, C.P.M.; Alou, M.T.; Daillère, R.; Fluckiger, A.; Messaoudene, M.; Rauber, C.; Roberti, M.P.; et al. Gut microbiome influences efficacy of PD-1–based immunotherapy against epithelial tumors. *Science* **2017**, *359*, 91–97. [CrossRef] [PubMed]
38. Wang, Q.; Zhang, J.; Tu, H.; Liang, D.; Chang, D.W.; Ye, Y.; Wu, X. Soluble immune checkpoint-related proteins as predictors of tumor recurrence, survival, and T cell phenotypes in clear cell renal cell carcinoma patients. *J. Immunother. Cancer* **2019**, *7*, 1–9. [CrossRef]
39. Kloten, V.; Lampignano, R.; Krahn, T.; Schlange, T. Circulating Tumor Cell PD-L1 Expression as Biomarker for Therapeutic Efficacy of Immune Checkpoint Inhibition in NSCLC. *Cells* **2019**, *8*, 809. [CrossRef]
40. Moher, D.; Liberati, A.; Tetzlaff, J.; Altman, D.G.; The PRISMA Group. Preferred Reporting Items for Systematic Reviews and Meta-Analyses: The PRISMA Statement. *PLoS Med.* **2009**, *6*, e1000097. [CrossRef]
41. Higgins, J.P.T.; Thompson, S.G.; Deeks, J.J.; Altman, U.G. Measuring inconsistency in meta-analyses. *BMJ* **2003**, *327*, 557–560. [CrossRef]
42. Egger, M.; Smith, G.D.; Schneider, M.; Minder, C. Bias in meta-analysis detected by a simple, graphical test. *BMJ* **1997**, *315*, 629–634. [CrossRef] [PubMed]
43. Peters, J.L.; Sutton, A.J.; Jones, D.R.; Abrams, K.R.; Rushton, L. Contour-enhanced meta-analysis funnel plots help distinguish publication bias from other causes of asymmetry. *J. Clin. Epidemiol.* **2008**, *61*, 991–996. [CrossRef] [PubMed]
44. Negrier, S.; Bushmakin, A.; Cappelleri, J.; Korytowsky, B.; Sandin, R.; Charbonneau, C.; Michaelson, M.D.; Figlin, R.; Motzer, R.J. Assessment of progression-free survival as a surrogate end-point for overall survival in patients with metastatic renal cell carcinoma. *Eur. J. Cancer* **2014**, *50*, 1766–1771. [CrossRef] [PubMed]
45. Haber, D.A.; Velculescu, V.E. Blood-Based Analyses of Cancer: Circulating Tumor Cells and Circulating Tumor DNA. *Cancer Discov.* **2014**, *4*, 650–661. [CrossRef] [PubMed]
46. Jin, X.; Chen, Y.; Chen, H.; Fei, S.; Chen, D.; Cai, X.; Liu, L.; Lin, B.; Su, H.; Zhao, L.; et al. Evaluation of Tumor-Derived Exosomal miRNA as Potential Diagnostic Biomarkers for Early-Stage Non–Small Cell Lung Cancer Using Next-Generation Sequencing. *Clin. Cancer Res.* **2017**, *23*, 5311–5319. [CrossRef]
47. Cohen, J.D.; Li, L.; Wang, Y.; Thoburn, C.; Afsari, B.; Danilova, L.V.; Douville, C.B.; A Javed, A.; Wong, F.; Mattox, A.; et al. Detection and localization of surgically resectable cancers with a multi-analyte blood test. *Science* **2018**, *359*, 926–930. [CrossRef]
48. Chen, G.; Huang, A.C.; Zhang, W.; Zhang, G.; Wu, M.; Xu, W.; Yu, Z.; Yang, J.; Wang, B.; Sun, H.; et al. Exosomal PD-L1 contributes to immunosuppression and is associated with anti-PD-1 response. *Nature* **2018**, *560*, 382–386. [CrossRef]

49. Diab, A.; Hurwitz, M.; Cho, D.; Papadimitrakopoulou, V.; Curti, B.; Tykodi, S.; Puzanov, L.; Ibrahim, N.K.; Tolaney, S.M.; Tripathy, D.; et al. NKTR-214 (CD122-biased agonist) plus nivolumab in patients with advanced solid tumors: Preliminary phase 1/2 results of PIVOT. *J. Clin. Oncol.* **2018**, *36*, 3006. [CrossRef]
50. Anderson, A.C.; Joller, N.; Kuchroo, V.K. Lag-3, Tim-3, and TIGIT: Co-inhibitory Receptors with Specialized Functions in Immune Regulation. *Immunity* **2016**, *44*, 989–1004. [CrossRef]
51. Ascierto, P.A.; Melero, I.; Bhatia, S.; Bono, P.; Sanborn, R.E.; Lipson, E.I.; Callahan, M.K.; Gajewski, T.; Gomez-Roca, C.A.; Hodi, F.S.; et al. Initial efficacy of anti-lymphocyte activation gene-3 (anti–LAG-3; BMS-986016) in combination with nivolumab (nivo) in pts with melanoma (MEL) previously treated with anti–PD-1/PD-L1 therapy. *J. Clin. Oncol.* **2017**, *35*, 9520. [CrossRef]
52. US National Library of Medicine. ClinicalTrials.gov. Available online: https://clinicaltrials.gov/ct2/show/NCT03470922 (accessed on 5 May 2020).
53. Brignone, C.; Escudier, B.; Grygar, C.; Marcu, M.; Triebel, F. A Phase I Pharmacokinetic and Biological Correlative Study of IMP321, a Novel MHC Class II Agonist, in Patients with Advanced Renal Cell Carcinoma. *Clin. Cancer Res.* **2009**, *15*, 6225–6231. [CrossRef] [PubMed]
54. US National Library of Medicine. ClinicalTrials.gov. Available online: https://clinicaltrials.gov/ct2/show/NCT03252938 (accessed on 5 May 2020).
55. US National Library of Medicine. ClinicalTrials.gov. Available online: https://clinicaltrials.gov/ct2/show/NCT03538028 (accessed on 5 May 2020).
56. US National Library of Medicine. ClinicalTrials.gov. Available online: https://clinicaltrials.gov/ct2/show/NCT03849469 (accessed on 5 May 2020).
57. Guillerey, C.; Harjunpää, H.; Carrié, N.; Kassem, S.; Teo, T.; Miles, K.; Krumeich, S.; Weulersse, M.; Cuisinier, M.; Stannard, K.; et al. TIGIT immune checkpoint blockade restores CD8+ T-cell immunity against multiple myeloma. *Blood* **2018**, *132*, 1689–1694. [CrossRef] [PubMed]
58. Solomon, B.L.; Garrido-Laguna, I. TIGIT: A novel immunotherapy target moving from bench to bedside. *Cancer Immunol. Immunother.* **2018**, *67*, 1659–1667. [CrossRef]
59. Harding, J.J.; Patnaik, A.; Moreno, V.; Stein, M.; Jankowska, A.M.; De Mendizabal, N.V.; Liu, Z.T.; Koneru, M.; Calvo, E. A phase Ia/Ib study of an anti-TIM-3 antibody (LY3321367) monotherapy or in combination with an anti-PD-L1 antibody (LY3300054): Interim safety, efficacy, and pharmacokinetic findings in advanced cancers. *J. Clin. Oncol.* **2019**, *37*, 12. [CrossRef]
60. US National Library of Medicine. ClinicalTrials.gov. Available online: https://clinicaltrials.gov/ct2/show/NCT02608268 (accessed on 5 May 2020).
61. US National Library of Medicine. ClinicalTrials.gov. Available online: https://clinicaltrials.gov/ct2/show/NCT03652077 (accessed on 5 May 2020).
62. US National Library of Medicine. ClinicalTrials.gov. Available online: https://clinicaltrials.gov/ct2/show/NCT03092856 (accessed on 5 May 2020).
63. US National Library of Medicine. ClinicalTrials.gov. Available online: https://clinicaltrials.gov/ct2/show/NCT02554812 (accessed on 5 May 2020).
64. Fyfe, G.; I Fisher, R.; A Rosenberg, S.; Sznol, M.; Parkinson, D.R.; Louie, A.C. Results of treatment of 255 patients with metastatic renal cell carcinoma who received high-dose recombinant interleukin-2 therapy. *J. Clin. Oncol.* **1995**, *13*, 688–696. [CrossRef]
65. US National Library of Medicine. ClinicalTrials.gov. Available online: https://clinicaltrials.gov/ct2/show/NCT03729245 (accessed on 5 May 2020).
66. Bennett, C.L. Venous Thromboembolism and Mortality Associated with Recombinant Erythropoietin and Darbepoetin Administration for the Treatment of Cancer-Associated Anemia. *JAMA* **2008**, *299*, 914. [CrossRef]

14

Predicting Response to Immunotherapy in Metastatic Renal Cell Carcinoma

Matthew D. Tucker and Brian I. Rini *

Department of Medicine, Division of Hematology and Oncology, Vanderbilt University Medical Center, Nashville, TN 37232, USA; matthew.tucker@vumc.org
* Correspondence: brian.rini@vumc.org

Simple Summary: Immunotherapy-based treatment options have become standard of care in metastatic renal cell carcinoma. Despite significant improvement in overall survival with these therapies, the tumors of many patients will eventually progress. This review highlights the ongoing efforts to develop biomarkers to help predict which patients are most likely to benefit from treatment with immunotherapy.

Abstract: Immunotherapy-based combinations, driven by PD-1, PD-L1, and CTLA-4 inhibitors, has altered the treatment landscape for metastatic renal cell carcinoma (RCC). Despite significant improvements in clinical outcomes, many patients do not experience deep or lasting benefits. Recent efforts to determine which patients are most likely to benefit from immunotherapy and immunotherapy-based combinations have shown promise but have not yet affected clinical practice. PD-L1 expression via immunohistochemistry (IHC) has shown promise in a few clinical trials, although variations in the IHC assays as well as the use of different values for positivity presents unique challenges for this potential biomarker. Several other candidate biomarkers were investigated including tumor mutational burden, gene expression signatures, single gene mutations, human endogenous retroviruses, the gastrointestinal microbiome, and peripheral blood laboratory markers. While individually these biomarkers have yet to explain the heterogeneity of treatment response to immunotherapy, using aggregate information from these biomarkers may inform clinically useful predictive biomarkers.

Keywords: biomarkers; immunotherapy; renal cell carcinoma; PD-L1

---

1. Introduction

An estimated 400,000 new renal cancers are diagnosed annually world-wide leading to over 175,000 deaths [1]. Early systemic therapies designed to target the immunogenicity of metastatic renal cell carcinoma (mRCC), such as interferon-alpha and high-dose IL-2, were effective in only a small percentage of patients [2,3]. While subsequent therapies designed against angiogenesis including tyrosine kinase inhibitors (TKI) targeting vascular endothelial growth factor (VEGF) and its receptor (VEGFR) improved response rates and progression-free survival, nearly all patients developed resistance [4].

The implementation of monoclonal antibodies against the immune checkpoint proteins programmed cell death 1 (PD-1), programmed death-ligand 1 (PD-L1), and anti-cytotoxic T-lymphocyte-associated protein-4 (CTLA-4) has dramatically changed the treatment paradigm for mRCC [5]. After demonstrating improved overall survival (OS) compared to the mammalian target of rapamycin (mTOR) inhibitor everolimus in the post-VEGF-R inhibitor setting, nivolumab (anti PD-1) became the first immune checkpoint inhibitor to gain FDA approval for advanced RCC in November of 2015 [6,7]. Subsequently, in April 2018, the immunotherapy combination nivolumab plus ipilimumab (anti-CTLA-4) gained approval in the first-line setting after demonstrating improved OS versus sunitinib [8]. In April and May of 2019, two additional immunotherapy-based combinations were approved in the first-line setting: pembrolizumab (anti-PD-1) plus the anti-VEGFR agent axitinib and avelumab (anti-PD-L1) plus axitinib [9–11]. Despite these advances, only a minority of patients treated with immunotherapy will have a durable response, prompting the search for predictive biomarkers. Since the early phases of development of immunotherapy in mRCC, tremendous efforts have been made towards understanding the biology of the tumor microenvironment (TME) to help identify candidate biomarkers, such as immunohistochemistry (IHC) expression of PD-L1, tumor mutational burden (TMB), polybromo-1 gene (*PBRM1*) mutations, human endogenous retroviruses (hERVs), gastrointestinal microbiota, sarcomatoid histology, and the neutrophil to lymphocyte ratio (NLR).

2. Programmed Death-Ligand 1

Expression of PD-L1 (historically denoted as B7 homolog 1) on tumor cells and tumor-infiltrating lymphocytes was initially shown to be a poor prognostic marker for patients with renal cell carcinoma based on IHC analyses performed in 2004 [12,13]. Furthermore, in 2006 Thompson et al. performed a retrospective analysis of over 300 patients with mRCC and found that the 5-year cancer-specific survival rate was 42% for patients expressing PD-L1 versus 83% for patients who were negative [14]. Subsequently, a post-hoc analysis of the phase III trial COMPARZ, comparing efficacy of pazopanib to sunitinib, found that patients treated with either agent had significantly worse OS and progression-free survival (PFS) if they were PD-L1+ compared to those who were PD-L1− [15]. Thus, tumor PD-L1 expression is a negative prognostic factor in RCC and predicts against response to anti-VEGFR therapy.

Early phase clinical trials with anti-PD-1 monotherapy showed potential for the use of PD-L1 expression as a predictive biomarker for immunotherapy in mRCC [16,17]. The phase III clinical trial CheckMate 025 demonstrated improved efficacy of nivolumab over everolimus regardless of PD-L1 status, i.e., the marker was prognostic but not predictive [6]. Interestingly, the prior association of worse prognosis was observed in both groups, as patients who were PD-L1+ had numerically lower OS compared with PD-L1- patients. PD-L1 expression has been evaluated in several randomized clinical trials (Table 1).

In the phase III CheckMate 214 trial, evaluating nivolumab in combination with ipilimumab versus sunitinib, 91% (1002/1096) of patients in the intention-to-treat (ITT) population had quantifiable tumor tissue available for PD-L1 testing [8]. Tumors were positive if they had tumor cells (from baseline tumor samples prior to therapy) with $> 1\%$ PD-L1 expression as assessed using the Dako PD-L1 IHC 28-8 pharmDx test. Multivariate analysis of baseline factors was presented in the 32-month extended follow-up report [18] and showed that PD-L1 expression was a negative predictor for survival among patients treated with sunitinib [hazard ratio (HR) 0.70; 95% CI 0.52-0.93 for patients negative for PD-L1 expression]. However, PD-L1 was not associated with survival among patients treated with nivolumab plus ipilimumab even in univariate analysis, suggesting that combination immunotherapy was able to overcome the negative prognostic effects associated with PD-L1 expression.

Table 1. Clinical outcomes by PD-L1 expression status from phase III clinical trials of immunotherapy in mRCC.

Trial Name	Treatment + Arms	mOS PD-L1+	mOS PD-L1-	mOS ITT	mPFS PD-L1+	mPFS PD-L1-	mPFS ITT	CR% in PD-L1+	CR% in PD-L1-	ORR in PD-L1+	ORR in PD-L1-
CheckMate 214 [8]	Nivolumab + ipilimumab vs. sunitinib (intermediate and poor-risk)	NR vs. 19.6 mo (HR 0.45)	NR vs. NR (HR 0.73)	NR vs. 26.0 mo (HR 0.63)	22.8 mo vs. 5.9 mo (HR 0.46)	11.0 mo vs. 10.4 mo (1.00 *)	11.6 mo vs. 8.4 mo (HR 0.82 *)	16% vs. 1%	7% vs. 1%	58% vs. 22%	37% vs. 28%
KEYNOTE-426 [9,10]	Pembrolizumab + axitinib vs. sunitinib	HR 0.54 (12-mo OS)	HR 0.59 * (12-mo OS)	NR vs. 35.7 (HR 0.68) [10]	15.3 mo vs. 8.9 mo (HR 0.62)	15.0 mo vs. 12.5 mo (HR 0.87 *)	15.4 mo vs. 11.1 mo (HR 0.71) [10]				
JAVELIN Renal 101 [19]	Avelumab + axitinib vs. sunitinib	HR 0.83 *		HR 0.80 *	13.8 mo vs. 7.0 mo (HR 0.62)		13.3 mo vs. 8.0 mo (HR 0.69)	5.6% vs. 2.4%	1% vs. 1%	55.9% vs. 27.2%	47.1% vs. 27.3%
IMmotion151 [20]	Atezolizumab + bevacizumab vs. sunitinib	HR 0.84		HR 0.93 *	11.2 mo vs. 7.7 mo (HR 0.74)	11.2 mo vs. 9.5 mo (HR 0.89 *)		9% vs. 4%	3% vs. 1%	43% vs. 35%	33% vs. 32%
CheckMate 025 [6]	Nivolumab vs. everolimus	21.8 mo vs. 18.8 mo (HR 0.79 *)	27.4 mo vs. 21.2 mo (HR 0.77)				4.6 mo vs. 4.4 mo (HR 0.88 *)				

* reported HR is not statistically significant

Among patients with International Metastatic RCC Database Consortium (IMDC) favorable-risk disease, only 11% (11/115) of those treated with nivolumab plus ipilimumab and 12% (13/111) of those treated with sunitinib were PD-L1+ compared to 26% (100/384) and 29% (114/392) of patients with IMDC intermediate- and poor-risk disease [8]. Exploratory analysis according to PD-L1 expression was performed in the intermediate- and poor-risk patient population. The median PFS for PD-L1+ patients was 22.8 months with nivolumab plus ipilimumab versus 5.9 months with sunitinib (HR 0.46; 95% CI, 0.31–0.67), while the median PFS between nivolumab plus ipilimumab versus sunitinib was not significantly different among those who were PD-1L− (HR 1.00; 95% CI, 0.80–1.26). While overall survival was significantly longer with nivolumab plus ipilimumab versus sunitinib in both the PD-L1+ and negative groups, the degree of improvement in overall survival was greater in the PD-L1+ patients: HR 0.45 (95% CI, 0.29–0.71) in the PD-L1+ group and HR 0.73 (95% CI, 0.56–0.96) in the PD-L1− population. Additionally, the difference in ORR between nivolumab plus ipilimumab versus sunitinib was numerically higher in the PD-L1+ group with ORR of 58% with nivolumab plus ipilimumab versus 22% with sunitinib ($p < 0.001$), compared with 37% versus 28% ($p = 0.03$) in the PD-L1− group. Complete responses were also more frequent in the PD-L1+ group with 16% CR with nivolumab plus ipilimumab versus 1% with sunitinib, compared to 7% and 1% among respective PD-L1− patients. Thus, PD-L1 expression enriches for clinical benefit with combination nivolumab plus ipilimumab but cannot be used as a predictive biomarker given the significant benefit observed in the PD-L1− group.

The role of PD-L1 expression has also been explored in combinations of anti-VEGF therapy with immunotherapy. IMmotion150, a randomized phase II trial, investigated the clinical activity of atezolizumab with or without bevacizumab against sunitinib in patients with treatment-naive mRCC [21]. This trial included numerous ancillary biomarker investigations, including PD-L1 expression. Co-primary end points were PFS in both the ITT and in the PD-L1+ patient populations. PD-L1 was measured using the Ventana SP142 IHC assay, and PD-L1 was considered positive if >1% tumor-infiltrating immune cells (ICs) expressed PD-L1. The percentage of patients considered PD-L1+ among the three treatment groups were 59% sunitinib, 52% atezolizumab, and 50% atezolizumab + bevacizumab. The initial stratification was based on PD-L1 status of >5% (instead of >1%), which is thought to explain some of the imbalance among the treatment arms. The median PFS in the PD-L1+ population was 14.7 months with atezolizumab + bevacizumab versus 7.8 months with sunitinib (HR 0.64; 95% CI, 0.38–1.08), while the median PFS in the ITT population was 11.7 months with atezolizumab + bevacizumab versus 8.4 months with sunitinib (HR 1.00; 95% CI, 0.69–1.45). Furthermore, the hazard ratios for improvement in PFS were numerically improved with increasing levels of PD-L1 expression among patients treated with atezolizumab plus bevacizumab. Thus, PD-L1 expression enriched for response to this combination, although the overall activity of this regimen is lower compared to other immunotherapy-based doublets in mRCC.

The randomized phase III trial, IMmotion 151 further explored these findings. IMmotion151 enrolled patients with clear cell or sarcomatoid histology randomized to atezolizumab plus bevacizumab versus sunitinib [20]. Co-primary end points included investigator assessed progression-free survival in PD-L1+ patients and overall survival in the intention-to-treat population. PD-L1 was measured using the Ventana SP142 IHC assay, and PD-L1 was considered positive if >1% tumor-infiltrating immune cells (ICs) expressed PD-L1. Among patients in the PD-L1+ subset, median PFS was 11.2 months in the atezolizumab plus bevacizumab arm compared with 7.7 months in the sunitinib arm; HR 0.74 (95 CI 0.57–0.96; $p = 0.0217$). Similar to IMmotion 150, the HRs for PFS were numerically improved with increasing levels of PD-L1 expression. However, overall survival in the ITT population did not cross the prespecified significance boundary, with median overall survival HR 0.93 (0.76–1.14; $p = 0.4751$) at interim analysis. The HR for median overall survival in the PD-L1+ patients was 0.84 (0.62–1.15; $p = 0.2857$). ORR was 43% (76/178) in the PD-L1+ atezolizumab plus bevacizumab group compared to 35% (64/184) in the PD-L1+ sunitinib group, per investigator assessment. This difference was not seen among the PD-L1- group; 33% (90/276) for atezolizumab plus bevacizumab versus 32% (89/276) for sunitinib. For investigator assessed PD-L1+ patients, CR was 9% with atezolizumab plus bevacizumab vs. 4% with sunitinib, while CR was only 3% and 1% in the respective PD-L1− groups.

In the phase III KEYNOTE-426 trial [9], in which the combination pembrolizumab plus axitinib was compared to sunitinib, PD-L1 expression was not incorporated into the primary endpoint; however, PD-L1 expression was tested and reported in the exploratory analysis. Expression was assessed using the PD-L1 IHC 22C3 pharmDx assay (Agilent Technologies) and was calculated using the combined positive score [CPS; calculated as the number of PD-L1+ cells (tumor cells, lymphocytes, and macrophages) divided by the total number of tumor cells, multiplied by 100]. Seventy-seven percent of patients (822/1062) had tumor samples evaluable for PD-L1 expression, and of these 60.5% had a combined positive score >1. The 12-month OS rates among PD-L1+ patients were 90.1% with pembrolizumab plus axitinib and 78.4% with sunitinib (HR 0.54, 95% CI, 0.34–0.84). In the PD-L1− group the 12-month OS rates were 91.5% versus 78.3% respectively (HR 0.59, 95% CI 0.34–1.02). The median PFS among PD-L1+ patients was 15.3 months with pembrolizumab plus axitinib versus 8.9 months with sunitinib (HR 0.62, 95% CI 0.47–0.80), and in the PD-L1- group median PFS was 15.0 months versus 12.5 months (HR 0.87, 95% CI 0.62–1.23). Given marked benefit in both PD-L1+ and PD-L1− patients over sunitinib, there was no signal for use of PD-L1 expression as a predictive biomarker for treatment with pembrolizumab plus axitinib. However, it is notable that the poor prognostic association of PD-L1 expression with sunitinib was not observed in this study as had been shown previously, with 12 months OS 78.4% in the PD-L1+ patients and 78.3% in those who were PD-L1−. This difference may be at least partly explained by the use of a different assay and different methodology, namely the combined positive score, for determining PD-L1 expression.

The phase III JAVELIN Renal 101 trial, evaluating the combination avelumab plus axitinib versus sunitinib, incorporated PD-L1 expression into the combined primary endpoints of PFS and OS among PD-L1+ patients [11]. Expression was considered positive if >1% of immune cells were positive within the sampled tumor area as assessed by the Ventana PD-L1 SP263 assay (Ventana Medical Systems). Similar to the KEYNOTE-426 trial, JAVELIN Renal 101 also had a large number (69%, 560/812) of patients with evaluable samples positive for PD-L1. With a median follow-up of at least 13 months, PD-L1+ patients had a median PFS of 13.8 months with avelumab plus axitinib versus 7.0 months with sunitinib (HR 0.62, 95% CI 0.49–0.77) compared with 13.3 months versus 8.0 months (HR 0.69, 95% CI, 0.57–0.83) in the ITT group [19]. The overall CR rate was 3.8% with the combination avelumab plus axitinib, and 15 of these 17 patients with CR were PD-L1+. The CR rate was only 2.0% overall in the sunitinib group. Interestingly, the majority of these patients (7/9) were also PD-L1+. A new analysis of JAVELIN Renal 101 reassessed PD-L1 expression using the percentage of tumor cell positivity and found only 27% (218/812) of patients had expression >1% [22], and by using this approach 92% (196/212) would have also been considered positive using the immune cell algorithm. While there was no difference in PFS among the avelumab plus axitinib group (HR 0.89; 95% CI 0.65–1.22), PFS was shorter among PD-L1+ patients in the sunitinib arm (HR 1.57; 95% CI 1.16–2.14). Increasing the expression cutoff to 5%, 10%, and 25% did not lead to statistical difference among the avelumab plus axitinib group. Similar to KEYNOTE-426, PD-L1 status alone does not appear to predict response to immunotherapy in combination with axitinib.

One of the biggest drawbacks for PD-L1 as a predictive biomarker, is the variety of available tests and different methodologies for determining positivity. New biomarker analysis from CheckMate 214 presented at ASCO 2020 compared the previously reported PD-L1 expression data as defined using tumor cell expression >1% to the combined positive score [23]. Most notably, the percentage of patients determined to be PD-L1+ increased from 23% (113/498) to 61% (298/487) in the nivolumab plus ipilimumab group and from 25% (125/494) to 60% (298/493) in the sunitinib group, comparable to KEYNOTE-426 and JAVELIN Renal 101. The combination nivolumab plus ipilimumab significantly improved OS compared to sunitinib in both PD-L1+ and PD-L1− patients regardless of which test was used. However, stratified overall survival within the nivolumab plus ipilimumab group by PD-L1 combined positive score was not reported. Therefore, it remains unclear at this time whether the enrichment for response seen with PD-L1 expression (as initially reported using >1% positive tumor cells) remains using the combined positive score with this immunotherapy combination.

3. Tumor Mutational Burden

Tumor mutational burden (TMB) has been theorized to predict response to immunotherapy given increased formation of neoantigens on the tumor surface which lead to enhanced immunogenicity [24]. In June of 2020, the FDA announced a tumor-agnostic approval for pembrolizumab in patients whose tumors harbor TMB > 10 mutations per megabase (muts/Mb) [25], though the utility of TMB for predicting response to immunotherapy in RCC remains unproven.

Genomic profiling on over 1600 tumor samples from a variety of solid tumor types was performed using the MSK-IMPACT assay to examine the association between TMB and response to immunotherapy [26,27]. Given the heterogeneity of TMB between different histologies [28], TMB was analyzed using pre-specified cutoff percentages within each histology. Using a binary cutoff of 20%, a significant improvement in OS was observed across the entire cohort; HR 0.061 ($p = 1.3 \times 10^{-7}$). Patients with RCC made up 9% ($N = 151$) of the cohort. When limiting the analysis to this subgroup, no significant difference was found in OS between the patients in the top 20% of TMB and those below (cutoff 5.9 muts/Mb), HR 0.569. Using a more stringent cutoff of 10% (7.9 muts/Mb) or a more inclusive cutoff of 30% (cutoff 4.9 muts/Mb), a difference in OS was still not found.

Numerous retrospective analyses in RCC evaluating TMB have since been conducted with little to no association found. Labriola et al. evaluated 34 patients with mRCC treated with immunotherapy (32 with nivolumab, 2 with nivolumab plus ipilimumab, and 1 with pembrolizumab) who underwent genomic profiling with the PGDx elio panel [29]. Patients were grouped as either progressive disease or disease control (defined as stable disease or partial response). There was no significant difference observed in the TMB score between the two groups ($p = 0.7682$), with a mean TMB of 3.01 muts/Mb among the progressive disease group versus 2.63 muts/Mb in the disease control group. There were three patients who had a TMB score > 10 muts/Mb; two had progressive disease and one was in the disease control group.

Wood et al. examined a cohort of 431 patients with melanoma, non-small cell lung cancer, and RCC who had publicly available whole exome sequencing [30]. They determined TMB status based on consensus calls in DNA variants. Overall survival data was available for 56 patients with RCC, 50 of whom had reported response data available (excluding combination immunotherapy). Separating patients into two binary groups: TMB high (defined as those exceeding the disease-matched 80th percentile) and TMB low, there was no significant difference in overall survival ($p > 0.05$). Using logistic regression to evaluate for response probability and TMB, they found that TMB was a partial predictor of response in melanoma and non-small cell lung cancer but they found no significant difference among patients with RCC ($p = 0.894$).

Dizman et al. evaluated 91 patients at the City of Hope Comprehensive Cancer Center with mRCC who had undergone genomic profiling with DNA whole exome sequencing and RNA next-generation sequencing using the GEM ExTra assay [31]. Only patients whose genomic profiling was performed prior to initiation of systemic treatment were included for analysis. One cohort of patients were treated with immunotherapy ($N = 32$) and the other with VEGF-TKI therapy ($N = 43$). Eleven patietns (34%) patients in the immunotherapy cohort were treated with first-line nivolumab plus ipilimumab, while the remaining patients were treated with nivolumab monotherapy in either the second- or third-line settings. Patients were defined as with clinical benefit if they achieved complete or partial response of any duration or stable disease for at least six months. Overall, the median TMB was low at 1.2 muts/Mb (range 0.03–4.0) and no significant difference was seen between patients with clinical benefit versus no clinical benefit in either the immunotherapy cohort ($p = 0.82$) or the VEGF-TKI cohort ($p = 0.091$).

Braun et al. performed extensive genomic analyses on tumor samples from patients enrolled on the randomized phase III CheckMate 025 trial, treated with nivolumab monotherapy or the mTOR inhibitor everolimus and on the phase II CheckMate 010 trial [32]. The data were combined with existing whole exome sequencing and RNA-seq data from CheckMate 009 [33]. Whole exome sequencing data was available for 261 patients treated with nivolumab and 193 patients treated with everolimus. Clinical benefit was defined as having complete or partial response or stable disease with tumor shrinkage and PFS of at least six months, and they calculated TMB as the calculated sum of all non-synonymous mutations in each sample. No differences were observed in the total mutation burden between the clinical benefit group ($N = 78$) and the no clinical benefit group ($N = 95$); $p = 0.81$.

Interestingly, Huang et al. performed analysis on available somatic mutation data and transcriptome profiles from patients with clear cell RCC in the TCGA cohort ($N = 537$) [34]. TMB was defined as the total number of variants divided by the whole length of exons, 38 million (including base substitutions, deletions, and insertions). Pearson correlation analysis was used to evaluate expression of PD-1, PD-L1, and CTLA-4 with TMB. While no significant association was found between TMB and CTLA-4 ($p = 0.270$) or PD-1 ($p = 0.493$), a significant negative correlation between TMB and PD-L1 expression was determined ($R = -1.51$ and $p = 0.006$). Analysis from CheckMate 214 presented at ASCO 2020, showed no difference in PFS or OS between high TMB and low TMB within either the nivolumab plus ipilimumab arm or in the sunitinib arm [23], and recently published data from JAVELIN Renal 101 showed that TMB did not differentiate PFS in either the avelumab plus axitinib group (HR 1.09; 95% CI 0.79–1.50) or in the sunitinib group (HR 0.79; 95% CI 0.60–1.05 [22]. Overall, despite recent tumor-agnostic FDA approval for immunotherapy in tumors with TMB > 10 muts/Mb [25], TMB does not appear to reliably predict response in mRCC.

4. RNA Gene Expression

Gene expression profiling using RNA sequencing was evaluated in several randomized control trials (Table 2). McDermott et al. conducted pre-specified exploratory genomic analysis of IMmotion 150, the phase 2 trial of atezolizumab + bevacizumab versus sunitinib, and atezolizumab monotherapy versus sunitinib [21]. Gene expression analysis was performed by generating whole transcriptome profiles for 263 patients using RNA sequencing, TruSeq RNA Access (Illumina). Gene expression signatures previously found to be associated with angiogenesis (*VEGFA, KDR, ESM1, PECAM1, ANGPTL4,* and *CD34*), immune activation (*CD8A, EOMES, PRF1, IFNG,* and *CD274*), and myeloid inflammation (*IL-6, CXCL1, CXCL2, CXCL3, CXCL8,* and *PTGS2*) were used to group patients into high and low expression categories for each signature, separated by the median expression score derived for each group [35–41]. They found that the Angio^{High} subgroup had increased vascular density as determined by CD31 IHC, and that the Teff^{High} subgroup was associated with increased expression of PD-L1 on immune cells by IHC and with increased CD8+ T-cell infiltration.

Table 2. Gene expression signatures evaluated from randomized controlled trials in mRCC.

Biomarker	Trial	Patient Population	Key Findings
IMmotion 150 Angio Signature (*VEGFA, KDR, ESM1, PECAM1, ANGPTL4, CD34*)	CheckMate 214 [23]	Within sunitinib arm	Improved PFS among Angio^{High} (0.58)
	IMmotion150 [21]	Within sunitinib arm	ORR Angio^{High} 46% vs. Angio^{Low} 9%
		Atezolizumab + bevacizumab vs. sunitinib	Improved PFS among Angio^{Low} with atezolizumab + bevacizumab (HR 0.59)
	IMmotion151 [42]	Within sunitinib arm	Improved PFS among Angio^{High} (0.59)
		Atezolizumab + bevacizumab vs. sunitinib	Improved PFS among Angio^{Low} with atezolizumab + bevacizumab (HR 0.68)
	JAVELIN Renal 101 [22,43]	Within sunitinib arm	Improved PFS among Angio^{High} (0.64)
		Avelumab + axitinib vs. sunitinib	Improved PFS among Angio^{Low} with avelumab + axitinib

Table 2. *Cont.*

Biomarker	Trial	Patient Population	Key Findings
IMmotion 150 Teff Signature (*CD8A, EOMES, PRF1, IFNG, CD274*)	CheckMate 214 [23]	Within sunitinib arm	No difference in OS or PFS
		Within ipilimumab + nivolumab arm	No difference in OS or PFS
	IMmotion150 [21]	Within atezolizumab + bevacizumab	ORR T_{eff}^{High} 49% vs. T_{eff}^{Low} 16%
		Atezolizumab + bevacizumab vs. sunitinib	Improved PFS among $Teff^{high}$ with atezolizumab + bevacizumab (HR 0.55)
	IMmotion151 [42]	Atezolizumab + bevacizumab vs. sunitinib	Improved PFS among $Teff^{high}$ PFS with atezolizumab + bevacizumab (HR 0.76)
	JAVELIN Renal 101 [22]	Within avelumab + axitinib	Trend toward improved PFS among $Teff^{high}$ (HR 0.79, 95% CI 0.58-1.08)
		Within sunitinib arm	No difference in PFS
IMmotion 150 Myeloid Signature (*IL6, CXCL1, CXCL2, CXCL3, CXCL8, PTGS2*)	CheckMate 214 [23]	Within sunitinib arm	No difference in OS or PFS
		Within ipilimumab + nivolumab arm	No difference in OS or PFS
	IMmotion150 [21]	Within atezolizumab arm	Reduced PFS among $Myeloid^{High}$ (HR 2.98)
		Within atezolizumab + bevacizumab arm	Reduced PFS among $Myeloid^{High}$ (HR 1.71)
		Atezolizumab vs. sunitinib	Reduced PFS among $Myeloid^{High}$ with atezolizumab (HR 2.03)
		Atezolizumab + bevacizumab vs. sunitinib	No difference in PFS
	JAVELIN Renal 101 [22]	Within sunitinib arm	No difference in PFS
		Within avelumab + axitinib arm	No difference in PFS
IMmotion 150 $Myeloid^{high}$ vs. $Myeloid^{low}$ in $Teff^{high}$	CheckMate 214 [23]	Within sunitinib arm	No difference in OS or PFS
		Within ipilimumab + nivolumab arm	No difference in OS or PFS
	IMmotion150 [21]	Within atezolizumab arm	Reduced PFS among $Teff^{High}Myeloid^{High}$ (HR 3.82)
		Atezolizumab vs. atezolizumab + bevacizumab	Improved PFS among $Teff^{High}Myeloid^{High}$ with atezolizumab + bevacizumab (HR 0.25)
	JAVELIN Renal 101 [22]	Within sunitinib arm	No difference in PFS
		Within avelumab + axitinib arm	No difference in PFS
JAVELIN Renal 101 Immuno (*CD3G, CD3E, CD8B, THEMIS, TRAT1, GRAP2, CD247, CD2, CD96, PRF1, CD6, IL7R, ITK, GPR18, EOMES, SIT1, NLRC3, CD244, KLRD1, SH2D1A, CCL5, XCL2, CST7, GFI1, KCNA3, PSTPIP1*)	CheckMate 214 [23]	Within sunitinib arm	No difference in OS or PFS
		Within ipilimumab + nivolumab arm	No difference in OS or PFS
	JAVELIN Renal 101 [22]	Within avelumab + axitinib	Improved PFS among $Immuno^{high}$ with avelumab + axitinib (HR 0.60)
		Within sunitinib arm	No difference in OS or PFS

Table 2. *Cont.*

Biomarker	Trial	Patient Population	Key Findings
Tumor Inflammation Signature (*PSMB10, HLA-DQA1, HLA-DRB1, CMKLR1, HLA-E, NKG7, CD8A, CCL5, CXCL9, CD27, CXCR6, IDO1, STAT1, TIGIT, LAG3, CD274, PDCD1LG2, CD276*)	CheckMate 214 [23]	Within sunitinib arm	No difference in OS or PFS
		Within ipilimumab + nivolumab arm	No difference in OS or PFS

When evaluated within the sunitinib treatment arm, high angiogenesis gene expression was associated with improved overall response (46% in Angio^{High} versus 9% in Angio^{Low}) and PFS (HR 0.31; 95% CI, 0.18–0.55). While there was no difference in PFS among patients within the Angio^{High} subgroup, whether evaluated between atezolizumab plus bevacizumab versus sunitinib or between atezolizumab monotherapy versus sunitinib, there was an improvement in PFS observed among patients in the Angio^{Low} subgroup who were treated with atezolizumab plus bevacizumab versus sunitinib (HR 0.59; 95% CI, 0.35–0.98).

Within the atezolizumab plus bevacizumab arm, high immune gene expression was associated with improved overall response (49% in Teff^{High} versus 16% in Teff^{Low}) and PFS (HR 0.50; 95% CI, 0.30–0.86). Additionally, when evaluated across treatment arms, Teff^{High} was associated with longer PFS with atezolizumab plus bevacizumab versus sunitinib (HR 0.55; 95% CI, 0.32–0.95).

High expression of genes involved in myeloid inflammation was associated with reduced PFS within the atezolizumab monotherapy arm (HR 2.98; 95% CI, 1.68–5.29) but not within the sunitinib arm. To further investigate the impact of myeloid inflammation and response to immunotherapy, the investigators examined the subgroup of patients with Teff^{High} and Myeloid^{High} tumors. Within this subgroup, patients treated with atezolizumab plus bevacizumab showed improved PFS versus those treated with atezolizumab alone (HR 0.25; 95% CI, 0.10–0.60). Interestingly, among patients in the Teff^{High}Myeloid^{Low} subgroup, no significant differences were seen between the atezolizumab plus bevacizumab arm and the atezolizumab monotherapy arm. Overall, while these findings require further validation, they suggest that the addition of anti-VEGF treatment to immunotherapy, may help mediate some of the immunosuppressive effects of myeloid inflammation and may provide further insight into the efficacy of other anti-VEGF plus immunotherapy combinations, such as pembrolizumab or avelumab in combination with axitinib. Additionally, they support that expression of angiogenesis genes increase tumor susceptibility to sunitinib and that immune gene expression is associated with response to immunotherapy.

These genomic profiles were further validated in the prospective randomized phase III clinical trial, IMmotion151 and presented at ESMO 2018 [42]. RNA sequencing was performed on 823 patients. Patients with Teff^{High} had improved PFS with atezolizumab plus bevacizumab compared to sunitinib (HR, 0.76; 95% CI 0.59–0.99). While Angio^{High} was associated with improved PFS within the sunitinib arm (HR, 0.59; CI 0.47–0.75), there was no significant difference in PFS across treatment arms. Notably, Angio^{High} expression was more prevalent among patients with favorable risk as compared with intermediate/poor-risk, and Teff^{High} was more frequent among patients in the intermediate/poor-risk group, providing a biologic correlate of the differential clinical effects observed in CheckMate 214.

RNA expression profiling was also prospectively evaluated in the phase III clinical trial JAVELIN Renal 101 [11,22,43]. Researchers created whole transcriptome profiles using RNA sequencing on 720 baseline tumor samples and developed a new gene expression signature, Renal 101 Immuno, derived from 26 genes involved in T-cell proliferation, natural killer cell activation, interferon gamma signaling, and others. Using this signature, patients treated with avelumab plus axitinib who had high levels of expression (at or above the median level of expression) had significantly longer PFS compared with patients with low levels of expression (HR, 0.60; 95% CI, 0.44–0.83). Evaluating this signature in an independent dataset from the phase 1b JAVELIN 100 trial [44], high expression was again associated with prolonged PFS (HR 0.36; 95% CI 0.16–0.81). Using the gene expression signatures from the previous IMmotion studies, they also showed that the Angio^{High} signature was again associated with improved PFS within the sunitinib arm but was not significantly different between the avelumab + axitinib arm versus the sunitinib arm. Among patients with Angio^{Low} gene expression, PFS was significantly longer in the avelumab + axitinib arm compared with sunitinib. These data reinforce data from IMmotion 150 that Angio^{low} patients have better outcome with an immunotherapy-based regimen versus sunitinib monotherapy.

The RNA expression profiles from IMmotion150 and JAVELIN Renal 101 were further examined in a pooled analysis of available data from CheckMate 009, 010, and 025 [32]; however, no associations between high expression of any gene signature and improved clinical benefit, PFS, or OS were observed. One potential explanation for this difference is that the majority of patients included were treated with nivolumab in the second-line setting after prior anti-VEGF therapy, whereas patients in both IMmotion studies and JAVELIN Renal 101 were treatment-naïve. A multicenter retrospective analysis of 86 patients with mRCC treated with immunotherapy evaluated both a large T-effector gene panel and a smaller 5-Gene panel (*FOXP3*, *CCR4*, *KLRK1*, *ITK*, and *TIGIT*) [45]. While there was no difference observed between high and low expression of the larger T-effector panel, there was a significant difference in the ORR between the cohort with high 5-Gene expression versus low [31% (14/45) versus 2% (1/41); $p = 0.001$].

Biomarker data from CheckMate 214 presented at ASCO 2020 also reported the breakdown of six different gene expression signatures [23]. Twenty percent (109/550) of patients in the nivolumab plus ipilimumab arm and 19% (104/546) of patients in the sunitinib arm had tumor tissue evaluable to perform RNA sequencing. While Angio^{High} score (as per IMmotion150) was significantly associated with improved PFS within the sunitinib arm, no other observed significant differences were observed between the remaining gene expression signatures. Of note, this was the first reported study to evaluate these signatures with the use of an anti-CTLA-4 agent in combination with anti-PD-1; additionally, the percentage of patients with tumor evaluable for testing was low. However, when dichotomizing patients to PFS < 18 months versus > 18 months, they found differences in several HALLMARK [46] gene signatures: TNFalpha signaling via NFkB, epithelial mesenchymal transition, and inflammatory response. Gene expression signatures have successfully defined several subtypes of RCC related to varying degrees of immune involvement and angiogenesis; however, these signatures require further prospective validation prior to clinical use as predictive biomarkers.

5. *Polybromo-1* Mutations

In addition to mutations in the *von Hippel-Lindau* (*VHL*) gene, the pathogenesis of clear cell RCC includes a several secondary mutations including in *Polybromo-1* (*PBRM-1*), which has recently been implicated as a potential biomarker for immunotherapy [47]. Whole exome sequencing was performed to analyze pre-treatment tumor samples from 35 patients with mRCC treated with nivolumab on the prospective open-label phase I study, CA209-009 [33]. Patients were grouped into three different response categories for analysis: clinical benefit (patients with complete or partial response along with patients with stable disease if they had any objective reduction in tumor size lasting at least six months), no clinical benefit (patients with progressive disease leading to treatment discontinuation within three months), and intermediate benefit (patients who did not fit into the clinical benefit or no clinical benefit categories).

Truncating or loss of function mutations in *PBRM1* were more frequent in the clinical benefit group (9/11) compared with the no clinical benefit group (3/13, $p = 0.012$) with an odds ratio for clinical benefit of 12.93 (95% CI 1.54–190.8). OS and PFS were both significantly improved in patients with *PBRM1* loss of function ($N = 19$) compared to those with *PBRM1* intact ($N = 16$); $p = 0.0074$ and $p = 0.29$ respectively. They also evaluated *PBRM1* loss of function in an additional 63 patients who were treated with anti-PD-1(L1) therapy either alone or in combination with anti-CTLA-4 therapy. Again, tumors from patients deriving clinical benefit were more likely to harbor loss of function mutations in *PBRM1* (17/27) compared to those with *PBRM1* intact (4/19, $p = 0.0071$) with an odds ratio for clinical benefit of 6.10 (95% CI 1.42–32.64).

Braun et al. sought to validate these findings using archival tumor tissue from patients treated with nivolumab or everolimus from the randomized phase III trial, CheckMate 025 [48]. Of note, archival specimens were obtained prior to any treatment (including anti-VEGF therapy.) *PBRM1* mutations were identified in 29% (55/189) treated with nivolumab and in 23% (45/193) of patients who received everolimus. Among those treated with nivolumab, *PBRM1* mutations were present in 39% (15/38) of responding patients (either complete or partial response) compared to 22% (16/74) of non-responding patients (odds ratio 2.34, $p = 0.04$). Overall survival (HR, 0.65; $p = 0.03$) and progression-free survival (HR, 0.067; $p = 0.03$) were both associated with the presence of *PBRM1* mutations. However, among those treated with everolimus there was no significant difference between responders who harbored *PBRM1* mutations (1/5) and non-responders who harbored *PBRM1* mutations (10/56; $p = 0.64$). There was no significant association of *PBRM1* mutation with OS (HR, 0.81; $p = 0.27$) or PFS (HR 0.83; $p = 0.32$) among those treated with everolimus.

The association of *PBRM1* mutations with anti-PD-1 therapy was further investigated using pooled data from patients treated with nivolumab in either CheckMate-009, CheckMate-010, or CheckMate-025 who underwent whole exome sequencing [32]. Collectively, there was a significant benefit in OS and PFS for patients harboring *PBRM1* mutations ($p < 0.001$ and $p = 0.0056$ respectively). They also evaluated the presence of *PBRM1* mutations along with the degree of T-cell infiltration present in the tumor. Using CD8 immunofluorescence on 153 tumor samples from nivolumab treated patients, they quantified the density of CD8+ cells in the tumor center and at the tumor margin. Tumors were classified as "immune excluded" if at least five-fold more CD8+ cells were present in the tumor margin compared to the tumor center, "immune desert" if they were not "excluded" but still had below the 25th percentile of CD8+ cells in the tumor center, and "immune infiltrate" if they were not "excluded" and had greater than the 25th percentile of CD8+ cells in the tumor center. The majority (73%) of samples were classified as "immune infiltrated." While there was no significant association between the degree of tumor infiltration and clinical benefit, there was an association observed between the presence of *PBRM1* mutations and lower T-cell infiltration ($p = 0.013$). *PBRM1* mutations were detected in 47% of immune "deserts" and 29% of immune "excluded" tumors, but only 22% of immune "infiltrated' tumors ($p = 0.01$ for non-infiltrated versus infiltrated tumors).

However, there are also data to suggest that *PBRM1* mutations are associated with an immunosuppressive and pro-angiogenesis tumor microenvironment. Using a murine model, Liu et al. observed that *PBRM1* inactivation was associated with a less immunogenic tumor microenvironment, which was validated using human gene expression data from the TCGA-KIRC dataset [49]. The IMmotion150 dataset [21] was also analyzed, showing that patients with *PBRM1* mutations had a significantly lower ORR with both atezolizumab monotherapy and atezolizumab plus bevacizumab. Gene expression data from IMmotion150, TCGA, and the International Cancer Genome Consortium showed increased angiogenesis signatures among patients with *PBRM1* mutations from all three cohorts [49]. Clinical data from mRCC patients with pancreatic metastases demonstrated *PBRM1* mutations were associated with improved response to anti-VEGF therapy, supporting that *PBRM1* mutant tumors may have a more angiogenic phenotype [50]. Additionally, biomarker data from CheckMate 214 presented at ASCO 2020 showed no significant difference in PFS or OS between *PBRM1* wild type or mutant within either the nivolumab plus ipilimumab arm or in the sunitinib arm [23]. Furthermore, analysis from JAVELIN Renal 101 showed no association of *PBRM1* with PFS in either treatment arm [22]. Given conflicting results from multiple analyses, *PBRM1* mutations are not ready for clinical use as a predictive biomarker and require further investigation to understand their role in the tumor microenvironment. Some of the discrepant results may be due to the different populations studied, such as treatment-naïve versus VEGF-refractory.

6. Human Endogenous Retroviruses

Human endogenous retroviruses (hERVs) represent a group of long terminal repeat retrotransposons that collectively make up about 8% of the human genome [51,52]. Despite being normally silenced in somatic tissue, their expression has been reported in multiple cancer types, including RCC [53]. Aberrant transcriptional activation of hERVs has been theorized to induce an antitumor immune response and up-regulation of immune checkpoint pathways, increasing sensitivity to immunotherapy [54].

Using a cohort of 24 mRCC patients, Panda et al. used RNA sequencing to investigate an association of hERV expression and response to single agent PD-1(L1) therapy [54]. The RNA level of *ERV3-2* was measured using real-time quantitative PCRs (RT-qPCRs) with two independent primers. Regardless of which primer was used, they found that *ERV3-2* expression was significantly higher in responders compared with non-responders. Patients were also classified as either *ERV3-2* high or low based on an optimal cutoff derived from the receiver operating characteristic curves. *ERV3-2* high patients were significantly more likely to respond and had significantly longer PFS.

Post-hoc analysis from patients treated with nivolumab on CheckMate 010 was performed using RT-qPCR on 99 formalin-fixed paraffin-embedded tissue (FFPE) pretreatment tumors to determine expression levels of pan-*ERVE4*, pan-*ERV3.2*, *hERV4700 GAG* or *ENV*, and the reference genes *18S* and *HPRT1* [55]. Patients were dichotomized as high or low expression using the 25th percentile as the cutoff. Using this cutoff, only *hERV4700 ENV* was significantly associated with PFS and response. PFS was 7.0 months among the high-*hERV4700 ENV* group versus 2.6 months among the low expression group ($p = 0.010$), and the ORR for high-*hERV4700 ENV* was 35.6% versus 12.5% ($p = 0.036$).

Using pooled data from CheckMate 009, CheckMate 010, and CheckMate 025, Braun et al. found that hERV expression determined using RNA sequencing correlated with expression obtained by RT-qPCR; however, the authors note that *ERV3-2* expression was not reliably inferred using this technique, which highlights a potential limitation of using RNA sequencing to measure hERV expression in FFPE tissue [32]. Despite this limitation, they did find two hERVs (*ERV2282* and *EVR3382*) that were weakly associated with response, PFS, and OS when using expression as a continuous variable; however, when divided into high and low expression (based on median expression of each hERV) these were no longer significant for both improved PFS and OS. hERV expression presents a relatively new candidate biomarker that requires further prospective validation as well as improved reproducibility of technique.

7. Gastrointestinal Microbiome

Recent studies have shown a link between the intestinal microbiome and cancer immunosurveillance, including a role in response to immunotherapy [56–58]. A small Japanese study evaluated 31 patients with mRCC treated with immunotherapy and retrospectively separated them by antibiotic use within 30 days of treatment or not [59]. The median PFS for patients treated with antibiotics ($N = 5$) was 2.8 months compared with 18.4 months ($p < 0.001$) in the group without antibiotics ($N = 26$). Subsequently, Lalani et al. performed a retrospective analysis on two cohorts to explore the association of antibiotic use and response to immunotherapy in mRCC: the first, a single center cohort of patients who received anti-PD-1(L1) therapy ($N = 146$), and the second, a trial-database from patients treated with interferon, anti-VEGF therapies, or mTOR inhibitors ($N = 4144$) [60]. Antibiotic use was defined as anytime from 8 weeks before the start of therapy through 4 weeks after initiation. In the anti-PD-1(L1) cohort, patients with antibiotic exposure ($N = 31$) had a significantly lower ORR (12.9% versus 34.8%, $p = 0.026$) and shorter PFS (HR, 1.96, 95% CI 1.20–3.20, $p = 0.007$) compared to the group without antibiotic exposure ($N = 115$). In the trial-database cohort ORR was significantly lower (19.3% versus 24.2%, $p = 0.005$), PFS significantly shorter (HR 1.16, 95% CI 1.04–1.30), and OS significantly shorter (HR 1.25, 95% CI 1.10–1.41) in the antibiotic group compared with the no antibiotic group. However, in subgroup analysis the authors note that the difference in the trial-database group was driven by patients treated with interferon ($N = 510$) and prior cytokine therapy ($N = 520$), while no difference in OS was observed between antibiotic users in either the anti-VEGF (no prior cytokines) group ($N = 2454$) or in the mTOR group ($N = 660$).

Baseline fecal samples were collected from patients with mRCC treated with nivolumab on the NIVOREN GETUG-AFU 26 phase 2 clinical trial to investigate the relationship between the microbiome and response to immunotherapy [61]. Patients were dichotomized by prior antibiotic exposure, namely those who had received antibiotics within the two months prior to treatment with nivolumab ($N = 11$) and those without prior antibiotic exposure ($N = 58$). The ORR was lower in the antibiotic group at 9% versus 28% in the group without prior antibiotics ($p < 0.03$). Median PFS and OS were also longer in the no antibiotic group (5 months and NR) compared with the antibiotic group (2 months and 25 months; $p = 0.03$ and $p = 0.04$). They subsequently performed analysis of the relative taxonomic abundance for prevalent fecal bacteria between the two groups and found overrepresentation of *Eubacterium rectale* ($p = 0.02$) in the no antibiotic group and overrepresentation of *Erysipelotrichaceae bacterium* and *Clostridium hathewayi* in the antibiotic group ($p < 0.02$).

Additionally, they separated the group without prior antibiotic exposure into responders ($N = 30$) and non-responders ($N = 28$) and compared the various taxonomical fecal bacterial profiles. Patients in the responder group were more likely to harbor overrepresentation of *Akkermansia muciniphila, Bacteroides salyersiae,* and *Eubacterium siraeum* compared with non-responders. Likewise, patients in the non-responder group were more likely to have overrepresentation of *Erysipelotrichaceae bacterium, Clostridium hathewayi,* and *Clostridium clostridioforme*.

Recently, Salgia et al. performed an observational study of 31 patients with mRCC treated with either nivolumab monotherapy (77%) or nivolumab plus ipilimumab (23%) and assessed the gut microbiota composition using metagenomic sequencing [62]. Of note, patients with antibiotic exposure within 14 days were excluded. Using the Shannon diversity index, greater microbial diversity was associated with clinical benefit ($p = 0.001$). Prospective and controlled studies are warranted to further explore and validate using the microbiome to predict response to immunotherapy, as well as to explore the role of alteration of the host microbiota to enhance therapeutic response.

8. Sarcomatoid Differentiation

Sarcomatoid differentiation, present in around 10% of patients with RCC, is associated with more aggressive clinical features, including shorter time to relapse, worse IMDC prognostic classification, and shortened PFS and OS with anti-VEGF therapies [63–65].

A comparison of 40 tumors with sarcomatoid histology present versus clear cell RCC without sarcomatoid features found that tumors with sarcomatoid histology were significantly more likely to have co-expression of PD-L1 on tumor cells and on tumor-infiltrating-lymphocytes [66], suggesting the potential for improved response to immunotherapy. In the IMmotion151 trial, 61% (86/142) of patients with sarcomatoid histology were positive for PD-L1 expression [67], and analysis presented at ESMO 2018 showed that tumors with sarcomatoid histology were more likely to be $\text{Angio}^{\text{Low}}$ and $\text{Teff}^{\text{High}}$ compared with non-sarcomatoid tumors [42]. The HR for PFS in the sarcomatoid subgroup was 0.45 (95% CI 0.26–0.77) in the PD-L1+ population and 0.52 (0.34–0.79) in the ITT population [67]. Given that PFS was improved in both the PD-L1+ and PD-L1− populations, sarcomatoid histology may be an independent predictor of response.

Post-hoc analysis of patients from CheckMate 214 identified sarcomatoid features in 16.4% (139/847) of patients with intermediate/poor-risk RCC [68]. Overall survival was significantly improved in this subgroup with nivolumab plus ipilimumab versus sunitinib (HR 0.45; 95% CI 0.3–0.7). The ORR was 60.8% with nivolumab plus ipilimumab versus 23.1% with sunitinib ($p < 0.0001$), and the CR rate was 18.9% versus 3.1% respectively. Of note, 52% (69/133) of patients with quantifiable PD-L1 expression were positive. Iacovelli et al. performed a meta-analysis of the four published phase III randomized combination immunotherapy clinical trials that included patients with sarcomatoid histology [69]. Collectively there were 467 patients included with sarcomatoid features present, 226 randomized to immunotherapy-based combination treatment and 241 randomized to sunitinib. Overall, PFS significantly favored treatment with immunotherapy-based combinations (HR 0.56; 95% CI, 0.43–0.71). Excluding JAVELIN Renal 101 (given OS data was not mature at time of analysis), OS also significantly favored treatment with immunotherapy-based combinations (HR 0.56; 95% CI 0.43–0.82). The ORR was 52.6% for combination therapy versus 20.7% with sunitinib, with CR rates of 11.5% and 0.8% respectively. Overall, this meta-analysis supports the use of immunotherapy-based combinations in the front-line setting for patients with mRCC with sarcomatoid features, although if a specific regimen has greater effect awaits further study. Additional work exploring the role of immunotherapy-based combinations in other distinct RCC histologies is necessary.

9. Neutrophil to Lymphocyte Ratio

The baseline neutrophil to lymphocyte ratio (NLR) has been shown to have a negative prognostic association with RCC and to predict a more aggressive phenotype [70–72]. While the poor prognostic association of PD-L1 expression appears to be mitigated by immunotherapy [8–10], this does not appear to be the case for NLR.

Zahoor et al. performed a retrospective analysis of 90 patients treated with nivolumab as second-line or later therapy for mRCC. After multivariate analysis, a higher baseline NLR was associated with an increased risk of progression (HR 1.86, 95% CI, 1.05–3.29) [73]. Additionally, Lalani et al. performed a retrospective review of 142 patients treated with anti-PD-1(L1) therapies and found that baseline NLRs were significantly higher in the poor IMDC risk group compared to those with favorable or intermediate risk ($p < 0.001$) [74]. Interestingly, the results indicate that the NLR between 4 to 8 weeks post treatment initiation was a more accurate predictor of response than at baseline, and an increase in NLR > 25% was associated with shorter PFS (HR 2.60, 95% CI 1.53–4.39).

Furthermore, exploratory analysis of the JAVELIN Renal 101 trial, presented at ASCO 2020, demonstrated significantly improved OS (HR 0.51; 95% CI 0.30–0.87) and a trend toward improved PFS (HR 0.85; 95% CI 0.63–1.15) among patients treated on the avelumab plus axitinib arm who had a baseline NLR < the median compared to patients with baseline NLR > the median [75]. While the overall differences between groups is somewhat modest, the ratio is cost-effective and easily performed in clinic without the need for additional testing. Additional prospective validation is needed for pre-treatment laboratory biomarkers such as NLR.

10. Conclusions

While immunotherapy-based combinations have become the standard of care for first-line mRCC, the majority of patients will eventually progress on these regimens. Additionally, immune-related adverse events can lead to serious toxicity and have the potential to be life-threatening [76]. Therefore, the ability to predict which patients are most likely to respond would have significant clinical impact. Despite tremendous investigation on numerous candidate biomarkers, none have yet proven ready for clinical practice.

PD-L1 expression has been shown to enrich for response, most notably in CheckMate 214; however, patients with negative expression can still respond and maintain the potential for complete response. Furthermore, the commercially available anti-PD-L1 clones currently in use are highly variable, and PD-L1 expression patterns have been shown to be heterogenous throughout different tumor regions [77]. Therefore, immunotherapy should not be withheld for patients who are known to be PD-L1−. New imaging modalities are being developed to quantify PD-1 and PD-L1, which may help reduce some of the variability in future studies [78,79]. TMB, while recently approved as a tumor-agnostic biomarker for response to pembrolizumab, has been shown to be an unreliable predictor in RCC and should not be used in clinical decision making for these patients.

Gene expression using RNA sequencing has generated new understanding into the biology of RCC and patterns of response to therapy. Improvement in PFS with atezolizumab plus bevacizumab were observed in both IMmotion150 and IMotion151 among $Teff^{High}$ patients; however, this improvement was not observed in updated analysis of CheckMate 214. Future prospective trials should incorporate pre-specified analyses of gene expression signatures to assess their potential for clinical utility.

Individual gene alterations, such as loss of function mutations in *PBRM1*, have demonstrated mixed results, and should not be used clinically at this time. Likewise, while antibiotic exposure has been associated with decreased response to immunotherapy, these data have yet to be prospectively validated and should neither prohibit patients who have recently required antibiotics from receiving immunotherapy nor should it limit clinicians' use of antibiotics for infected patients. Given the enhanced efficacy observed among patients with sarcomatoid differentiation, these patients should receive upfront immunotherapy-based combinations instead of VEGF-TKI alone when systemic therapy is warranted.

While data regarding the NLR as a predictive biomarker is limited and is impacted by the known poor prognostic associations in RCC. However, such peripheral blood biomarkers have the benefit of being cost-effective and readily available; continued efforts toward identifying laboratory biomarkers is warranted.

In addition to developing biomarkers associated with radiographic response, there are several other facets of clinical practice that may be improved with the addition of biomarkers. Biomarkers that predict durability may help identify patients who can safely discontinue therapy after achieving a clinical response, and biomarkers that predict immune-related adverse events may help determine which patients should be observed more closely and potentially for which immunotherapy should be avoided or limited. While some candidate biomarkers may only enrich for response, these insights also help with developing novel therapies and combinations which may lead to improved outcomes with immunotherapy.

Author Contributions: M.D.T. and B.I.R. performed data research, wrote, and edited this review. All authors have read and agreed to the published version of the manuscript.

References

1. Bray, F.; Ferlay, J.; Soerjomataram, I.; Siegel, R.L.; Torre, L.A.; Jemal, A. Global cancer statistics 2018: GLOBOCAN estimates of incidence and mortality worldwide for 36 cancers in 185 countries. *CA Cancer J. Clin.* **2018**, *68*, 394–424. [CrossRef] [PubMed]
2. Coppin, C.; Porzsolt, F.; Awa, A.; Kumpf, J.; Coldman, A.; Wilt, T. Immunotherapy for advanced renal cell cancer. *Cochrane Database Syst. Rev.* **2005**, CD001425. [CrossRef]
3. Klapper, J.A.; Downey, S.G.; Smith, F.O.; Yang, J.C.; Hughes, M.S.; Kammula, U.S.; Sherry, R.M.; Royal, R.E.; Steinberg, S.M.; Rosenberg, S. High-dose interleukin-2 for the treatment of metastatic renal cell carcinoma: A retrospective analysis of response and survival in patients treated in the surgery branch at the National Cancer Institute between 1986 and 2006. *Cancer* **2008**, *113*, 293–301. [CrossRef] [PubMed]
4. Mantia, C.M.; McDermott, D.F. Vascular endothelial growth factor and programmed death-1 pathway inhibitors in renal cell carcinoma. *Cancer* **2019**, *125*, 4148–4157. [CrossRef]
5. Rini, B.I.; Battle, D.; Figlin, R.A.; George, D.J.; Hammers, H.; Hutson, T.; Jonasch, E.; Joseph, R.W.; McDermott, D.F.; Motzer, R.J.; et al. The society for immunotherapy of cancer consensus statement on immunotherapy for the treatment of advanced renal cell carcinoma (RCC). *J. Immunother. Cancer* **2019**, *7*, 354. [CrossRef]
6. Motzer, R.J.; Escudier, B.; McDermott, D.F.; George, S.; Hammers, H.J.; Srinivas, S.; Tykodi, S.S.; Sosman, J.A.; Procopio, G.; Plimack, E.R.; et al. Nivolumab versus Everolimus in Advanced Renal-Cell Carcinoma. *N. Engl. J. Med.* **2015**, *373*, 1803–1813. [CrossRef]
7. Xu, J.X.; Maher, V.E.; Zhang, L.; Tang, S.; Sridhara, R.; Ibrahim, A.; Kim, G.; Pazdur, R. FDA Approval Summary: Nivolumab in Advanced Renal Cell Carcinoma After Anti-Angiogenic Therapy and Exploratory Predictive Biomarker Analysis. *Oncologist* **2017**, *22*, 311–317. [CrossRef]
8. Motzer, R.J.; Tannir, N.M.; McDermott, D.F.; Arén Frontera, O.; Melichar, B.; Choueiri, T.K.; Plimack, E.R.; Barthélémy, P.; Porta, C.; George, S.; et al. Nivolumab plus Ipilimumab versus Sunitinib in Advanced Renal-Cell Carcinoma. *N. Engl. J. Med.* **2018**, *378*, 1277–1290. [CrossRef]

9. Rini, B.I.; Plimack, E.R.; Stus, V.; Gafanov, R.; Hawkins, R.; Nosov, D.; Pouliot, F.; Alekseev, B.; Soulières, D.; Melichar, B.; et al. Pembrolizumab plus Axitinib versus Sunitinib for Advanced Renal-Cell Carcinoma. *N. Engl. J. Med.* **2019**, *380*, 1116–1127. [CrossRef]
10. Plimack, E.R.; Rini, B.I.; Stus, V.; Gafanov, R.; Waddell, T.; Nosov, D.; Pouliot, F.; Soulieres, D.; Melichar, B.; Vynnychenko, I.; et al. Pembrolizumab plus axitinib versus sunitinib as first-line therapy for advanced renal cell carcinoma (RCC): Updated analysis of KEYNOTE-426. *J. Clin. Oncol.* **2020**, *38*. [CrossRef]
11. Motzer, R.J.; Penkov, K.; Haanen, J.; Rini, B.; Albiges, L.; Campbell, M.T.; Venugopal, B.; Kollmannsberger, C.; Negrier, S.; Uemura, M.; et al. Avelumab plus Axitinib versus Sunitinib for Advanced Renal-Cell Carcinoma. *N. Engl. J. Med.* **2019**, *380*, 1103–1115. [CrossRef] [PubMed]
12. Thompson, R.H.; Gillett, M.D.; Cheville, J.C.; Lohse, C.M.; Dong, H.; Webster, W.S.; Krejci, K.G.; Lobo, J.R.; Sengupta, S.; Chen, L.; et al. Costimulatory B7-H1 in renal cell carcinoma patients: Indicator of tumor aggressiveness and potential therapeutic target. *Proc. Natl. Acad. Sci. USA* **2004**, *101*, 17174–17179. [CrossRef] [PubMed]
13. Thompson, R.H.; Gillett, M.D.; Cheville, J.C.; Lohse, C.M.; Dong, H.; Webster, W.S.; Chen, L.; Zincke, H.; Blute, M.L.; Leibovich, B.C.; et al. Costimulatory molecule B7-H1 in primary and metastatic clear cell renal cell carcinoma. *Cancer* **2005**, *104*, 2084–2091. [CrossRef] [PubMed]
14. Thompson, R.H.; Kuntz, S.M.; Leibovich, B.C.; Dong, H.; Lohse, C.M.; Webster, W.S.; Sengupta, S.; Frank, I.; Parker, A.S.; Zincke, H.; et al. Tumor B7-H1 is associated with poor prognosis in renal cell carcinoma patients with long-term follow-up. *Cancer Res.* **2006**, *66*, 3381–3385. [CrossRef] [PubMed]
15. Choueiri, T.K.; Figueroa, D.J.; Fay, A.P.; Signoretti, S.; Liu, Y.; Gagnon, R.; Deen, K.; Carpenter, C.; Benson, P.; Ho, T.H.; et al. Correlation of PD-L1 tumor expression and treatment outcomes in patients with renal cell carcinoma receiving sunitinib or pazopanib: Results from COMPARZ, a randomized controlled trial. *Clin. Cancer Res.* **2015**, *21*, 1071–1077. [CrossRef]
16. Topalian, S.L.; Hodi, F.S.; Brahmer, J.R.; Gettinger, S.N.; Smith, D.C.; McDermott, D.F.; Powderly, J.D.; Carvajal, R.D.; Sosman, J.A.; Atkins, M.B.; et al. Safety, activity, and immune correlates of anti-PD-1 antibody in cancer. *N. Engl. J. Med.* **2012**, *366*, 2443–2454. [CrossRef]
17. Choueiri, T.K.; Fishman, M.N.; Escudier, B.; McDermott, D.F.; Drake, C.G.; Kluger, H.; Stadler, W.M.; Perez-Gracia, J.L.; McNeel, D.G.; Curti, B.; et al. Immunomodulatory Activity of Nivolumab in Metastatic Renal Cell Carcinoma. *Clin. Cancer Res.* **2016**, *22*, 5461–5471. [CrossRef]
18. Motzer, R.J.; Rini, B.I.; McDermott, D.F.; Arén Frontera, O.; Hammers, H.J.; Carducci, M.A.; Salman, P.; Escudier, B.; Beuselinck, B.; Amin, A.; et al. Nivolumab plus ipilimumab versus sunitinib in first-line treatment for advanced renal cell carcinoma: Extended follow-up of efficacy and safety results from a randomised, controlled, phase 3 trial. *Lancet Oncol.* **2019**, *20*, 1370–1385. [CrossRef]
19. Choueiri, T.K.; Motzer, R.J.; Rini, B.I.; Haanen, J.; Campbell, M.T.; Venugopal, B.; Kollmannsberger, C.; Gravis-Mescam, G.; Uemura, M.; Lee, J.L.; et al. Updated efficacy results from the JAVELIN Renal 101 trial: First-line avelumab plus axitinib versus sunitinib in patients with advanced renal cell carcinoma. *Ann. Oncol.* **2020**, *31*, 1030–1039. [CrossRef]
20. Rini, B.I.; Powles, T.; Atkins, M.B.; Escudier, B.; McDermott, D.F.; Suarez, C.; Bracarda, S.; Stadler, W.M.; Donskov, F.; Lee, J.L.; et al. Atezolizumab plus bevacizumab versus sunitinib in patients with previously untreated metastatic renal cell carcinoma (IMmotion151): A multicentre, open-label, phase 3, randomised controlled trial. *Lancet* **2019**, *393*, 2404–2415. [CrossRef]
21. McDermott, D.F.; Huseni, M.A.; Atkins, M.B.; Motzer, R.J.; Rini, B.I.; Escudier, B.; Fong, L.; Joseph, R.W.; Pal, S.K.; Reeves, J.A.; et al. Clinical activity and molecular correlates of response to atezolizumab alone or in combination with bevacizumab versus sunitinib in renal cell carcinoma. *Nat. Med.* **2018**, *24*, 749–757. [CrossRef] [PubMed]
22. Motzer, R.J.; Robbins, P.B.; Powles, T.; Albiges, L.; Haanen, J.B.; Larkin, J.; Mu, X.J.; Ching, K.A.; Uemura, M.; Pal, S.K.; et al. Avelumab plus axitinib versus sunitinib in advanced renal cell carcinoma: Biomarker analysis of the phase 3 JAVELIN Renal 101 trial. *Nat. Med.* **2020**. [CrossRef]
23. Motzer, R.J.; Choueiri, T.K.; McDermott, D.F.; Yao, J.; Ammar, R.; Pappillon-Cavanagh, S.; Saggi, S.S.; McHenry, B.M.; Ross-Macdonald, P.; Wind-Rotolo, M.; et al. Biomarker analyses from the phase III CheckMate 214 trial of nivolumab plus ipilimumab (N+I) or sunitinib (S) in advanced renal cell carcinoma (aRCC). *J. Clin. Oncol.* **2020**, *38*, 5009. [CrossRef]

24. Rizvi, N.A.; Hellmann, M.D.; Snyder, A.; Kvistborg, P.; Makarov, V.; Havel, J.J.; Lee, W.; Yuan, J.; Wong, P.; Ho, T.S.; et al. Cancer immunology. Mutational landscape determines sensitivity to PD-1 blockade in non-small cell lung cancer. *Science* **2015**, *348*, 124–128. [CrossRef]
25. FDA Approves Pembrolizumab for Adults and Children with TMB-H Solid Tumors. News Release. FDA. 17 June 2020. Available online: https://bit.ly/30QEt40 (accessed on 11 August 2020).
26. Samstein, R.M.; Lee, C.H.; Shoushtari, A.N.; Hellmann, M.D.; Shen, R.; Janjigian, Y.Y.; Barron, D.A.; Zehir, A.; Jordan, E.J.; Omuro, A.; et al. Tumor mutational load predicts survival after immunotherapy across multiple cancer types. *Nat. Genet.* **2019**, *51*, 202–206. [CrossRef] [PubMed]
27. Cheng, D.T.; Mitchell, T.N.; Zehir, A.; Shah, R.H.; Benayed, R.; Syed, A.; Chandramohan, R.; Liu, Z.Y.; Won, H.H.; Scott, S.N.; et al. Memorial Sloan Kettering-Integrated Mutation Profiling of Actionable Cancer Targets (MSK-IMPACT): A Hybridization Capture-Based Next-Generation Sequencing Clinical Assay for Solid Tumor Molecular Oncology. *J. Mol. Diagn.* **2015**, *17*, 251–264. [CrossRef] [PubMed]
28. Alexandrov, L.B.; Nik-Zainal, S.; Wedge, D.C.; Aparicio, S.A.; Behjati, S.; Biankin, A.V.; Bignell, G.R.; Bolli, N.; Borg, A.; Børresen-Dale, A.L.; et al. Signatures of mutational processes in human cancer. *Nature* **2013**, *500*, 415–421. [CrossRef] [PubMed]
29. Labriola, M.K.; Zhu, J.; Gupta, R.; McCall, S.; Jackson, J.; Kong, E.F.; White, J.R.; Cerqueira, G.; Gerding, K.; Simmons, J.K.; et al. Characterization of tumor mutation burden, PD-L1 and DNA repair genes to assess relationship to immune checkpoint inhibitors response in metastatic renal cell carcinoma. *J. Immunother. Cancer* **2020**, *8*. [CrossRef] [PubMed]
30. Wood, M.A.; Weeder, B.R.; David, J.K.; Nellore, A.; Thompson, R.F. Burden of tumor mutations, neoepitopes, and other variants are weak predictors of cancer immunotherapy response and overall survival. *Genome Med.* **2020**, *12*, 33. [CrossRef]
31. Dizman, N.; Lyou, Y.; Salgia, N.; Bergerot, P.G.; Hsu, J.; Enriquez, D.; Izatt, T.; Trent, J.M.; Byron, S.; Pal, S. Correlates of clinical benefit from immunotherapy and targeted therapy in metastatic renal cell carcinoma: Comprehensive genomic and transcriptomic analysis. *J. Immunother. Cancer* **2020**, *8*. [CrossRef]
32. Braun, D.A.; Hou, Y.; Bakouny, Z.; Ficial, M.; Sant' Angelo, M.; Forman, J.; Ross-Macdonald, P.; Berger, A.C.; Jegede, O.A.; Elagina, L.; et al. Interplay of somatic alterations and immune infiltration modulates response to PD-1 blockade in advanced clear cell renal cell carcinoma. *Nat. Med.* **2020**, *26*, 909–918. [CrossRef] [PubMed]
33. Miao, D.; Margolis, C.A.; Gao, W.; Voss, M.H.; Li, W.; Martini, D.J.; Norton, C.; Bossé, D.; Wankowicz, S.M.; Cullen, D.; et al. Genomic correlates of response to immune checkpoint therapies in clear cell renal cell carcinoma. *Science* **2018**, *359*, 801–806. [CrossRef] [PubMed]
34. Huang, J.; Li, Z.; Fu, L.; Lin, D.; Wang, C.; Wang, X.; Zhang, L. Comprehensive characterization of tumor mutation burden in clear cell renal cell carcinoma based on the three independent cohorts. *J. Cancer Res. Clin. Oncol.* **2020**, 1–13. [CrossRef] [PubMed]
35. Brauer, M.J.; Zhuang, G.; Schmidt, M.; Yao, J.; Wu, X.; Kaminker, J.S.; Jurinka, S.S.; Kolumam, G.; Chung, A.S.; Jubb, A.; et al. Identification and analysis of in vivo VEGF downstream markers link VEGF pathway activity with efficacy of anti-VEGF therapies. *Clin. Cancer Res.* **2013**, *19*, 3681–3692. [CrossRef]
36. Fehrenbacher, L.; Spira, A.; Ballinger, M.; Kowanetz, M.; Vansteenkiste, J.; Mazieres, J.; Park, K.; Smith, D.; Artal-Cortes, A.; Lewanski, C.; et al. Atezolizumab versus docetaxel for patients with previously treated non-small-cell lung cancer (POPLAR): A multicentre, open-label, phase 2 randomised controlled trial. *Lancet* **2016**, *387*, 1837–1846. [CrossRef]
37. Scheller, J.; Chalaris, A.; Schmidt-Arras, D.; Rose-John, S. The pro- and anti-inflammatory properties of the cytokine interleukin-6. *Biochim. Biophys. Acta* **2011**, *1813*, 878–888. [CrossRef]
38. Russo, R.C.; Garcia, C.C.; Teixeira, M.M.; Amaral, F.A. The CXCL8/IL-8 chemokine family and its receptors in inflammatory diseases. *Expert Rev. Clin. Immunol.* **2014**, *10*, 593–619. [CrossRef]
39. Ha, H.; Debnath, B.; Neamati, N. Role of the CXCL8-CXCR1/2 Axis in Cancer and Inflammatory Diseases. *Theranostics* **2017**, *7*, 1543–1588. [CrossRef]
40. Zelenay, S.; van der Veen, A.G.; Böttcher, J.P.; Snelgrove, K.J.; Rogers, N.; Acton, S.E.; Chakravarty, P.; Girotti, M.R.; Marais, R.; Quezada, S.A.; et al. Cyclooxygenase-Dependent Tumor Growth through Evasion of Immunity. *Cell* **2015**, *162*, 1257–1270. [CrossRef]

41. Powles, T.; Nickles, D.; Van Allen, E.; Chappey, C.; Zou, W.; Kowanetz, M.; Kadel, E.; Denker, M.; Boyd, Z.; Vogelzang, N.; et al. Immune biomarkers associated with clinical benefit from atezolizumab (MPDL3280a; anti-PD-L1) in advanced urothelial bladder cancer (UBC). *J. Immunother. Cancer* **2015**, *3*. [CrossRef]
42. Rini, B.I.; Huseni, M.; Atkins, M.B.; McDermott, D.F.; Powles, T.B.; Escudier, B.; Banchereau, R.; Liu, L.; Leng, N.; Fan, J.; et al. Molecular correlates differentiate response to atezolizumab (atezo) + bevacizumab (bev) vs. sunitinib (sun): Results from a phase III study (IMmotion151) in untreated metastatic renal cell carcinoma (mRCC). *Ann. Oncol.* **2018**, *29* (Suppl. 8), LBA31. [CrossRef]
43. Choueiri, T.K.; Albiges, L.; Haanen, J.B.; Larkin, J.M.; Uemura, M.; Pal, S.K.; Gravis, G.; Campbell, M.T.; Penkov, K.; Lee, J.L.; et al. Biomarker analyses from JAVELIN Renal 101: Avelumab + axitinib (A + Ax) versus sunitinib (S) in advanced renal cell carcinoma (aRCC). *J. Clin. Oncol.* **2019**, *37*, 101. [CrossRef]
44. Choueiri, T.K.; Larkin, J.; Oya, M.; Thistlethwaite, F.; Martignoni, M.; Nathan, P.; Powles, T.; McDermott, D.; Robbins, P.B.; Chism, D.D.; et al. Preliminary results for avelumab plus axitinib as first-line therapy in patients with advanced clear-cell renal-cell carcinoma (JAVELIN Renal 100): An open-label, dose-finding and dose-expansion, phase 1b trial. *Lancet Oncol.* **2018**, *19*, 451–460. [CrossRef]
45. Zhu, J.; Pabla, S.; Labriola, M.; Gupta, R.T.; McCall, S.; George, D.J.; Dressman, D.; Glenn, S.; George, S.; Morrison, C.; et al. Evaluation of tumor microenvironment and biomarkers of immune checkpoint inhibitor (ICI) response in metastatic renal cell carcinoma (mRCC). *J. Clin. Oncol.* **2019**, 607. [CrossRef]
46. Liberzon, A.; Birger, C.; Thorvaldsdóttir, H.; Ghandi, M.; Mesirov, J.P.; Tamayo, P. The Molecular Signatures Database (MSigDB) hallmark gene set collection. *Cell Syst.* **2015**, *1*, 417–425. [CrossRef] [PubMed]
47. Network, C.G.A.R. Comprehensive molecular characterization of clear cell renal cell carcinoma. *Nature* **2013**, *499*, 43–49. [CrossRef]
48. Braun, D.A.; Ishii, Y.; Walsh, A.M.; Van Allen, E.M.; Wu, C.J.; Shukla, S.A.; Choueiri, T.K. Clinical Validation of PBRM1 Alterations as a Marker of Immune Checkpoint Inhibitor Response in Renal Cell Carcinoma. *JAMA Oncol.* **2019**, *5*, 1631–1633. [CrossRef]
49. Liu, X.D.; Kong, W.; Peterson, C.B.; McGrail, D.J.; Hoang, A.; Zhang, X.; Lam, T.; Pilie, P.G.; Zhu, H.; Beckermann, K.E.; et al. PBRM1 loss defines a nonimmunogenic tumor phenotype associated with checkpoint inhibitor resistance in renal carcinoma. *Nat. Commun.* **2020**, *11*, 2135. [CrossRef]
50. Singla, N.; Xie, Z.; Zhang, Z.; Gao, M.; Yousuf, Q.; Onabolu, O.; McKenzie, T.; Tcheuyap, V.T.; Ma, Y.; Choi, J.; et al. Pancreatic tropism of metastatic renal cell carcinoma. *JCI Insight* **2020**, *5*. [CrossRef]
51. Balestrieri, E.; Pica, F.; Matteucci, C.; Zenobi, R.; Sorrentino, R.; Argaw-Denboba, A.; Cipriani, C.; Bucci, I.; Sinibaldi-Vallebona, P. Transcriptional activity of human endogenous retroviruses in human peripheral blood mononuclear cells. *Biomed. Res. Int.* **2015**, *2015*, 164529. [CrossRef]
52. Lander, E.S.; Linton, L.M.; Birren, B.; Nusbaum, C.; Zody, M.C.; Baldwin, J.; Devon, K.; Dewar, K.; Doyle, M.; FitzHugh, W.; et al. Initial sequencing and analysis of the human genome. *Nature* **2001**, *409*, 860–921. [CrossRef] [PubMed]
53. Rooney, M.S.; Shukla, S.A.; Wu, C.J.; Getz, G.; Hacohen, N. Molecular and genetic properties of tumors associated with local immune cytolytic activity. *Cell* **2015**, *160*, 48–61. [CrossRef] [PubMed]
54. Panda, A.; de Cubas, A.A.; Stein, M.; Riedlinger, G.; Kra, J.; Mayer, T.; Smith, C.C.; Vincent, B.G.; Serody, J.S.; Beckermann, K.E.; et al. Endogenous retrovirus expression is associated with response to immune checkpoint blockade in clear cell renal cell carcinoma. *JCI Insight* **2018**, *3*. [CrossRef] [PubMed]
55. Pignon, J.C.; Jegede, O.; Shukla, S.A.; Braun, D.A.; Horak, C.; Wind-Rotolo, M.; Ishii, Y.; Catalano, P.J.; Freeman, G.J.; Jennings, R.B.; et al. Association of human endogenous retrovirus (hERV) expression with clinical efficacy of PD-1 blockade in metastatic clear cell renal cell carcinoma (mccRCC). *J. Clin. Oncol.* **2019**, 4568. [CrossRef]
56. Zitvogel, L.; Ayyoub, M.; Routy, B.; Kroemer, G. Microbiome and Anticancer Immunosurveillance. *Cell* **2016**, *165*, 276–287. [CrossRef] [PubMed]
57. Zitvogel, L.; Daillère, R.; Roberti, M.P.; Routy, B.; Kroemer, G. Anticancer effects of the microbiome and its products. *Nat. Rev. Microbiol.* **2017**, *15*, 465–478. [CrossRef]
58. Routy, B.; Le Chatelier, E.; Derosa, L.; Duong, C.P.M.; Alou, M.T.; Daillère, R.; Fluckiger, A.; Messaoudene, M.; Rauber, C.; Roberti, M.P.; et al. Gut microbiome influences efficacy of PD-1-based immunotherapy against epithelial tumors. *Science* **2018**, *359*, 91–97. [CrossRef]

59. Ueda, K.; Yonekura, S.; Ogasawara, N.; Matsunaga, Y.; Hoshino, R.; Kurose, H.; Chikui, K.; Uemura, K.; Nakiri, M.; Nishihara, K.; et al. The Impact of Antibiotics on Prognosis of Metastatic Renal Cell Carcinoma in Japanese Patients Treated with Immune Checkpoint Inhibitors. *Anticancer. Res.* **2019**, *39*, 6265–6271. [CrossRef]
60. Lalani, A.A.; Xie, W.; Braun, D.A.; Kaymakcalan, M.; Bossé, D.; Steinharter, J.A.; Martini, D.J.; Simantov, R.; Lin, X.; Wei, X.X.; et al. Effect of Antibiotic Use on Outcomes with Systemic Therapies in Metastatic Renal Cell Carcinoma. *Eur. Urol. Oncol.* **2020**, *3*, 372–381. [CrossRef]
61. Derosa, L.; Routy, B.; Fidelle, M.; Iebba, V.; Alla, L.; Pasolli, E.; Segata, N.; Desnoyer, A.; Pietrantonio, F.; Ferrere, G.; et al. Gut Bacteria Composition Drives Primary Resistance to Cancer Immunotherapy in Renal Cell Carcinoma Patients. *Eur. Urol.* **2020**, *78*, 195–206. [CrossRef]
62. Salgia, N.J.; Bergerot, P.G.; Maia, M.C.; Dizman, N.; Hsu, J.; Gillece, J.D.; Folkerts, M.; Reining, L.; Trent, J.; Highlander, S.K.; et al. Stool Microbiome Profiling of Patients with Metastatic Renal Cell Carcinoma Receiving Anti-PD-1 Immune Checkpoint Inhibitors. *Eur. Urol.* **2020**. [CrossRef] [PubMed]
63. Shuch, B.; Bratslavsky, G.; Linehan, W.M.; Srinivasan, R. Sarcomatoid renal cell carcinoma: A comprehensive review of the biology and current treatment strategies. *Oncologist* **2012**, *17*, 46–54. [CrossRef] [PubMed]
64. Kyriakopoulos, C.E.; Chittoria, N.; Choueiri, T.K.; Kroeger, N.; Lee, J.L.; Srinivas, S.; Knox, J.J.; Bjarnason, G.A.; Ernst, S.D.; Wood, L.A.; et al. Outcome of patients with metastatic sarcomatoid renal cell carcinoma: Results from the International Metastatic Renal Cell Carcinoma Database Consortium. *Clin. Genitourin. Cancer* **2015**, *13*, e79–e85. [CrossRef] [PubMed]
65. Golshayan, A.R.; George, S.; Heng, D.Y.; Elson, P.; Wood, L.S.; Mekhail, T.M.; Garcia, J.A.; Aydin, H.; Zhou, M.; Bukowski, R.M.; et al. Metastatic sarcomatoid renal cell carcinoma treated with vascular endothelial growth factor-targeted therapy. *J. Clin. Oncol.* **2009**, *27*, 235–241. [CrossRef]
66. Joseph, R.W.; Millis, S.Z.; Carballido, E.M.; Bryant, D.; Gatalica, Z.; Reddy, S.; Bryce, A.H.; Vogelzang, N.J.; Stanton, M.L.; Castle, E.P.; et al. PD-1 and PD-L1 Expression in Renal Cell Carcinoma with Sarcomatoid Differentiation. *Cancer Immunol. Res.* **2015**, *3*, 1303–1307. [CrossRef]
67. Rini, B.I.; Motzer, R.J.; Powles, T.; McDermott, D.F.; Escudier, B.; Donskov, F.; Hawkins, R.; Bracarda, S.; Bedke, J.; De Giorgi, U.; et al. Atezolizumab plus Bevacizumab Versus Sunitinib for Patients with Untreated Metastatic Renal Cell Carcinoma and Sarcomatoid Features: A Prespecified Subgroup Analysis of the IMmotion151 Clinical Trial. *Eur. Urol.* **2020**. [CrossRef]
68. Tannir, N.M.; Signoretti, S.; Choueiri, T.K.; McDermott, D.F.; Motzer, R.J.; Flaifel, A.; Pignon, J.C.; Ficial, M.; Arén Frontera, O.; George, S.; et al. Efficacy and Safety of Nivolumab Plus Ipilimumab versus Sunitinib in First-Line Treatment of Patients with Advanced Sarcomatoid Renal Cell Carcinoma. *Clin. Cancer Res.* **2020**. [CrossRef]
69. Iacovelli, R.; Ciccarese, C.; Bria, E.; Bracarda, S.; Porta, C.; Procopio, G.; Tortora, G. Patients with sarcomatoid renal cell carcinoma-re-defining the first-line of treatment: A meta-analysis of randomised clinical trials with immune checkpoint inhibitors. *Eur. J. Cancer* **2020**, *136*, 195–203. [CrossRef]
70. Arda, E.; Yuksel, I.; Cakiroglu, B.; Akdeniz, E.; Cilesiz, N. Valuation of Neutrophil/Lymphocyte Ratio in Renal Cell Carcinoma Grading and Progression. *Cureus* **2018**, *10*, e2051. [CrossRef]
71. Zhao, H.; Li, W.; Le, X.; Li, Z.; Ge, P. Preoperative Neutrophil-to-Lymphocyte Ratio Was a Predictor of Overall Survival in Small Renal Cell Carcinoma: An Analysis of 384 Consecutive Patients. *Biomed. Res. Int.* **2020**, *2020*, 8051210. [CrossRef]
72. Shao, Y.; Wu, B.; Jia, W.; Zhang, Z.; Chen, Q.; Wang, D. Prognostic value of pretreatment neutrophil-to-lymphocyte ratio in renal cell carcinoma: A systematic review and meta-analysis. *BMC Urol.* **2020**, *20*, 90. [CrossRef] [PubMed]
73. Zahoor, H.; Barata, P.C.; Jia, X.; Martin, A.; Allman, K.D.; Wood, L.S.; Gilligan, T.D.; Grivas, P.; Ornstein, M.C.; Garcia, J.A.; et al. Patterns, predictors and subsequent outcomes of disease progression in metastatic renal cell carcinoma patients treated with nivolumab. *J. Immunother. Cancer* **2018**, *6*, 107. [CrossRef] [PubMed]
74. Lalani, A.A.; Xie, W.; Martini, D.J.; Steinharter, J.A.; Norton, C.K.; Krajewski, K.M.; Duquette, A.; Bossé, D.; Bellmunt, J.; Van Allen, E.M.; et al. Change in Neutrophil-to-lymphocyte ratio (NLR) in response to immune checkpoint blockade for metastatic renal cell carcinoma. *J. Immunother. Cancer* **2018**, *6*, 5. [CrossRef] [PubMed]

75. Bilen, M.A.; Rini, B.I.; Motzer, R.J.; Larkin, J.M.; Haanen, J.B.; Albiges, L.; Pagliaro, L.C.; Voog, E.; Lam, E.T.; Kislov, N.; et al. Association of neutrophil to lymphocyte ratio (NLR) with efficacy from JAVELIN Renal 101. *J. Clin. Oncol.* **2020**, *38*, 5061. [CrossRef]
76. Postow, M.A.; Sidlow, R.; Hellmann, M.D. Immune-Related Adverse Events Associated with Immune Checkpoint Blockade. *N. Engl. J. Med.* **2018**, *378*, 158–168. [CrossRef]
77. Nunes-Xavier, C.E.; Angulo, J.C.; Pulido, R.; López, J.I. A Critical Insight into the Clinical Translation of PD-1/PD-L1 Blockade Therapy in Clear Cell Renal Cell Carcinoma. *Curr. Urol. Rep.* **2019**, *20*, 1. [CrossRef]
78. Sánchez-Magraner, L.; Miles, J.; Baker, C.L.; Applebee, C.J.; Lee, D.J.; Elsheikh, S.; Lashin, S.; Withers, K.; Watts, A.G.; Parry, R.; et al. High PD-1/PD-L1 checkpoint interaction infers tumor selection and therapeutic sensitivity to anti-PD-1/PD-L1 treatment. *Cancer Res.* **2020**. [CrossRef]
79. Niemeijer, A.N.; Leung, D.; Huisman, M.C.; Bahce, I.; Hoekstra, O.S.; van Dongen, G.A.M.S.; Boellaard, R.; Du, S.; Hayes, W.; Smith, R.; et al. Whole body PD-1 and PD-L1 positron emission tomography in patients with non-small-cell lung cancer. *Nat. Commun.* **2018**, *9*, 4664. [CrossRef]

Permissions

All chapters in this book were first published by MDPI; hereby published with permission under the Creative Commons Attribution License or equivalent. Every chapter published in this book has been scrutinized by our experts. Their significance has been extensively debated. The topics covered herein carry significant findings which will fuel the growth of the discipline. They may even be implemented as practical applications or may be referred to as a beginning point for another development.

The contributors of this book come from diverse backgrounds, making this book a truly international effort. This book will bring forth new frontiers with its revolutionizing research information and detailed analysis of the nascent developments around the world.

We would like to thank all the contributing authors for lending their expertise to make the book truly unique. They have played a crucial role in the development of this book. Without their invaluable contributions this book wouldn't have been possible. They have made vital efforts to compile up to date information on the varied aspects of this subject to make this book a valuable addition to the collection of many professionals and students.

This book was conceptualized with the vision of imparting up-to-date information and advanced data in this field. To ensure the same, a matchless editorial board was set up. Every individual on the board went through rigorous rounds of assessment to prove their worth. After which they invested a large part of their time researching and compiling the most relevant data for our readers.

The editorial board has been involved in producing this book since its inception. They have spent rigorous hours researching and exploring the diverse topics which have resulted in the successful publishing of this book. They have passed on their knowledge of decades through this book. To expedite this challenging task, the publisher supported the team at every step. A small team of assistant editors was also appointed to further simplify the editing procedure and attain best results for the readers.

Apart from the editorial board, the designing team has also invested a significant amount of their time in understanding the subject and creating the most relevant covers. They scrutinized every image to scout for the most suitable representation of the subject and create an appropriate cover for the book.

The publishing team has been an ardent support to the editorial, designing and production team. Their endless efforts to recruit the best for this project, has resulted in the accomplishment of this book. They are a veteran in the field of academics and their pool of knowledge is as vast as their experience in printing. Their expertise and guidance has proved useful at every step. Their uncompromising quality standards have made this book an exceptional effort. Their encouragement from time to time has been an inspiration for everyone.

The publisher and the editorial board hope that this book will prove to be a valuable piece of knowledge for researchers, students, practitioners and scholars across the globe.

List of Contributors

Judikaël Saout
Université Rennes, Inserm, EHESP (Ecole des Hautes Etudes en Santé Publique), IRSET (Institut de recherche en santé, environnement et travail), UMR 1085, 35000 Rennes, France

Antoine Deleuze
Université Rennes, Inserm, EHESP (Ecole des Hautes Etudes en Santé Publique), IRSET (Institut de recherche en santé, environnement et travail), UMR 1085, 35000 Rennes, France
Department of Medical Oncology, Centre Eugene Marquis, 35000 Rennes, France

Laurence Crouzet and Brigitte Laguerre
Department of Medical Oncology, Centre Eugene Marquis, 35000 Rennes, France

Marc-Antoine Belaud-Rotureau and Frédéric Dugay
Université Rennes, Inserm, EHESP (Ecole des Hautes Etudes en Santé Publique), IRSET (Institut de recherche en santé, environnement et travail), UMR 1085, 35000 Rennes, France
Department of Cytogenetics, University Hospital, 35000 Rennes, France

Romain Mathieu
Université Rennes, Inserm, EHESP (Ecole des Hautes Etudes en Santé Publique), IRSET (Institut de recherche en santé, environnement et travail), UMR 1085, 35000 Rennes, France
Department of Urology, University Hospital, 35000 Rennes, France

Benoit Peyronnet, Gregory Verhoest and Karim Bensalah
Department of Urology, University Hospital, 35000 Rennes, France

Nathalie Rioux-Leclercq and Solène-Florence Kammerer-Jacquet
Université Rennes, Inserm, EHESP (Ecole des Hautes Etudes en Santé Publique), IRSET (Institut de recherche en santé, environnement et travail), UMR 1085, 35000 Rennes, France
Department of Pathology, University Hospital, 35000 Rennes, France

Soo-Youl Kim
Division of Cancer Biology, National Cancer Center, Goyang 10408, Korea

Jeffrey W. Keillor
Department of Chemistry and Biomolecular Sciences, University of Ottawa, Ottawa, ON K1N 6N5, Canada

Alexandr Poprach, Milos Holanek, Radek Lakomy and Igor Kiss
Department of Comprehensive Cancer Care, Masaryk Memorial Cancer Institute, 656 53 Brno, Czech Republic
Department of Comprehensive Cancer Care, Faculty of Medicine, Masaryk University, 625 00 Brno, Czech Republic

Renata Chloupkova
Institute of Biostatistics and Analyses, Faculty of Medicine, Masaryk University, 625 00 Brno, Czech Republic

Michal Stanik
Department of Urologic Oncology, Masaryk Memorial Cancer Institute and Masaryk University, 656 53 Brno, Czech Republic

Ondrej Fiala
Department of Oncology, University Hospital, 323 00 Pilsen, Czech Republic

Bohuslav Melichar
Department of Oncology, Palacky University Medical School and Teaching Hospital, 779 00 Olomouc, Czech Republic
University Hospital in Hradec Kralove, 500 05 Hradec Kralove, Czech Republic

Katerina Kopeckova
Department of Oncology, Motol University Hospital and 2nd Faculty of Medicine Charles University, 150 06 Prague, Czech Republic

Milada Zemanova
Department of Oncology, First Faculty of Medicine Charles University and General University Hospital, 120 00 Prague, Czech Republic

Igor Penka
Department of Surgery, University Hospital Bohunice, Faculty of Medicine, Masaryk University, 625 00 Brno, Czech Republic

Julia Bohosova
Central European Institute of Technology (CEITEC), University Campus Bohunice, Masaryk University, 625 00 Brno, Czech Republic

Tomas Buchler
Department of Oncology, First Faculty of Medicine, Thomayer Hospital and Charles University, 140 59 Prague, Czech Republic

Ying Zhang and Ingo G. H. Schmidt-Wolf
Department of Integrated Oncology, CIO Bonn, University Hospital Bonn, Venusberg-Campus 1, D 53127 Bonn, Germany

Jörg Ellinger and Manuel Ritter
Department of Urology, University Hospital Bonn, Venusberg-Campus 1, D 53127 Bonn, Germany

Ilaria Grazia Zizzari, Chiara Napoletano, Alessandra Di Filippo, Aurelia Rughetti and Marianna Nuti
Laboratory of Tumor Immunology and Cell Therapy, Department of Experimental Medicine, Policlinico Umberto I, "Sapienza" University of Rome, 00161 Rome, Italy

Andrea Botticelli, Alain Gelibter, Federica Urbano, Giulia Pomati, Simone Scagnoli and Salvatore Caponnetto
Division of Oncology, Department of Radiological, Oncological and Pathological Science, Policlinico Umberto I, "Sapienza" University of Rome, 00161 Rome, Italy

Fabio Calabrò
Division of Medical Oncology B, San Camillo Forlanini Hospital Rome, 00149 Rome, Italy

Ernesto Rossi and Giovanni Schinzari
Department of Medical Oncology, Fondazione Policlinico A.Gemelli Rome, 00168 Rome, Italy

Paolo Marchetti
Division of Oncology, Department of Radiological, Oncological and Pathological Science, Policlinico Umberto I, "Sapienza" University of Rome, 00161 Rome, Italy
Division of Oncology, Department of Clinical and Molecular Medicine, Ospedale Sant'Andrea, "Sapienza" University of Rome, 00189 Rome, Italy

Magdalena Rudzińska, Alessandro Parodi, Neonila V. Gorokhovets and Vladimir A. Makarov
Institute of Molecular Medicine, Sechenov First Moscow State Medical University, 119991 Moscow, Russia

Valentina D. Maslova
Faculty of Bioengineering and Bioinformatics, Moscow State University, 119992 Moscow, Russia

Yuri M. Efremov
Institute for Regenerative Medicine, Sechenov University, 119991 Moscow, Russia

Evgeni Y. Zernii and Andrey A. Zamyatnin Jr.
Belozersky Institute of Physico-Chemical Biology, Lomonosov Moscow State University, 119992 Moscow, Russia

Vasily A. Popkov
Belozersky Institute of Physico-Chemical Biology, Lomonosov Moscow State University, 119992 Moscow, Russia

Andrey V. Golovin
Institute of Molecular Medicine, Sechenov First Moscow State Medical University, 119991 Moscow, Russia
Faculty of Bioengineering and Bioinformatics, Moscow State University, 119992 Moscow, Russia
Shemyakin-Ovchinnikov Institute of Bioorganic Chemistry, Russian Academy of Sciences, 117997 Moscow, Russia

Yasir Khan, Timothy D. Slattery and Lisa M. Pickering
The Royal Marsden Hospital NHS Foundation Trust, Fulham Road, London SW3 6JJ, UK

María T. Bourlon
Hemato-Oncology Department, Instituto Nacional de Ciencias Médicas y Nutrición Salvador Zubirán, 14080 Mexico City, Mexico

Nicola Longo, Marco Capece, Giuseppe Celentano, Roberto La Rocca, Gianluigi Califano, Claudia Collà Ruvolo, Fabio Esposito, Luigi Napolitano, Francesco Mangiapia, Vincenzo Mirone and Massimiliano Creta
Department of Neurosciences, Science of Reproduction and Odontostomatology, University of Naples Federico II, 80131 Naples, Italy

Carlo Buonerba
Department of Clinical Medicine and Surgery, University of Naples Federico II, 80131 Naples, Italy

Ferdinando Fusco
Department of Woman, Child and General and Specialized Surgery, Urology Unit, University of Campania 'Luigi Vanvitelli', 80131 Naples, Italy

Łukasz Szylberg
Department of Clinical Pathomorphology, Collegium Medicum in Bydgoszcz, Nicolaus Copernicus University in Torun, 85-067 Bydgoszcz, Poland
Department of Tumor Pathology and Pathomorphology, Oncology Centre-Prof. Franciszek Łukaszczyk Memorial Hospital, 85-796 Bydgoszcz, Poland

Adam Kowalewski and Dariusz Grzanka
Department of Clinical Pathomorphology, Collegium Medicum in Bydgoszcz, Nicolaus Copernicus University in Torun, 85-067 Bydgoszcz, Poland

Marek Zdrenka
Department of Tumor Pathology and Pathomorphology, Oncology Centre-Prof. Franciszek Łukaszczyk Memorial Hospital, 85-796 Bydgoszcz, Poland

Sascha D. Markowitsch, Patricia Schupp, Julia Lauckner, Olesya Vakhrusheva, Kimberly S. Slade, René Mager, Axel Haferkamp and Eva Juengel
Department of Urology and Pediatric Urology, University Medical Center Mainz, Langenbeckstraße 1, 55131 Mainz, Germany

Thomas Efferth
Institute of Pharmaceutical and Biomedical Sciences, Johannes Gutenberg University Mainz, Staudingerweg 5, 55128 Mainz, Germany

Reza Elaidi and Letuan Phan
ARTIC (Association pour la Recherche sur les Thérapeutiques Innovantes en Cancérologie), Hôpital Européen Georges Pompidou, 75015 Paris, France

Delphine Borchiellini
Department of Medical Oncology, Centre Antoine-Lacassagne, 06100 Nice, France

Philippe Barthelemy
Department of Medical Oncology, Hôpital civil, 67091 Strasbourg, France

Alain Ravaud
Department of Medical Oncology, Hôpital St Andre, 33000 Bordeaux, France

Stéphane Oudard and Yann Vano
Department of Medical Oncology, Hôpital Européen Georges Pompidou, 75015 Paris, France

Trace M. Jones, Jennifer S. Carew and Steffan T. Nawrocki
Division of Translational and Regenerative Medicine, Department of Medicine and The University of Arizona Cancer Center, Tucson, AZ 85724, USA

Alberto Carretero-González, Daniel Castellano and Guillermo de Velasco
Medical Oncology Department, University Hospital 12 de Octubre, 28041 Madrid, Spain

David Lora
Clinical Research Unit, IMAS12-CIBERESP, University Hospital 12 de Octubre, 28041 Madrid, Spain

Isabel Martín Sobrino and Irene Sáez Sanz
School of Medicine, Universidad Complutense de Madrid, University Hospital 12 de Octubre, 28040 Madrid, Spain

Urbano Anido Herranz
Medical Oncology Department, University Clinical Hospital of Santiago de Compostela, 15076 Santiago de Compostela, Spain

Nieves Martínez Chanzá
Medical Oncology Department, Jules Bordet Institute, Université Libre de Bruxelles, 1000 Brussels, Belgium

Matthew D. Tucker and Brian I. Rini
Department of Medicine, Division of Hematology and Oncology, Vanderbilt University Medical Center, Nashville, TN 37232, USA

Index

www.ingramcontent.com/pod-product-compliance
Lightning Source LLC
LaVergne TN
LVHW080947210926
848485LV00004B/795